contents

To Joe, Leo, and Chernet with love

—Hope

To Elise and Kate with love

—Monique

acknowledgments

Sometimes a team comes together that's a writer's dream. Christine Tomasino of the Tomasino Agency led our team, along with Eric Lupfer of the William Morris Agency, and brought us together with Ten Speed Press. Editorial director Julie Bennett and senior editor Clancy Drake became the perfect publisher: mentor, editor, guide, and that funny friend. The entire Ten Speed team was truly dedicated to the book: Toni Tajima, who designed it; Molly Feuer, who illustrated it; Kristi Hein, who served as copy editor; and Jasmine Star, who was responsible for proofreading.

We wanted women to find this book to be a constant reference they could turn to over many years. The first step was to make sure we sought the best expertise we could find. We therefore send many thanks to social worker Jane Morgenstern MSW. Her unique understanding of the complex issues facing young women was invaluable.

We wish we could thank all of our friends and families by name. They offered their own experiences, which added important sections, and their support and enthusiasm, which carried us through writing a lengthy and evidence-based book. Family and friends make everything possible!

Hope is very grateful to the many women who have allowed her the privilege of caring for their health and sharing in their lives, and in so doing, have taught her so much about the many strengths of a woman. As a writer, Monique says the most important requirement is that you have a friend who is part inspiring mentor and part terrifying critic, preferably a Marine, for which she thanks Mr. Ed Fouhy.

Many, many thanks.

Hope Ricciotti, MD, and
Monique Doyle Spencer

welcome to the real life body book!

Good news: Even if you've taken less than stellar care of yourself until now, you can move in the direction of better health, regardless of your age. And you can start right now.

A healthy body makes life easier. It's like having a new car all day, every day—one that has new tires, windshield wiper fluid filled to the top, and that new car smell. You can count on a healthy body to give you the energy you need to live well for a very long time.

When we're young, though, we tend to take health for granted, and it's easy to feel like nothing really bad could ever happen to you or your body. The younger you are, the more invincible you feel. But if you haven't been taking care of your body, maybe you can already feel that you need to make some changes.

Well, we understand the body better now than ever and we learn more with each passing year. If your mother reads this book, she'll be stunned by how much we now know about preventing illness. Today an ounce of prevention isn't worth a pound of cure—it's worth a *ton* of it. Opening *The Real Life Body Book* is a great first step.

How do you make decisions about your body? Think about your body and your health for a minute and then let's look at how you find information and make choices.

Maybe you're the research type. As a medical student I loved having access to unlimited medical information. All of those expensive subscription websites and reference books that I could hardly lift were now mine to explore. It was a gold mine to a young aspiring doctor. So what was the problem?

Within a week, I had diagnosed myself with bacterial meningitis, dengue fever, and a dozen different kinds of cancer, all of them so rare that to this day I have never seen a case. I ruled out rattlesnake bite, but just barely. It's irresistible: the more unfiltered information you have, the more scary diseases you'll find in yourself. You're not alone—if you get a group of doctors talking about medical school, ask them if they've ever had the plague. The room will fall silent. Feet will shuffle. Someone will make an embarrassed cough. They're all remembering those nights of shivering fear from doing too much research.

Maybe you rely on the Favorite Four: best friends, Mom, magazines, and the Internet. You already know the problem there: the information may be old (Mom, God bless her) or faddish (magazines) or based on rumors (best friends) or downright crazy talk (the Internet).

So what's the big deal with getting to know the real life facts about your body?

It's this: the decisions you make today will make your future body healthy, sturdy, and energetic—or vulnerable, sickly, and sedentary. Look around at the older people you know. By the time you've read this book, you'll recognize the good or bad decisions they made when they were your age!

You don't need any more stress in your life and a little knowledge can relieve a lot of anxiety. We hope you keep this book for a long time: for the day that you find a lump . . . or develop a zit the day before a job interview.

You can read the book straight through or bounce around or just look up something you need to know today. Right now you might be worried about that discharge you've got, but later you might be more interested in learning about fertility—or adult acne, or what it really feels like to get a mammogram.

Throughout these pages, when we write "I," that's Hope speaking, and when we write "we," we're referring to doctors in general. You'll also find three different types of sidebars that give you more essential information about your health. A *Real Life Fact* highlights important things that we want to emphasize or that we didn't cover elsewhere in the text, a *Real Life Question* answers the questions that Hope commonly gets from her patients, and a *Note to Self* covers details that you'll want to remember. Words that appear in **blue** are defined in the glossary (see page 430).

Knowledge is the first step if you want to lead a healthy life. This book answers, in full detail, the basic questions: How does your body work? How can you keep it healthy?

It will also help you to become an equal partner with your doctors—a skill that's useful for a lifetime.

Here's to good health!

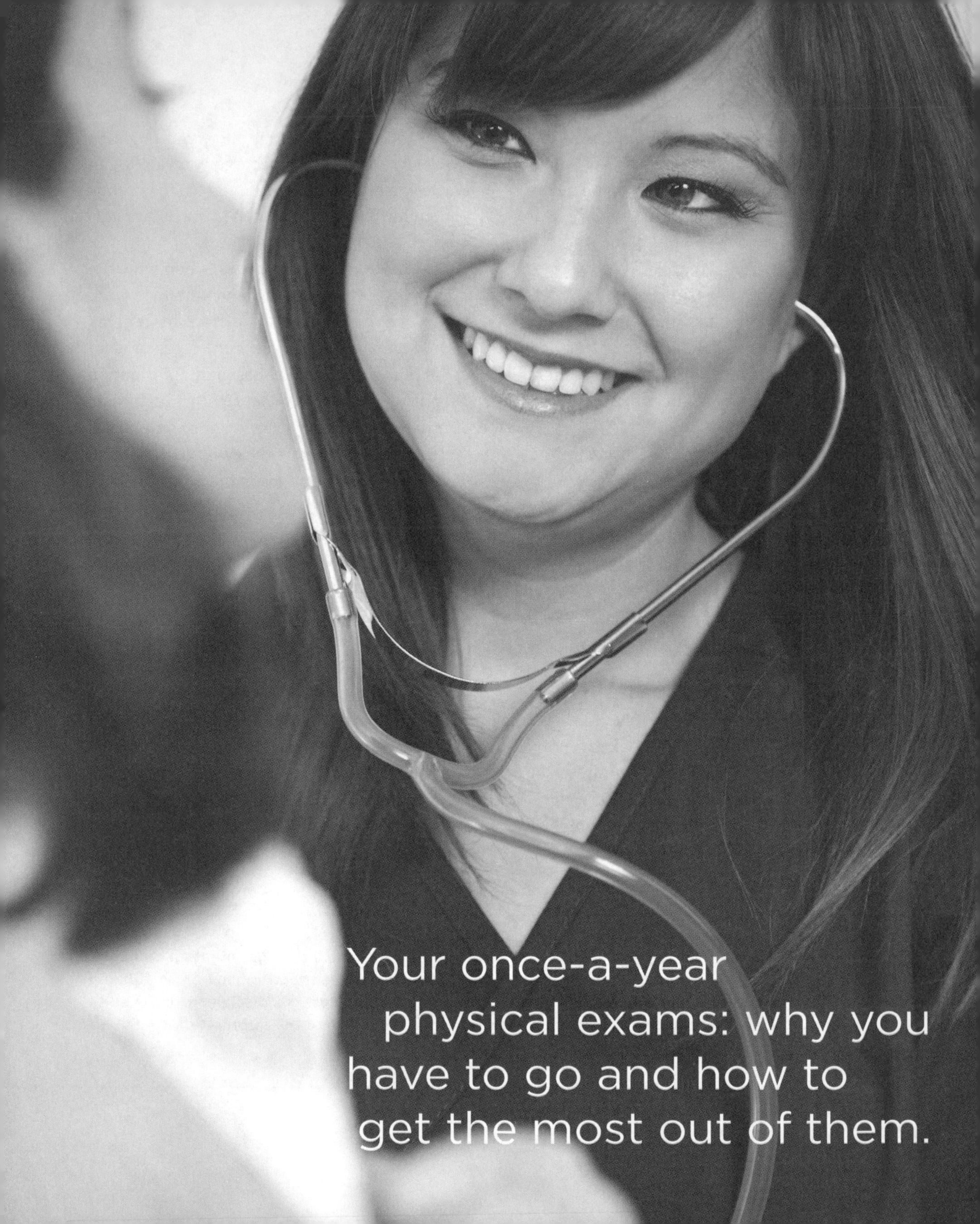
Your once-a-year
physical exams: why you
have to go and how to
get the most out of them.

meet your body and your doctor

You really want to cancel your appointment for a physical today.

You haven't shaved your legs since your cousin's wedding. It's a busy day at work. You're not even sick. Your best friend agrees. Cancel, she says, because that gives her permission to cancel hers too.

You've had physical exams before, but as you've matured, your body has entered a different category. It has stopped growing, you're out of training bras, and your doctor wants to take a look at you from the inside out. No more sweet pediatricians with a teddy bear on the stethoscope. Now there are stirrups involved.

Why bother keeping this appointment? Because your annual physical (also called a preventive-care visit) is one of the most important things you can do for your future health. If you want your first car to look great in five years, you take it in for regular maintenance checks. If you want your face to look great in ten years, you wear sunscreen. Your body needs the same care, so you really need to see your doctor at least once a year, even if you feel fine.

This chapter tells you exactly what an adult woman's physical and gynecologic exams are like, exactly what tests they will do and why you have them, and exactly how to collect a urine sample and whether or not you should carry your sample back to the reception desk. (No, you shouldn't.)

Your annual examination with a family practice doctor or general practitioner is preventive maintenance. Many older women regret that they didn't do a better job with preventive medicine

REAL LIFE FACT: Living on the Edge

The Centers for Disease Control says that the leading causes of death in women ages nineteen to thirty-nine are accidents, cancer, violence, HIV, heart diseases, and suicide. So as you get ready for your annual physical, think about these issues and expect your doctor to discuss them with you and offer advice.

when they were young. Now they look older and feel older than they should, and they know it. Just watch any TV show aimed at older people; almost all of the commercials are for prescription drugs. So many of those ailments could have been prevented years ago. And prevention is always easier than cure.

Many young women only see a **gynecologist** (or "gyn" for short) once a year, and that's it for health care. As long as you are young and healthy, that can work for you. However, if you have health issues such as **asthma**, high blood pressure, **diabetes**, or a significant family history of heart attacks or **cancer**, you'll also want to have a primary care doctor, who can refer you to specialists as needed. If you rely on your gyn as your primary doctor, it's very important that you tell him or her that! You don't want him or her to assume that somebody else is taking care of your high blood pressure problem.

In the following sections, I'm going to explain what you'll experience during your annual exam with a general practitioner and what to expect during a gynecology exam. The two exams can be pretty similar, so why don't you read both sections, especially if your primary doc is your gynecologist.

Some good news: Today we understand a lot about which exams and tests are necessary for health and which are a waste of your time and energy. You don't have to worry about issues you can't control or those that are unlikely to affect you. Instead, you can focus your efforts on the health strategies that can really make a difference for your future well-being.

Getting Ready for Your Annual Visit

Your annual visit should include a physical exam, getting your questions answered, and, if needed, a recommendation for some blood testing and ultrasound or other imaging. You should expect questions and conversation about your mental health and any issues of abuse in your life. You'll be asked questions about your own health and the health of your family members. And you may be asked if there's any special reason for your visit. If you're having any health concerns, now is the time to bring them up.

Before the Visit: Planning Ahead

To get the most out of your annual visit, spend some time on a few issues in advance. Start by thinking carefully about your body and any questions you have about it. Be prepared to discuss any health problems you have now or have had in the past. Is your period a problem for you, perhaps giving you abnormal pain or arriving on an irregular schedule? Is the vaginal discharge you have normal, or should you be concerned? What should you do about a persistent headache? What's your sex life like? Are you at a healthy weight and fitness level? How do you handle stress? Any rashes? How's your mood? Your doctor will ask you about smoking, alcohol, and other drug use. S/he wants to make sure you're driving safely and soberly and using protective gear for sports, such as a bicycle helmet.

Take the time to find out about the health of your immediate family members—mother, father, brothers and sisters, and grandparents. Your personal risk for illness is often influenced by the health history of your family. When your health history is complete, tests and exams can be tailored for any risk factors for illnesses.

This counseling and education part of your annual physical is as important as the physical examination and laboratory testing in many ways. Improving your health knowledge and talking openly with your doctor are two of the biggest reasons to come for an annual exam. It's worth taking the time to build a

REAL LIFE FACT: Family Checklist

Before your first annual physical with a doctor, one of your jobs is to research your family's health history. Sometimes it's nearly impossible to collect an accurate family history, for many reasons. You may be adopted, or your parents may be. You may come from a family that rarely talks about illness, so nobody knows the health problems of your aunts and uncles or grandparents. Just do your best to gather what is known. It helps to have as many pieces of information as possible, but screening tests can fill in many blanks. Your doctor can still take very good care of you!

Use this checklist to review your immediate family's medical history. Does anyone (parents, grandparents, brothers, or sisters) have any of the following?

- ___ Alcoholism/addiction
- ___ Breast cancer
- ___ Colon cancer
- ___ Depression
- ___ Diabetes
- ___ Heart attacks before the age of sixty
- ___ High blood pressure
- ___ High cholesterol
- ___ Obesity
- ___ Ovarian cancer
- ___ Thyroid disease

comfortable, trusting relationship with your doctor. This can be hard for a healthy person to do, as you may see your doctor only once a year. So make the most of each physical to connect and communicate.

Confidentiality: Is It Really Safe to Talk?

Your visit with your doctor is confidential. If you don't speak openly about any issues you have, you might not get the right counseling and screening done at your appointment. You really can tell your doctor that you have used drugs or had unsafe sex, and your news must be kept confidential. If you share openly, your doctor will have better information, which means better medical care for you.

To safeguard the privacy of your health care information in our electronic world, in 1996 Congress passed the Healthcare Insurance Portability and Accountability Act (HIPAA). This is incredibly complex legislation, but it basically means this: your health care information is private. Under **HIPAA**, no one, not even your family members, can view your medical records or obtain information from your doctor (there are some exceptions for patients under eighteen, which vary by state). HIPAA can sometimes cause you some extra red tape, as you have to sign release forms to allow your information to be transferred to your insurance company and other health care systems, but generally it's worth it to maintain your privacy.

But Why Does the Doctor Have to Ask That?

Expect some open discussions about sexuality and contraception. Your physical is a good place to be completely honest about your sex life. Your doctor needs to know if you're having sex and what protection you use against disease and, if you want to avoid it, pregnancy. These can have a big impact on your health. You can also expect to discuss these issues with your gynecologist during your annual exam; see the section later in this chapter for more information about your gyn visit.

If you feel that your doctor isn't being as thorough as we're describing here, you should raise these issues yourself, or perhaps think about changing doctors! Your doctor is not being nosy—well, maybe s/he is in his or her private life, but in this meeting it's his or her job to understand your life and background so that s/he can partner with you in your health care. In fact, one of the most important messages to you in this book is to encourage you to be an equal partner in your health care!

Remember that I'm talking about your visit with your own doctor. Some employers require physicals with a doctor *they* choose. I'm not a lawyer, but in my opinion that is not the place to share every little detail about your health or your lifestyle.

Is This You? "I Would Go If They Didn't Weigh Me."

Your doctor should also ask about your diet and physical activity. S/he hopes that your weight is in a healthy range, but also knows that for many of us, it's not. Some heavy women even delay their doctor appointments out of fear of feeling uncomfortable about being weighed. As tough as this may be for you, try to put these feelings aside. Make and keep the appointments you need to maintain a healthy body, whatever weight it is.

I want to repeat this. Don't ever let your weight keep you from seeing the doctor. Please.

The Physical Exam—What Actually Happens?

Maybe you've already had a physical someplace besides the school infirmary, but we'll start with a refresher course. You'll check in at the front desk and will be handed forms to fill out. These may include a detailed health questionnaire about your family medical history, plus your insurance information and HIPAA form. If you have insurance, bring your insurance card with you. You may be required to make a co-payment.

What Are My Vitals and Why Are They Being Checked?

Then you'll be called to have your "vitals" checked: your height, weight, and blood pressure. Some people hate being weighed. Try to remember that everyone who examines you has had the same experience, because they all have to have annual physicals too.

NOTE TO SELF

If you're uninsured, you may be asked to pay a portion, or even all, of your bill at your appointment. If your income is low, you may qualify for Medicaid. If you can't afford the care you need, consider looking for a community-based health center that offers care on a sliding scale based on your income. If you have an emergency and require hospital care, some nonprofit hospitals offer free or discounted care as part of their mission or tax status.

Low-cost health care differs by state or region. You can do research on the Internet or by calling toll-free to see what assistance is available in your area. Work with the finance staff at the hospital or clinic to help you navigate the system. Be sure to read the appendix, Tools to Use, for a lot more information.

To check your blood pressure, the medical assistant will put a cuff around your upper arm and put a stethoscope under it. Then s/he will pump air into the cuff until it feels extremely tight. Don't worry; this lasts for only a few seconds. Sometimes it's done by a little machine. S/he'll release the air and record the results. (More on blood pressure in chapter 5, Your Heart.)

NOTE TO SELF

If your blood pressure tests high, ask that it be taken again later in the exam. Many people (including one of the authors!) have "white coat" hypertension (high blood pressure), which is when the anxiety you feel during the exam causes a high result that's not typical for you.

Top Off Your Tank: The Urine Sample

Step two may be a urine sample, so be sure you've had some water before your appointment. Someone will hand you a cup and send you to the bathroom to collect it.

All you have to do is sit on the toilet, pee into the cup, put the cap on, and wipe the spills off with toilet paper. Sometimes, though, s/he will ask you to do what's called a clean catch test. S/he will hand you some wipes that you'll clean yourself with before peeing, wiping from front to back, from around the **urethra** where you pee, back past the **vagina**. S/he will want your midstream pee, which is not the first few drops, so you pee for a second or two, stop if you can, then start catching the pee. S/he will tell you where to leave the collected sample. If s/he doesn't, ask someone. Don't stay in the bathroom wondering what on earth to do. Everybody has been in your shoes, including the front desk staff, the nurses, and the doctors.

The Gown

Next, you'll be shown to a small exam room with a table or platform that you sit on. They'll ask you to get undressed and then leave the room while you do. You'll be given an unattractive gown (also called a johnny) to keep you covered. Some are cotton, others are made of thick paper that make you feel wrapped like the fish you bought for dinner. If you're cold, keep your socks on, unless you've noticed anything unusual about your feet that you want to show the doctor.

The johnny opens in the back, so put it on that way unless you're told to put the opening in the front. It lets the doctor look at one body part at a time. We think that makes it more comfortable for you.

As you know from the movies, some patients have a habit of walking around in a gown without closing the back. You'll notice

NOTE TO SELF

If you need a plus-size gown, ask for it. Many doctors have them. If s/he doesn't, you can ask for two gowns. Put one on with the opening at the back, and then drape the other one over your shoulders and down your back. Or do whatever makes you feel most comfortable. And remember that many, many people before you have had the same problem.

REAL LIFE QUESTION: Why do you want to see my pee?

Pee tells us a lot about your health in a quick snapshot. It's an easy way to find anything that shouldn't be there—like excess sugar, blood, protein, or bacteria—that might alert us to a health problem. It can also be used to test for pregnancy.

REAL LIFE FACT: Three Vital Signs

Your doctor may want to know your three vital signs. Vitals are how we can look at your health from the outside.

Pulse: The number of times your heart beats in a minute while you are at rest. A normal resting pulse is between 60 and 100 beats per minute. Your pulse may not be taken in a routine preventive-care visit.

Blood pressure: The pressure your blood makes against the walls of your arteries when your heart pumps. If you squeeze a water balloon in the middle, you can see how the skin of it stretches. That's like blood pressure. Blood pressure changes frequently but can be a good indicator of your health. It's best if your numbers are below 120 over 80. (More about blood pressure in chapter 5, Your Heart.)

Body temperature: Usually taken with a thermometer placed under your tongue. A high temperature can be a sign of illness. Your temperature changes all day and during your monthly cycle. We don't call it a fever until it starts to reach above 100 degrees Fahrenheit. Low temperatures cause concern below 95 degrees Fahrenheit. This probably won't be checked unless you are seeing the doctor for an illness.

that the system for closing a gown is actually a brainteaser of strings that you won't figure out anytime soon. It doesn't matter. Cover yourself and hop up on the table.

The Doctor Will See You Now: The Exam

While you're sitting up, the doctor will examine your skin, listen to your heart and lungs with a stethoscope, and feel your neck. The doctor also looks into your ears, eyes, and nose. You'll lie down. The doctor will press on your belly. S/he is actually feeling for any problems with your **intestines**, spleen, **liver**, or **kidneys**.

Next is often the breast exam, which sounds fun but usually isn't, but it's not uncomfortable either. The doctor uses the tips of the fingers to check for lumps throughout your breasts and armpits. (This will also be done if you see a gynecologist; see the section on the breast exam, page 17, for the details.) Even though breast cancer is uncommon in young women, it's a good idea to check. A monthly self-exam in the shower is a good habit to get into. (More on that in chapter 12, Your Breasts.)

Do you need a pelvic examination? You do if you're having any menstrual problems, if you're sexually active, or if you're twenty-one or older. You should have a Pap smear beginning at age twenty-one and then every two years until age twenty-nine. Once you turn thirty, you can decrease this schedule to every three years if you haven't had any abnormal Paps and your HPV testing is negative. Recent scientific data supports decreasing the frequency of **Pap tests** as you get older for women at low risk for cervical cancer. But speak to your doctor about the schedule that is right for you because some women need to have them more often, especially if they've had abnormal results in the past. These exams can be done by your primary care doctor or by your gynecologist (see the section on the pelvic exam, page 13, for the details).

Grooming: Shouldn't I Be Minty Fresh?

Back to the shaving issue. Many women feel they need to be perfectly groomed and shaved for a physical exam, as if it's a really big date or something. Your doctor, seriously, doesn't care. Twenty years from now, your husband or partner will also tell you that it doesn't matter. Before going to the doctor, just take your usual shower. That's it. It's usually best to have your physical when you're not having your period, but you can't always predict that. When you make the appointment, check to find out what your doctor wants you to do if you happen to have your period on the same day as your appointment.

Questions and Follow-Up

The doctor will ask you all of the questions that your mother is dying to ask you: Are you having sex? If so, how often? Are you smoking? And so on. As I've already stressed, this part is important—you have to spill the beans, no matter what.

Next come any follow-up measures that your doctor recommends. One may be a blood test. Sometimes the doctor has this done right in the office. Sometimes you have to go to a lab. The doctor fills out a form, listing all of the blood tests s/he wants. You sit outside the lab, reading the form, secretly sure that your doctor thinks you're dying. Why else would s/he be asking for all of these tests? Relax. In fact, these are just a routine check of your basic blood health.

Blood Test

To give you a blood test, a technician will put a tight band around your upper arm to get a **vein** to stand out. You might be asked to make a fist to help your veins perk up. S/he'll clean the area and then gently insert a needle, using a tube to collect blood. With the best technicians you may feel next to nothing; with others, there may be a sting on insertion. Sometimes more than one tube will be filled, but for you there's no difference between filling one and filling five. You don't have to watch! In fact, in many labs there will be distracting pictures on the wall for you to look at instead.

If you have a really hard time with needles and blood tests, ask for a butterfly needle. Seriously. These are tiny and gentle and used on kids—and on those with small, hard-to-stick veins. Some adults who hate going to the dentist go to kids' dentists for the same reason. (Plus you get stickers.)

Your Gynecology Exam—What Actually Happens

A typical appointment with a gynecologist should start with the general physical described above—your vital signs, an external exam of your internal organs, some blood tests, family history, reviewing any issues that you or your doctor want to discuss—plus the breast exam and the pelvic exam. There are also some special issues that you'll discuss during your gyn appointment:

- Your reproductive health, including fertility and sexuality
- Family planning
- Preventing sexually transmitted infections
- Infertility
- Menstrual (period) disorders
- Breast disorders and pain
- Mental health

Why Am I Seeing an Obstetrician/Gynecologist?

Obstetrics and gynecology are always linked together because you have to study both if you really want to understand a woman's body over her lifetime. Many gynecologists are also **obstetricians**, doctors who specialize in fertility, pregnancy, and childbirth, and spend most of their career delivering babies. Some hardly ever do.

Why Am I Having This Exam?

If you are having any menstrual problems, if you are sexually active, or if you are twenty-one or older, you should have an annual pelvic exam. It helps your doctor to identify problems with your sexual and reproductive organs, to diagnose sexually transmitted diseases, and to make sure that you are using effective measures to prevent disease and unwanted pregnancy. You should have a Pap smear (a test for cervical cancer) beginning at age twenty-one and then every two years unless you have an abnormal result.

Try to schedule your exam for a time when you're not having your period, though this can be difficult when you need to schedule months in advance.

The Pelvic Exam: Not the Fun Part

I don't know any woman, of any age, who likes having a pelvic exam, including me. But understanding what's going on down there can help you make a lot more sense of the exam.

I've read a lot of books on this subject, and they usually take one of two approaches. The first is the "baby doll" view, which is that you will be terribly scared, everything will hurt, and the exam room is a torture chamber. The second is the "what's the matter with you?" view, which tells you that nobody else has a problem with this exam, except crazy women and a few women who have what doctors call "mild discomfort." Those aren't helpful extremes. You won't like it and you might be uncomfortable, but as you become more experienced you'll be less and less bothered.

During the exam, you will be asked to lie on your back and move down so your bottom is at the end of the table. Moving your bottom down helps make the exam easier. You'll put your feet in special stirrups—metal foot holders at the end of the table that let you rest your legs while keeping them apart and out of the way. Do they really look like stirrups? Only if they were designed by horses for the discomfort of the rider.

The exam goes easiest if you can relax and allow your legs to fall open so that the doctor can examine your external genitalia and vagina. This is embarrassing for everyone at first, but the more times you do it, the easier it gets. The doctor will drape a sheet across your knees to keep you a bit more covered up and as much at ease as possible—but if you'd rather be able to see the doctor's face during the process, speak up. It's your choice.

Next, the doctor will use a **speculum** to look inside your vagina. A speculum is a two-sided slender metal or plastic instrument held together with a hinge, a bit like smooth salad tongs. Metal speculums are often kept at a warm temperature in a heated drawer to make the exam more comfortable. Some doctors use plastic ones, which feel warm at room temperature. Most doctors find it helpful to give you a running commentary on what is going on, so you know what to expect: "I'm going to touch you on the outside to examine you. Now I am inserting the speculum," and so on.

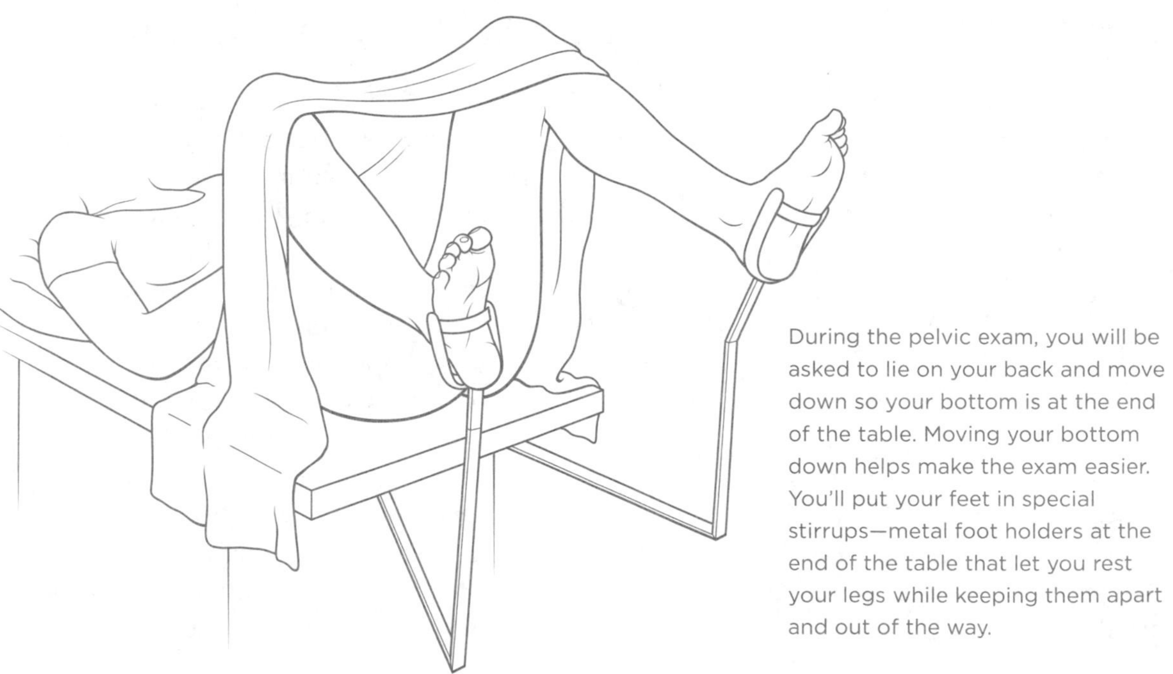

During the pelvic exam, you will be asked to lie on your back and move down so your bottom is at the end of the table. Moving your bottom down helps make the exam easier. You'll put your feet in special stirrups—metal foot holders at the end of the table that let you rest your legs while keeping them apart and out of the way.

The speculum is closed when it is inserted into your vagina. Then it is opened, which spreads your vagina a bit to allow your **cervix** and vagina to be viewed. This feels like pressure, and although you won't like it, it shouldn't be terribly painful.

Having the speculum inside you may make you want to tense your muscles, which usually makes this exam more uncomfortable. It helps a lot to breath slowly, like the breathing you do during yoga exercises, which helps you to relax your pelvic muscles. Every doctor has his or her own way of interacting with you during the exam. Some chat to keep you occupied; others leave that to the assistant. Some put posters on the ceiling so you have something else to focus on. Some ask you general questions so you'll be talking instead of tensing up. Be sure to let the doctor know if you prefer small talk or would rather be left alone with your iPod.

Once the speculum is in place, the doctor can see the cervix at the top of the vagina. S/he will use a special brush to take a few cells from the cervix to perform a Pap test for precancerous changes of the cervix. Some women don't feel this. Some feel a crampy feeling that goes away as soon as the test is done. Remind yourself that this is a powerful, lifesaving test.

The cells that have been collected are put into a liquid or spread onto a slide, which is sent to a special lab for processing. The cells are examined under the microscope by a specialist who looks for changes that might be precancerous.

When your doctor collects specimens with the speculum exam, s/he is also looking for sexually transmitted infections (**STIs**).

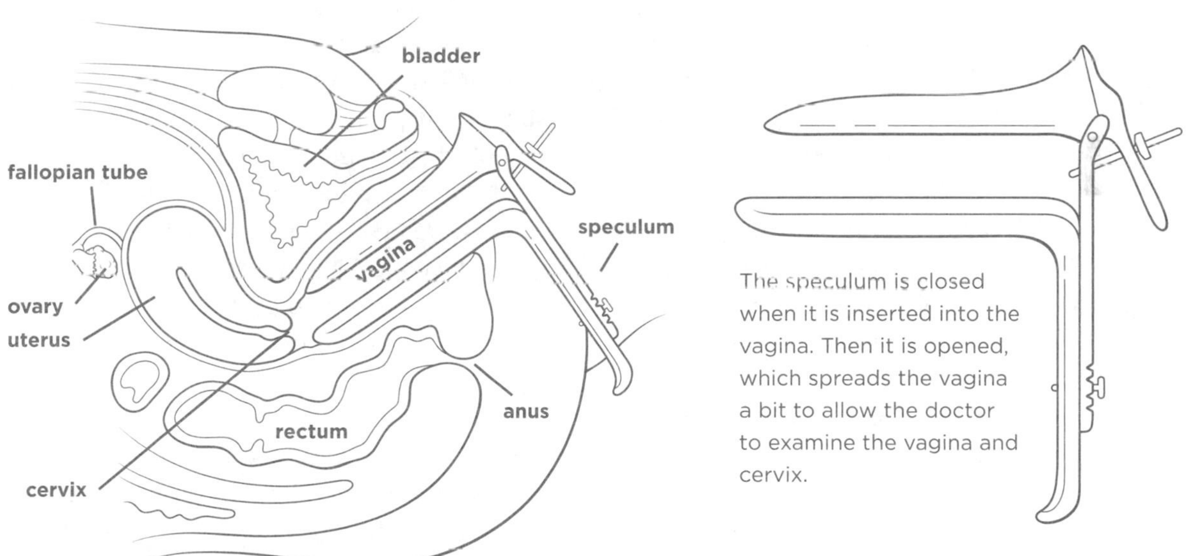

The speculum is closed when it is inserted into the vagina. Then it is opened, which spreads the vagina a bit to allow the doctor to examine the vagina and cervix.

REAL LIFE FACT: Most STIs Are Treatable

Because sexually transmitted infections (STIs) in women commonly cause no symptoms, it's important to be tested for STIs if you are sexually active, even if you feel fine. If left untreated, STIs can lead to pelvic inflammatory disease, a widespread infection of the pelvic organs. This can cause problems down the road due to scarring, such as infertility and chronic pelvic pain. If you are twenty-five or younger and you are having sex, please be checked routinely for chlamydia infections, even if you have no symptoms.

According to the Guttmacher Institute, STIs are diagnosed in fifteen million people each year in the United States. Not enough young adults are getting screened. In fact, other than testing for HIV/AIDS, fewer than half of adults eighteen to forty-four years of age have ever been tested for an STI. Is that untested person your partner? Maybe. That's why it's important for you to get the facts and ask for the right tests to be done. Be an equal partner in your health care by asking for testing.

This is an important point to be clear about, as many women think they are having a Pap test when they are tested for STIs, or vice versa. Be sure you know which tests are being done. Remember that this exam will not catch all STIs and does not replace blood tests you may need.

Out comes the speculum, in go two (gloved) fingers. The doctor will feel around the whole area, looking for anything out of the ordinary. S/he will press through the lower abdomen for the **uterus** and ovaries, and then check your **anus** and **rectum** too. S/he'll be using lots of lubricant to keep it as comfortable as possible, so when you're done, before you get dressed, you'll want to do lots of wiping with the gown.

Try to tolerate this exam as well as you can. Deep breathing can be relaxing. You want a thorough exam, not a quick one, and now that you're here and in the stirrups, you may as well get what you came for.

If everything is normal, most likely you will not need to be seen again for a year. Remember that yearly pelvic exams are an important part of preventive health, so you should go for annual exams even if all is well.

Preventive health care means detecting diseases early—before you have any symptoms. If you feel like the doctor or nurse practitioner was not the right one for you, don't let that prevent you from continuing your annual gynecologic examinations—*with someone else*. Not every doctor-patient relationship is perfect, and sometimes you just need to seek a better fit with a new health care provider. And remember, although no one loves having a pelvic exam, each time you do it gets easier.

NOTE TO SELF

Your gynecologist can take care of your preventive health care needs when you are young and healthy, but at some point it's a good idea to have a primary care doctor take charge of your care—either an internal medicine doctor or a family doctor. Doctors, including your gynecologist, are highly specialized today. It's good to have someone with more general knowledge on your team. Your gynecologist likely knows a good one, so ask. Good doctors know good doctors.

The Breast Exam: Details, Details

Part of the physical examination, either with your primary care physician or your gynecologist, is an examination of your breasts. If you are a teenager, this includes an evaluation of your development to make sure you have reached the normal level of maturity for your age. For all women, it includes checking whether there are any abnormal lumps, dimples, or discharge, or problems in the nearby **lymph nodes**.

Why Am I Having This Exam?

Breast exams by your doctor may detect lumps that can be felt yet can't be seen on mammography. Studies show that breast exams by health care providers can detect about 15 percent of tumors not seen on mammograms and are effective in reducing death rates from breast cancer. In fact, a Canadian study shows that exams are as effective as mammograms. But don't interpret the results to mean that mammograms don't matter—it seems they are most effective when both breast exam and mammogram are done together.

You don't need to start mammograms until you are at least forty, unless you are at high risk for breast cancer, but breast exams should start in your twenties. (Please see chapter 12, Your Breasts, for more about mammograms and breast health.)

One of the most important issues for breast health is to know what normal breasts feel like. Normal breasts are not perfectly smooth; they are a bit lumpy and bumpy. This is called physiologic modularity and is nothing to be concerned about. During your exam, your doctor will help you become familiar with the way your healthy breasts feel, so that you will be aware when something changes.

Some women's breasts are lumpier than others. They are also lumpier in the second half of your menstrual cycle. Lumpy breasts are not a risk factor for developing breast cancer, but they can make examining your breasts a bit more confusing.

What Does a Breast Exam Feel Like?

Are you worried that a breast exam will feel sexual? You're not alone in that worry—but here's the good news: it doesn't feel sexual at all. It just feels medical.

When the doctor examines your breasts, you lie on your back with your hands above your head. This helps spread out the breast tissue, making it easier to do a thorough exam. Breast tissue extends from your clavicle (collar bone) to your sternum (breast bone) and out to your armpit.

Your doctor will use his or her fingertips and go methodically over and around your breasts. Studies show that a breast examination is most effective when the doctor spends about two minutes on it. So don't get nervous if s/he spends some time poking around. It usually means the doctor is trying to be thorough, not that s/he has found anything abnormal!

Breast Self-Examination: The Controversy

There will be quite a few topics in this book where science and experience tell us conflicting things. The breast self-exam is a big one.

For years, doctors would show patients how to examine their breasts themselves. Until recently, breast self-exam was thought to be a good way for women to examine themselves for early signs of breast cancer.

Then came a 2002 study in Shanghai that showed no difference in overall deaths from breast cancer between women who did self-exams and women who did not. Also, the self-examiners would find **benign** lumps that would then have to be looked at with a **biopsy**, which can be stressful for any patient.

Since then, some doctors have stopped pushing the monthly self-exam. "Wait a minute," you say. "My mother found her cancer as she was doing a self-exam in the shower." And there's the controversy. We know from experience, not science, that many women find their own lumps. Statistically there may be no difference in the death rate, but for many individual women finding the lump is lifesaving.

What to do? Get to know your breasts as a first step. Examine them after your period when they are least lumpy. The shower is a good place to check them. Check again on a schedule that is easy to remember—the first day of each season, for example, or monthly.

Become familiar with your breasts. If you come across something that doesn't feel right, have the doctor check it out. No reason to panic now—almost all of the time, lumps are benign.

Know Your Family

Your health is influenced by your lifestyle, your behaviors, and your genetics. While you can't control your genes, you can make choices that will keep you healthy. I remember an angry patient who once told me, "I exercise every day, I don't smoke or drink, and I eat well. And because I carry a gene mutation, I still got breast cancer at age forty-two." I said, "Well, that's true, but you were diagnosed with stage I breast cancer, and your treatment was lumpectomy with radiation. You never needed chemotherapy, and you've had no recurrence in ten years." Her healthy lifestyle, along with sticking to her mammogram schedule and doctors' appointments, enabled early detection of her cancer and excellent tolerance of the treatment. This is a good example of nurture winning over nature, of lifestyle over genes.

Your Health: The Big Picture

Some people just like to worry. They often think they're dying, or that something awful is bound to happen. The truth is, you're likely to live to be so old that you start looking like your grandfather. But you still may want to know: What are women your age most likely to die of? What are women your age most likely to get sick from?

The real causes of sickness and death that affect your age group are listed below. These will probably scare you, but not nearly as much as the evening news does. On the news, you'll hear crazy stories about young people dying from things like mixing breath mints and diet soda. The media covers medical news in ways that are designed to shock you into watching the whole story. They give you the shocking headline ("News You Must Know to Survive!") during your 9:00 p.m. show so that you'll stay up and watch the news at 11:00 p.m.

The facts are usually much less dramatic and sensational. Knowing the facts, some of which may surprise you, can help you and your doctor to decide what you need to do for preventive maintenance.

The Centers for Disease Control keeps track of the leading causes of illness and death by age group. As you'll see, whether you're in

REAL LIFE FACT: Most Common Conditions, Illnesses, and Health Risks for Women Ages 19 to 39

- Acne
- Appendicitis
- Arthritis
- Back symptoms
- Cancer
- Chlamydia
- Depression
- Diabetes mellitus
- Gynecologic disorders
- Headache/migraine
- Hypertension
- Infectious, viral, and parasitic diseases
- Joint disorders
- Menstrual disorders
- Nose, throat, ear, and upper respiratory infections
- Obesity
- Sexual assault and domestic violence
- Sexually transmitted diseases
- Skin rash or dermatitis
- Substance abuse
- Urinary tract infections

Leading Causes of Death for Women Ages 19 to 39

- Cancer
- Accidents
- Heart diseases
- Suicide
- Human immunodeficiency virus (HIV)
- Homicide

REAL LIFE FACT: Expect to Talk with Your Doctor about . . .

Smoking	**Abuse**	**Diet**
Drinking and drug use	**Safer sex***	**Exercise**
Mental health	**Contraception***	**Family health issues**

***Can also be discussed with your gynecologist.**

your teens, twenties, or thirties, many of these leading health problems are preventable. No matter how many things in life are out of your control, you can still influence how long you live and how healthy you'll be by making the right health and lifestyles choices now.

Screening Tests

Screening and prevention are extremely important parts of your health care. Screening means using tests to detect a condition even if you have no signs or symptoms, or if you have early warning symptoms that can give your doctor a clue to a potential disease. So it is extremely important to share everything you are experiencing in your body with your doctor, even if you think it's not important.

Screening for cancer, for example, can us help to find it at an early and potentially curable stage. In some cases, cancer can be completely prevented by finding and removing the early stage cancer. A screening **colonoscopy**, usually given to people in middle age, can detect and painlessly remove colonic **polyps** that might eventually have become cancerous. A colonic polyp is a growth on the inside of the **colon**. Most polyps don't turn into cancer, but some do if they are allowed to grow. While most people do not need this test until after age fifty, if colon cancer runs in your family it may be important to have it at a younger age.

Screening tests for **heart disease** in young women, for example, include taking your blood pressure and checking your blood lipid levels. Lipid screening, done through blood testing, should include a total **cholesterol** level and an **HDL** level. You probably thought these tests were for middle-aged people because that's who's in the TV commercials for prescription drugs—but young women can have heart problems too.

If this test is normal, it should be repeated every five years. Screening tests such as EKGs, echocardiograms, or heart monitors should be reserved for symptoms such as chest pain or abnormal heartbeat rhythms. They have not been shown to be useful for young women otherwise. We'll talk more about this in chapter 5, Your Heart.

REAL LIFE FACT: Basic Tests to Have for Good Health

Here's a list of the tests you should have according to your age. Your doctor may follow this same schedule, or adjust according to your personal or family health history. If you have any questions about these tests or when you should start having them, be sure to ask your doctor.

AGE 20–29

- Annual physical, including breast and pelvic exams, blood tests, skin checks, and blood pressure.
- Fasting cholesterol and HDL (every five years if the tests are normal or more often according to your doctor's recommendations).
- Pap smear (and HPV testing if your Pap is abnormal) every two years (or more often according to your doctor's recommendations).
- Screening for HIV, chlamydia, and gonorrhea (yearly if you are sexually active).
- Dental exam and cleaning (at least once a year, but preferably every six months if your insurance covers it).
- Eye exam (if needed).

AGE 30–39

All of the above tests, plus:

- Thyroid stimulating hormone (TSH) starting at age 35 (and every five years after that, or according to your doctor's recommendations).
- Decrease the frequency of your Pap tests to every three years if your Paps have been normal and you are HPV negative. If you've had abnormal tests, discuss the right schedule with your doctor.
- Continue annual screening for HIV, chlamydia, and gonorrhea if you've had new partners (you don't need the screenings if you and your partner have tested negative and you're certain that you've only been with each other).

AGE 40–49

All of the above tests, plus:

- Mammogram (every one to two years, or more or less often according to your doctor's recommendations and your personal or family health history).
- Glucose testing for diabetes (every three years, but your doctor may recommend that you have it more often if you have personal or family risks factors).
- Talk to your doctor about the recommended schedule for eye exams. These aren't only to check your vision, but also to detect eye conditions such as glaucoma.

AGE 50 AND UP

All of the above tests, plus:

- Colonoscopy (every five to ten years or more often according to your doctor's recommendations and your personal and family health history).
- Bone density scan (every five years beginning after menopause if you have risk factors for osteoporosis, and by age sixty-five if you don't.

Not every disease can be screened at a time that makes a difference to your health. Even if you have regular checkups, have every blood test—heck, even if you have a medical degree—some diseases are not detectable until they've advanced to later stages. Ovarian cancer is a classic example. It's called the "silent killer" because the disease can grow without any signs. Even if you find ovarian cancer before you have symptoms, perhaps shown on an ultrasound, it may already be advanced. (See chapter 14, Your Ovaries, for more about ovarian cancer. There are some promising new screening techniques.)

Be sure to have the screening tests recommended for you, for those diseases that can be found early, and for which early detection can mean the healthiest possible result. Some diseases—including brain cancer, for example—are uncommon among young people. Not everyone needs the screening test, and the tests have not proven to be effective tools for detecting disease.

Sometimes you'll have these tests if you have a family history that warrants it—again, a good reason to educate yourself by asking your family questions, then writing down the answers and sharing this information with your doctor.

So now you know that information is a big key to the quality of your health care. Someday your children will thank you for writing down the family history. (Well, they may never actually say those words, but you'll know they are thinking it.)

What to Expect from Additional Medical Tests

Here's a quick description of how you'll *experience* some of the most common tests recommended by your doctor. If you're interested in the technical or medical details of these tests, check out www.radiologyinfo.org, a service of the Radiological Society of North America (RSNA).

For many of these tests, you'll have to change into a gown again. Just like for your annual exam, the doctor or nurse will tell you which way to put it on and what clothing to take off. For many tests, you should leave your jewelry at home, especially if you have body piercings.

X-Ray

X-rays are the original, magical look inside the body, first discovered in 1895. X-rays allow doctors to look at your bones. This is what your doctor will order up if s/he thinks you've broken a bone or if an employer requires a chest X-ray as part of a health exam.

To have an X-ray, you'll put on your gown and the X-ray technician will position you and a giant camera together. You might be sitting, standing, or lying down on a table. S/he will ask you if you are or think you might be pregnant, in which case s/he would take special care to protect the baby from the X-ray machine's radiation. Most likely, the technician will also cover the part of you that isn't being scanned with a lead blanket to protect you from exposure. Your job is to stay completely still for the one second it takes to capture the image of your bones.

Why are you being exposed to radiation? Many routine tests require that you have a tiny dose of radiation, which refers to waves or rays of energy. Practically everything sends out radiation—even *you*. There are many types of radiation, but it all falls into two categories: natural and artificial. Natural radiation is in cosmic rays from space, the earth itself, everything. Artificial radiation, which is manufactured, is used in medical testing.

Safety depends on dose. If we look at ordinary rocks from your backyard, the radiation levels will be so tiny we won't even be able to measure them. If we measure uranium, we'll see a lot of radiation. In small doses, radiation is fine. In big doses, it's poison. Over your lifetime, ordinary tests are believed to be safe, but don't ask for unnecessary testing. People were crazy for X-rays in the early twentieth century. Shoe stores offered X-rays to help people choose their shoes!

Ultrasound

An ultrasound lets a doctor take a live look at your insides and is often used to view a developing pregnancy or to check for lumps or cysts. Ultrasounds are a very important tool if you have an ovarian cyst, for example, or a breast lump, because the breast tissue of young women is often too dense for a mammogram to be reliable.

To have an ultrasound, you'll put on your gown and lie on a table or platform. The ultrasound technician will apply some gel to the area s/he is going to test (usually your pelvic area or your breasts) and roll a wand over the area to get an in-depth look. An ultrasound wand can also be inserted into parts of your body such as your vagina. In this case, for cleanliness, the technician will cover the wand with something that looks exactly like a **condom** and then use some gel for your comfort. The picture of your insides will show up on a little TV screen. It's exciting to watch if you're pregnant, but otherwise won't reveal much to you.

For some ultrasound tests, you'll need to have a full **bladder** during the examination, which helps the technician to get a better view. When you make your appointment, the doctor's office will tell you to drink about a year's worth of water before you arrive. You have to hold it through the exam. Don't worry, you'll make it—but you'll run to the bathroom when the test is done.

The ultrasound technician is performing the test for a radiologist, who will study your pictures and report back to your doctor. The technician has been instructed not to tell you anything because s/he has not been trained in reading the results. Asking or pressuring the technician for feedback on the exam is a bad idea, and it usually won't work anyway.

Mammogram

Although mammograms generally aren't recommended for women under the age of forty, we're including a description here because you may be asked to have a mammogram at an earlier age if you have a history of breast cancer in your family, or if you find a lump in your breast.

Don't use deodorant or powder before your mammogram. You'll remove your shirt and bra and put on a gown. You stand in front of the mammogram machine and have one breast tested at a time. The technician will position your breast on a tray and then move another tray down on top of your breast. The machine will squeeze and flatten your breast until it looks like it's been run over by a cartoon steamroller.

Does it hurt? Yes, but only for a couple of seconds and then it's over. At least until you do the other breast. But then you're finished for another year. In the end, it's worth a few seconds of pain for a test that could save your life. When it's that time, please go. All of those walks and marches and races for a breast cancer cure mean nothing if women don't have mammograms.

CT and PET Scans

CT and PET scans are used to look for problems ranging from appendicitis to cancer. Both are a bit like extremely high-resolution X-rays. To have a scan, you might have to prepare in advance by fasting before the appointment. (Try to schedule fasting tests for early in the morning!)

When you arrive at the doctor's office, you might have to drink a test liquid that will show up on the scan. It tastes pretty gross, but you'll be able to get it down. You might also need to have a contrast dye, which is given **intravenously** (by IV). Pay close attention to the questions they ask you about allergies because some people are allergic to contrast dye if they are allergic to other things, such as shellfish.

You'll lie down on a table, wearing a gown as usual. The scanner looks like a big metal doughnut and you'll be moved through it. This process usually doesn't bother people, but still, it's a big metal doughnut and it's a little weird. During the scan you'll be given instructions to take a deep breath, hold it in, and then release it. Try to hold still while you do that.

You might also be scanned twice. The technician may pass you through the doughnut once and take a scan, and then give you an IV of contrast dye and run you through the doughnut one more time. Your first scan will seem strange, but overall it's not bad.

MRI

MRI stands for *magnetic resonance imaging*, which means we use a big tube and magnets to look at your insides instead of radiation. Let's be real. For many people, an MRI is a difficult test. Not because it hurts, but because you're inside a tube that's making a whole lot of noise.

For anyone who's claustrophobic, MRIs are awful. If that's you, here's how to make it okay. First, ask your hospital if they have an MRI machine for large patients. In the past, these were old machines that didn't work so well, but the newer ones work fine, so be sure to ask about what is available. Obviously, also

REAL LIFE FACT: Getting Your Test Results

When you've had any type of test, your doctor—and normally no one else—will be the one to give you the results. It could take days or weeks to get a report, especially if you are young and healthy! But if the doctor already knows that you have cancer, for example, your scans may go to the top of the pile and you could know the results in a couple of days. If you are healthy and the doctor wants to rule something out, it's going to take longer.

ask for these machines if you're large. And ask well in advance to make sure you get scheduled for the right machine.

To have an MRI, you'll remove anything made of metal from your body, including piercings. Don't hide anything because you can easily be injured if the gigantic magnet inside the machine pulls the metal out of you. You'll put on a gown and then lie down on a table. Usually the technician will cover you with a blanket to keep you warm because you might be lying in the machine for ten minutes to an hour, depending on the test.

The easiest MRI test for many people is of your legs, because only your legs go inside the machine. The most challenging test is an MRI of the brain, because you have to keep your head completely still. Sometimes your head is secured in a kind of cage. It's not quite as bad as a hockey mask, but it's awkward.

The technician will give you disposable earplugs to wear. You can bring your own if you prefer. Once you're inside and the test starts, stay as still as you can and practice relaxation techniques such as measured breathing and visualization. The machine will make a series of loud banging noises all around you and then go quiet. Then it will start again with a different series of banging noises and then go quiet. This repeats until the test is finished.

If you are really anxious about claustrophobia, you can take a sedative in advance of the test as long as you have a buddy to drive you to and from the appointment. If you forget to take your sedative, you can put it under your tongue right before the test to get some immediate relief. Always arrange this in advance. The MRI technicians don't have any sedatives to give you.

And keep reminding yourself that it will be over soon.

Top Ten Real Life Questions Patients Want to Ask Me

Now you've scheduled your physical or your annual gyn exam. Before you head in, here are the top ten questions that I find young women want to know about. Some of them might seem silly at first look, but there's important information to be found by asking each one. Think of this as a head start!

1. How Can I Get Rid of PMS?

There are more jokes about **PMS** than about any other female condition. While you're in the middle of it, none of them are funny. You've got bloating, sore breasts, food cravings, cramps, irritability, and mood swings. You can probably add a few of your own favorite symptoms and complaints to this list.

There are many effective ways to reduce PMS. Exercise and calcium, which are good for you whether you have PMS or not, can help. A daily 1,000 mg calcium supplement has been shown to be helpful in several studies. Cutting back on caffeine may reduce irritability and mood swings. Cutting your salt intake may decrease bloating and swelling. There's lots more about PMS and other period-related problems later in this book.

2. Does What I Eat Really Make Any Difference?

Yes. If you eat and drink based on TV commercials and supermarket coupons, you could have a shorter life than your prehistoric ancestors did. Feeding your body well is crucial for good health—especially heart health—at any age. As you'll see in the chapter on your heart, the number one killer of women is heart disease. More women die from heart disease than from all types of cancer—including breast cancer—combined.

Our Western culture struggles with weight in every way. You may already know that every low-calorie diet you go on can actually make you heavier. We stress that the best way to eat for most people is a diet high in vegetables, fruit, whole grains, healthy fats (like olive oil), and lean **protein**, and low in **saturated fats** and highly processed foods. Notice we said "low," not "zero." Life really can include chocolate. In fact, you'll learn later in the book that it actually has some health benefits.

In the meantime, just keep in mind that you really are what you eat. I'll help you to learn how to eat well, and in a way that's realistic and enjoyable for your own way of life.

4. Do I Have to Exercise?

Your body needs to be moving. Every day. Lack of physical activity is a risk factor for heart

REAL LIFE QUESTION: 3. I'm thin, so I don't have to exercise, right?

An overweight active person is healthier than a skinny couch potato. Or a skinny recliner potato. Or a skinny computer potato.

disease, which you already know is the leading killer of women. Regular, moderate-to-vigorous exercise for thirty to forty minutes a day not only will help your body avoid heart disease, but also can help control cholesterol, diabetes, obesity, and high blood pressure.

Physical activity also builds muscle, a big variable in weight control. Fat tissue has much lower metabolic activity—meaning it burns fewer calories, even at rest—than muscle does. If you build and maintain muscle, your resting **metabolic rate** increases and your body requires more calories every day to perform its basic functions. So if you exercise regularly, you can even lose weight while you sleep!

And did you know that exercise also protects your bones and keeps you from slouching when you're older? (See chapter 7, Your Bones and Joints, for details.)

5. *How Can I Have Better Sex?*

Not in the mood for sex? You've got plenty of company. Unlike what you see on TV, many people do not have a roaring good sex life. Surveys show that 43 percent of all women eighteen to fifty-nine years old have some type of sexual dysfunction. *Sexual dysfunction* is a medical term used to describe a condition in people who have one or more of these characteristics: lack of desire for sex, problems getting excited or aroused, difficulty achieving orgasm, or inability to achieve orgasm. Comedians, on the other hand, may call sexual dysfunction "a medical term that means having children."

Your interest in sex changes with your monthly cycle, with relationship challenges, with many life changes, and as a normal result of aging. In some cases a medical condition can alter it. Many commonly prescribed drugs, including ones for blood pressure, depression, and birth control, can interfere with sex drive, arousal, and orgasm. For example, antidepressants known as **selective serotonin reuptake inhibitors** (SSRIs such as Prozac, Paxil, and Zoloft) combat depression by increasing the production of **serotonin** in the brain. Lower sexual desire is a common side effect of that increase.

Sexual changes are common in everyone's life. Don't let anybody tell you that you have "sexual dysfunction" just because you've lost interest for now. Just remember that there are many ways to rekindle your sexuality, as you will see in later chapters. Your doctor just might be able to help you have a better sex life!

6. *Do I Really Have to Tell You Everything?*

I must keep your information confidential—and I have to know everything. A doctor's job is to put together the whole puzzle that is your body, and I can't do that if you're hiding some of the pieces, including smoking and drug use. So see your doctor once a year, even if you're not sick, and be open about your real life. Depending on your family history, age, and lifestyle, you may be at risk for disease. With full information from you, we may catch disease in its early stages, when treatment is most effective. When it comes to your health, knowledge is power!

7. Can a Pap Test Detect Sexually Transmitted Infections?

Yes, but only one of them. A Pap test can detect **HPV**, the human papillomavirus, which can cause cervical cancer (cancer of the cervix). The cervix is the narrow passageway between your vagina and uterus.

There are at least twenty-five other diseases, including **AIDS**, that are spread mostly through sexual activity. Together these infections are called sexually transmitted infections (STIs). Although many **STIs** are treatable, some are not. If you're sexually active, you should be tested separately from your Pap test for STIs, such as **chlamydia** and **gonorrhea**—two common sexually transmitted infections that often show no symptoms in young women. STIs can affect your life and fertility in the future. Be tested early and often. It's easy and confidential (see page 8 for more information about how your privacy is protected).

8. Can My Underwire Bra Cause Breast Cancer?

Let's get rid of three common myths about breast cancer: Large-breasted women are not at increased risk, bras do not cause breast cancer, and deodorants and antiperspirants are not known to cause breast cancer. (More details in chapter 12, Your Breasts.)

9. Is a Manicure Good or Bad for My Health?

It can be good for your health if you are a mani-pedi person and having them relaxes you. Life is filled with stress, and too much

REAL LIFE QUESTION: Get rid of my period? That's a myth, right?

You've seen the commercials. Can you really use the Pill to change your menstrual cycle or even cut down on how often you get it? Yes.

Look at a pack of birth control pills. For three weeks, you take a combination of estrogen and progestin. For one week, you take a different colored pill that doesn't actually do anything. The drug companies provide this because they've learned that it reinforces the habit of daily pill taking during this week that the body is allowed to have a period.

A growing number of women are taking birth control without the seven days of "period pills." Result? They keep taking the estrogen-progestin and skip their period. Talk with your doctor about this first—and in any case, do not take the Pill if you smoke and you're over thirty-five.

stress can give you health problems: headaches, upset stomach, high blood pressure, and even **stroke** or heart disease. Stress can also make you feel depressed, angry, and anxious. It can affect relationships at home and at work. Sometimes even positive events (a new partner, new job, or vacation) can trigger stress. Of course, negative events, such as a failed test, the end of a relationship, the death of a loved one, or the loss of a job can worsen stress and anxiety too.

Chapter 2, Your Head, provides details about the toll stress takes on your health and offers "stress busters" to help alleviate both stress and its effects. Sneak preview: exercise, laughter, massage, manicure, music, friendship, love, napping, and reading.

If a good mani-pedi relieves stress for you, go ahead. Of course, a mani-pedi treatment for stress is helpful only if your nail tech practices safe, sanitary care of the tools and environment. Many women bring their own kit of tools to the salon to be sure. No doctor will advise you to have your cuticles cut, but we know you might do it anyway, so be watchful about germs.

10. *What Does That Vaginal Discharge Mean?*

It's normal to have vaginal discharge, also called secretions. Discharge is a liquid, creamy, or gel-like goop that you'll notice on toilet paper or your underwear. Its color, quantity, and consistency change with the phases of your monthly cycle.

The chapter on your vagina and cervix describes a healthy vagina, which has a small to moderate amount of discharge that ranges from clear to white and from thin to thick. Cells in the vagina produce normal discharges that provide lubrication and clean the vagina. The vaginal secretions provide a naturally acidic environment that prevents infections. (One of the surprising things you might learn: Bag the douche! The vagina is like a self-cleaning oven; it does not need to be cleaned out!)

If you have concern about a discharge, particularly if it's dark in color or has a fishy smell, ask your doctor about it.

What About Other Questions I'm Afraid to Ask?

This first chapter has offered you just a taste of what comes in the rest of the book. After years of seeing patients, I've learned what young women are thinking about, worried about, and even afraid to ask. Every chapter in this book has the answers you are looking for about your body and your health. In this chapter, we talked about how to get the best care from your doctor. In the rest of the book, we'll cover your body, from head to toe, with a long journey to everything else in between.

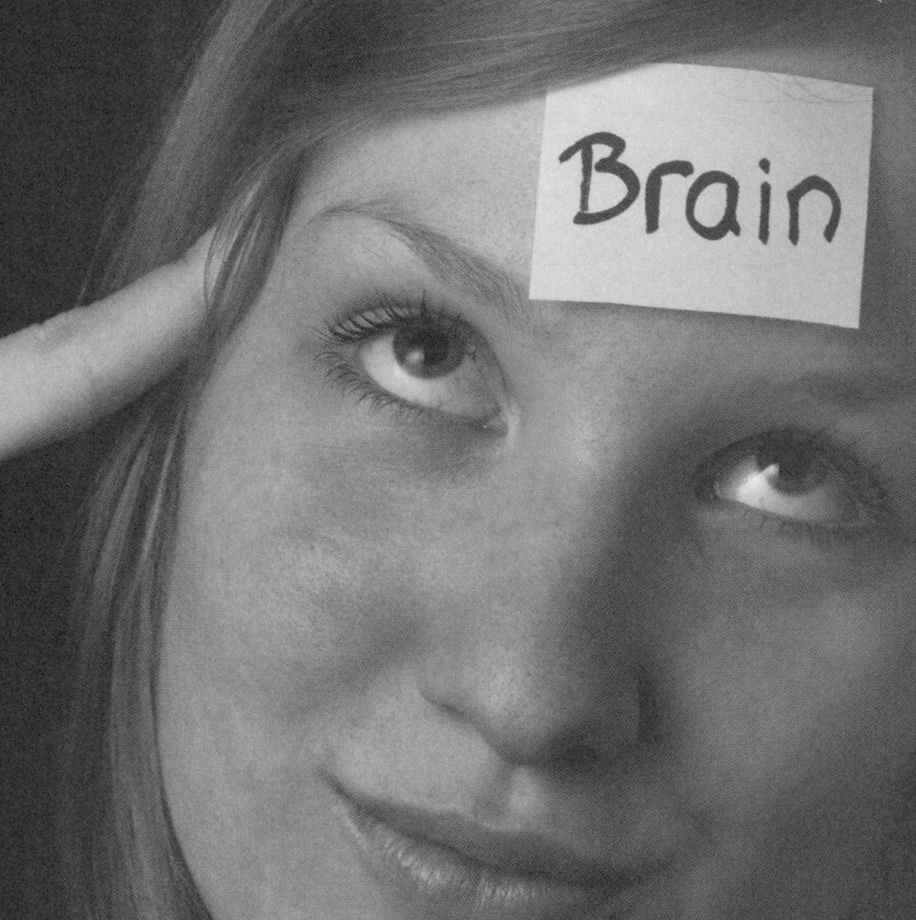

What's going on in your head—
and why does it need your body?

your head

Your brain and your body are like an old married couple. They take care of each other, they fight, they love each other, and they could wring each other's necks. What happens to one happens to the other. They can't get away from each other, so to keep one happy you have to make both happy.

Everything starts and ends here in the brain and in its connection to your body. The happiness you feel, the energy that gets you up every morning, the calm that allows you to sort through your ideas, the creativity that makes your life exciting, the joy and love you feel for your friends and family. It's also where you keep fury, anger, depression (that feeling that nothing matters), anxiety, irritability, headaches, **migraines** . . . oh, and **PMS**.

In this chapter we talk about the connections between your mind and your body. For example, you'll learn to recognize the role your hormones play in your emotions and how your diet can affect your energy level. You probably already know that your mind feels sharper when you are sleeping well and that you feel better about the world when you are exercising most days of the week. We'll talk about why these things are true, and also show you how to keep it all humming.

Sleep Your Way to a Healthy Brain

One of your most important jobs is to get a good night's sleep. Young women, especially, don't sleep as much as they need to. Having a good sleep life—meaning you sleep for seven and a half to eight hours every night, beginning and ending at about the same time every day—can make you feel wonderful.

Even if you are in a profession or situation that requires sleep deprivation, such as working occasional double shifts or regular overtime or caring for a newborn, make it a high priority to regularize or fix your sleep habits. Your mind will be sharper, your body will feel healthier, and your mood will be more even.

If you are laughing at the idea of a good night's sleep, you're in trouble. Shocked? Then you must not yet be aware of the impact that sleep deprivation has on your mind and body. Before you decide to skip this advice, remember one unavoidable fact: all over the world, people who torture other people use sleep deprivation as a major weapon. Lab rats that are deprived of sleep die within days or weeks. And countless car accidents are caused by those two seconds of drowsiness you feel. Two seconds is all it takes to hit a tree.

So I don't know why so many of us feel proud of our lack of sleep. We like to talk about how little sleep we get by on as if that's an achievement. Unfortunately, we are not able to see the damage this does to our brain and body. We don't connect it with the brain fog, the mood swings, or the decline in reaction time that makes us a walking accident risk. Instead, we try to jump-start ourselves with caffeine, which makes it harder to get to sleep at night, increasing our sleep deprivation. Soon, getting behind the wheel is as risky as driving drunk. Not convinced to get to bed on time tonight? How about this incentive? Not getting enough sleep increases your risk of **diabetes** and weight gain.

How is your sleep? Health problems, stress, and even joyful things can cause you to have a hard time falling asleep, staying asleep, or sleeping soundly. Let's look at the most common sleep issues and some simple tips for making them better.

Restless Legs

If your legs move on their own and disrupt your sleep and you have a "creepy crawly" feeling in your legs when sitting or lying down, you may have **restless legs syndrome** (RLS). There is no test for RLS, but your doctor can help you find ways to ease the restlessness. You'll start by looking for causes such as medications or vitamin deficiencies. For some people, diet and exercise changes can help, and for others, prescription medications can quiet the legs down. If you have the symptoms of RLS, see your doctor and educate yourself about this syndrome. You need a good night's sleep!

Sleep Apnea

The most serious sleep disorder is sleep apnea, in which you stop breathing many times in a night. Clues that you might have apnea: You are probably a loud snorer, as your body takes a big breath in when you wake up slightly from the lack of oxygen. You are probably drowsy during the day. Untreated, sleep apnea can lead to heart problems.

The first step in diagnosing sleep apnea is a talk with your doctor. S/he may recommend that you spend the night at a sleep clinic, where technicians will monitor you to determine if you are getting enough sleep or if you have a problem like apnea.

Sleep apnea is most common among overweight men, but plenty of people get it, and women of all sizes and shapes can be affected. If someone you love makes gasping snoring noises at night, please encourage him or her to talk to a doctor. Getting this problem corrected will make *your* life a whole lot better, too.

One Sheep, Two Sheep: Insomnia

Do you envy anyone who turns out the light and is asleep five minutes later? Can you read a whole book before you doze off? If you always have a hard time falling and staying asleep, then you might have insomnia. It might happen all the time, it might come and go, and it might be yet another problem caused by stress. No matter what causes your insomnia, it's so important to sleep well that we'll look at some basic solutions below. There are many, and it can take some time to figure out what's best for you.

Sleep experts recommend that you start to solve your problem with basic "sleep hygiene." First, wake up and get up at the same time every day (yes, including weekends). Go to bed at the same time every night. Reserve your bedroom for sleeping and sex—no TV, no work. Keep the room dark, quiet, and cool. Avoid caffeine. Exercise earlier in the day, not near bedtime.

Try meditating before you go to bed. Aromatherapy, especially the scent of lavender, helps some people sleep. There are many ways to get a scent into your room, including pillow sachets, silky eye masks, scented lotions and sprays, and even professional aromatherapy diffusers. (Please do not use candles or other flame-lit methods! Seriously.)

By creating regular and calming sleep habits, you are training your body to fall asleep naturally. Think about the method you might use to put a toddler to bed and try to create a similar routine. Yours might be reading, brushing your teeth, listening to some quiet music, and then lights out. Do yourself a favor and always make a last trip to the toilet before bedtime, even if you don't have to go. (This is a good lifetime habit to get into that might even help you during and after pregnancy.) If you pee right before you go to bed, you might avoid having to get up later.

Light box therapy may also help you. Many people with insomnia have an internal clock that's just set to the wrong time. When it's noon, your body thinks its dawn! It's hard for you to fall asleep and almost impossible to get up in the morning, like having jet lag that never gets better.

With light box therapy, you buy a special light box and sit near it first thing in the morning to tell your body that it's time to wake up. Set up the box in a spot that's easy for you to use. Some people check their email and have their morning drink while they spend thirty minutes sitting in the light. Light boxes can also help if you get especially depressed in the winter, which is called seasonal affective disorder (SAD).

Don't stare right at the light, and follow the directions that come with your box. To find one, try searching the Internet for "light therapy box." You may even find that your insurance company will help cover the cost.

If you are truly desperate, talk with your doctor about taking an over-the-counter sleep aid, such as those pain reliever "PM" medicines or melatonin. You might also talk about the benefits of going to a sleep clinic. As a last resort, your doctor can prescribe medication to help you sleep.

Why are pills the last resort? Sleep medications are habit-forming and have side effects. Some people have very vivid dreams or start sleepwalking. Others do things at night that they don't remember, including driving and having sex. Despite all of the happy, reassuring commercials you see on TV, you should try other methods before considering prescription medications.

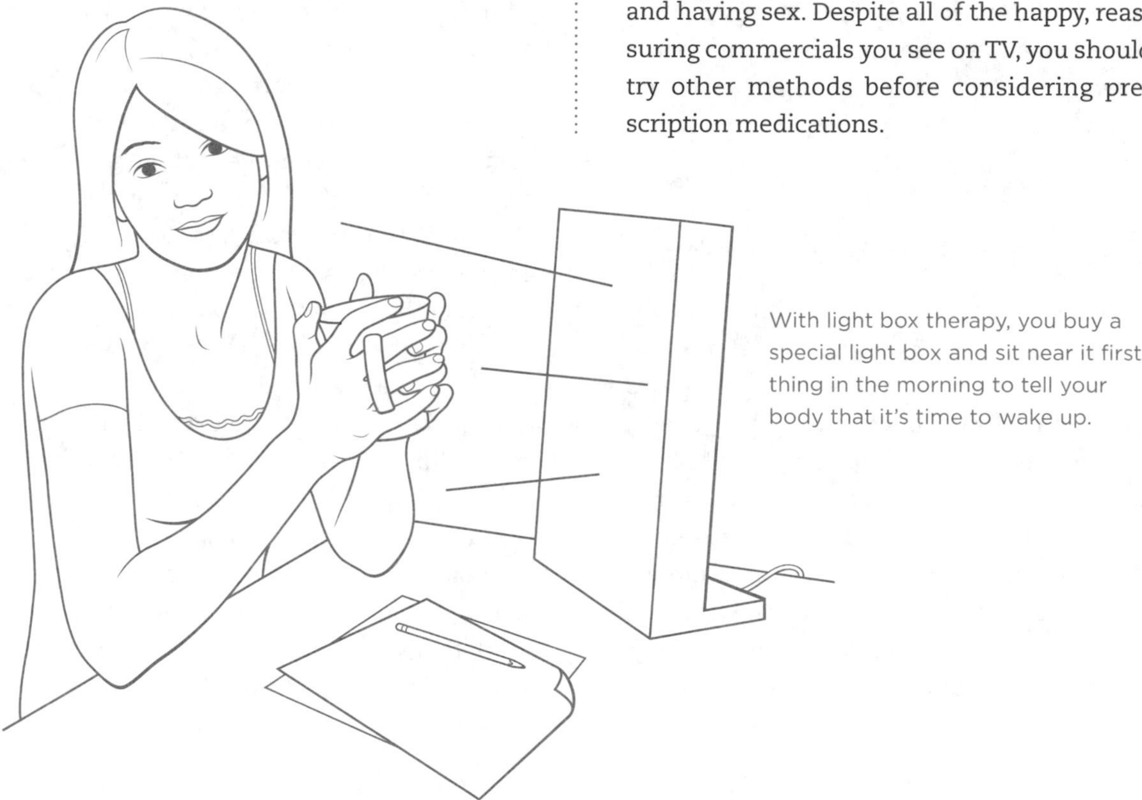

With light box therapy, you buy a special light box and sit near it first thing in the morning to tell your body that it's time to wake up.

Still lying awake at night? Sleep experts usually recommend that you get up. I don't think this works for everybody. If you actually *enjoy* getting up and getting a few things done, the method is wrong for you. Better to stay in bed, practice relaxation techniques, and hate lying there so darn much that you'll be motivated to improve your sleep hygiene.

NOTE TO SELF

Sleep deprivation causes car accidents every day. Fixing your sleep problems will make you a safer driver!

Feed Your Brain by Eating a Healthy Diet

Grandma always said it: eat carrots for your eyes and fish for your brain. Those are old myths, really, but the advice is great: your brain needs a healthy diet!

Chapter 17, Your Diet, is near the end of the book, but you'll notice that we bring up food and nutrition in every chapter. Every part of your body is affected by the food you eat. You've probably already noticed that your **bowels** tell you a lot about your diet, right? When you're eating well, everything moves along. When you aren't, you have trouble. Constipation, diarrhea, and gas are all signs that your diet needs a tune-up.

Your brain is just the same. It needs a diet filled with good food containing plenty of healthy stuff. Fruit, vegetables, whole grains, lean **protein**, fiber, and healthy fats such as olive oil are great for your brain.

What you eat affects way more than what you weigh or how you look. It gives you a healthy body with plenty of energy and hard-working organs, including your brain! Everything you do for a healthy body is also good for your brain.

Your Workout Exercises Your Brain, Too

If you ever find yourself on a desert island with no pharmacy, start exercising. Of all of the antidepressants in the world, only this one works for everybody. Psychopharmacologists know it, even when they are prescribing antidepressants: lots of physical exercise helps decrease depression. Exercise is also a great antianxiety solution.

For your general good health, exercise for half an hour most days, with enough energy to elevate your heart rate. For your brain, however, it can take even more exercise to manage depression, so I'm not recommending that you stop therapy just because you've started walking every day! Think of exercise as a partner to therapy.

A brief note on exercise: What's the best heart rate for you? Unless your doctor wants you to, you don't have to take your pulse; just keep your exercise at an intensity level where you can still talk in short sentences but not sing or chat.

If you have any health issues or a family history of health problems, ask your doctor before you start any exercise program that elevates your heart rate. If you have a healthy heart and your doctor has cleared you, start your sessions with a warm-up and always end with a cooldown.

Keep Those Stress Levels Down

Stress puts your body and brain through a shredder. If you lead a high-stress life and you feel you cannot or will not change it, it is essential that you find ways to reduce the impact stress has on your health.

Where can you start? Make a list of the things you like to do that let some air out of your big stress balloon. A warm bath, a long walk with the dog, exercise, quiet reading, a visit to your house of worship, a massage, spending time with a friend, a relaxing swim—all of these are good ideas.

Ask your friends what helps them relax, and then try a few of their ideas, too. Only use the activities that will cut down on stress—you either love a long bath or you don't. It's not a stress reducer if you end up staring at the dirty grout.

You can also reduce your stress by taking some classes. There are meditation groups and teachers who can show you the basics in just about every town in the United States. Self-hypnosis can help, too; check out a book on the subject from your local library. Yoga can also be a great stress reducer, but please find a good instructor who will make sure that your progress is gradual. Check out your local community's night classes, ask your friends or your doctor for a recommendation, or search the newspaper for ads. Health clubs and the YWCA or YMCA might offer classes too. You can even find stress reduction ideas, courses, and groups on the Internet that may be a good fit for your life.

So make your list and try them all! But first, let's look closely at your life to see if your stress can be reduced. List the problems that cause you stress, then start with a single one. Take that problem and break it down into its smallest parts. See if you can solve the small parts until the big problem starts to be easier to solve.

Let's say that you are part of a carpool to work that was great until you had children. Now one driver, who is unpredictable and likes to work late, is a big problem for you. As you wait for this driver to show up, you get steaming mad as the minutes tick by and you lose that precious time with your baby before bedtime. To tackle this stress, start with a small solution: talk to the driver to see if s/he can commit to leaving work at a time that works for both of you. If this doesn't work, then go to the next level: look for another carpool. No luck? Can you drive yourself? How about taking public transportation? If the small solutions don't work, then take a look at the big picture: Do you have career options? Location options? Telecommuting options?

Reducing stress is so important that it's worth it to make major changes in your life. If you really, honestly, truly believe that you can't, then head down the coping road: exercise, meditation, breathing exercises, yoga, self-hypnosis, music, reading, a satisfying hobby. These techniques don't just relax you; they also can clear your mind of all of the fog that makes it hard for you to set new priorities. Stress actually makes it *harder* for you to relieve stress.

Use the marriage of your mind and body to create a healthy life in which you think clearly, react to change or crises strongly, and make reasonable decisions. If you are a sleep-deprived young woman living a high-stress life, getting no physical activity, and eating a poor diet, you shouldn't even do a simple thing like driving!

We'll talk more about stress in chapter 3, Stress and Your Body.

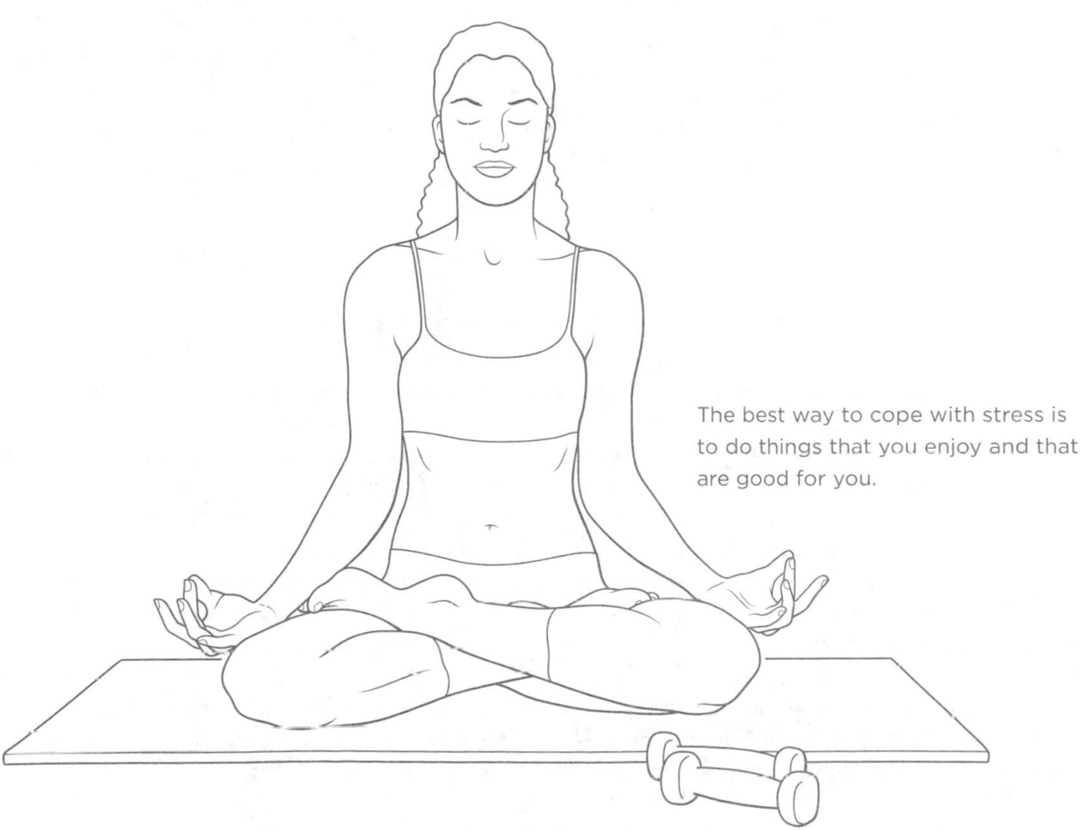

The best way to cope with stress is to do things that you enjoy and that are good for you.

What Can Go Wrong with Your Brain?

Here's the truth: relatively speaking, we know very little about the brain. It's the biggest frontier of medicine. The very best psychiatrists and neurologists in the world will tell you that we know ten times more than we did five years ago, but that still only totals a small amount of overall knowledge about the brain. The good news: We know enough about the brain to help you when things go wrong.

The Whole You

Before you medicate a problem you are having with your brain, let's map out what the rest of your body can do to help.

Did you know that your body will protect your brain first, above all other body parts? Look at cold weather as an easy way to understand this. Your mother told you to wear a hat when it's cold outside because heat leaves the body through your head. She's right—it's just a little more complicated than that. You should wear a hat because your body will do anything to keep your brain heated, so it sends all of its heat there. The fingers are the first to sacrifice their warmth, then the toes. The brain is drawing heat from your hands and feet to protect itself.

Your body and brain can work together on problems, and in most cases it's a good idea to consider solutions that take the whole body into account. Sure, you can take a pill that will adjust your brain chemistry, but that's not necessarily a perfect solution because the

REAL LIFE FACT: Prescription Drug Advertising

Before we start, I want to make sure you know this: You are in the first generation of Americans to grow up with prescription drugs advertised on television and in magazines. If you grab the remote and do some channel flipping, you'll notice how closely the drugs being advertised match the demographic of the show.

***Matlock*? Constipation, diabetes, "final expense" insurance, and scooters. Now switch to a show that *you* like. Depression, PMS, birth control, anxiety, insomnia, antacid. Watch the commercials carefully. First, ten seconds of black-and-white misery. Next, after the pill is taken, full color, and the world is sunshine, love, happiness, and health. Then the fine print, read by the speediest voice they can find. It says *Thisdrugisnotforeveryone.Sideeffectsmayincludedeath.Seeyourdoctorifyouhavethissideeffect*.**

Many of these are very good drugs. I'm a physician, not a faith healer, and I believe some medications can be very good choices. You just have to be aware that anything involving the brain is a complex medical problem for which a simple pill is not always the best solution.

other factors in your life that are causing you problems—work stress, lack of physical activity, a poor diet, and so on—are still going to be there.

So let's talk about some of the most common conditions that affect young women that could be considered disorders of the brain: depression, anxiety, PMS, eating disorders, and migraines.

Depression

First, there is garden-variety depression. You've lost a job. You got dumped. Usually, this depression will go away with "tincture of time." You'll start to feel a little better one day, when you have five minutes that you don't think about it. Soon it's ten minutes, and after a few weeks, maybe a few months, you just feel pangs. Painful pangs, but just pangs. Pangs are life companions, but specific pangs fade with time.

But what about having depression when you're leading a normal life with normal problems? A little stress, the occasional problem, maybe these are all things you can handle—and you mostly do. But underneath that, in the privacy of your mind, it's a different story. It's dark. The future is grim. You think you're a fraud—that you've fooled everybody into thinking you are better than you are. Getting out of bed is like climbing a mountain. You read the TV section every day to mark how the week is passing by, so grateful when it's finally halfway done on Wednesday night. You feel a general sense of pain inside. It's like grieving all the time, like being at a funeral—only you're not.

You watch the commercials describing the symptoms, and you know it's depression you're feeling. You can recognize what's happening.

What happens next?

You can go to the doctor and get antidepressants. In a couple of weeks maybe you'll feel better. In a few months, though, the medication might not work so well, and then you'll have to fiddle with the dosage. Often you'll be working with a new doctor, recommended by your general doctor, called a psychopharmacologist. If you are feeling such intense mental pain that you cannot function or you have active suicidal thoughts, then medication is likely the best the way to go. Don't hesitate. You need some relief now!

However, treating depression with medication requires an active partnership between you and your doctor to be certain that your mental health is improving, and to help you manage any side effects you might have from the medications. Be sure that you communicate clearly with your doctor about your progress and what you are feeling, so that your doctor hears and understands your situation. It often takes some adjusting and tinkering with doses and different medications to optimize the medical treatment of depression.

NOTE TO SELF

Exercise can be one of the most powerful treatments for depression.

But what if we enlist *all of you* in treating your depression?

Here's what we'd look at:

- **Sleep:** If you are depressed, good sleep hygiene is essential. Start tonight! Sleep deprivation may be causing a good bit of your depression.
- **Stress:** The mental shredder. For the depressed person, de-stressing has to happen. Start with coping mechanisms such as meditation and deep breathing.
- **Problems:** Now we've got to look at how you got to this point. Many people who have long-term, painful depression got there through a combination of challenges: illness, stress, sleep deprivation, and outside events.

Talk, Walk, and Other Therapies

If you are feeling depressed, a good talk therapist is a lifeline. Unfortunately, your psychopharmacologist is unlikely to be that person, and you will have to look around a little bit to find a talk therapist you like.

How do I define a good talk therapist? Somebody who helps you identify your vulnerable areas, cope with them, take small steps to free yourself from them, and keep moving forward.

A bad therapist is someone who fosters a feeling of victimhood instead of energetic survival. Someone who will let you talk, talk, talk about the same problem at work, week after week, without ever helping you to change it. Instead of teaching you how to find your strength, this therapist lets you coast.

It can be tough to find a good therapist. Ask trusted friends or family members. Ask your doctor. Don't be surprised if it takes a few appointments with different people before you find a good match. It's not like getting married, but it is a bit like finding a good carpool buddy.

There are a number of different approaches to general therapy. Following are basic layperson's descriptions of these fields.

REAL LIFE FACT: One Little Problem with Therapy

Many therapists don't take insurance! They could, but they don't. It would take years of putting them on the couch to figure out why.

Of course, some patients are concerned about their privacy and don't want it on their medical record that they received mental health support. HIPAA should protect your privacy, though, so if you have health insurance and your therapist accepts it, use it. Before you make an appointment, be sure to ask about billing. Therapy will cost $100 and up for a fifty-minute hour, depending on your area. Psychopharms are even more. Ask about cancellation policies, too.

PSYCHIATRY refers to a traditionally Freudian approach. It used to be called "being in analysis." It looks carefully at your past and your subconscious.

COGNITIVE BEHAVIORAL THERAPY AND DIALECTICAL BEHAVIORAL THERAPY aren't too interested in how you got to this state; they're more interested in helping you to find a way out. They can help you change a negative view of the world by changing patterns of thinking or behavior. These are practical approaches that work for many.

GROUP THERAPY helps you to create healthy and stable relationships. You'll work on how you communicate, express emotions, and deal with conflict. Group therapy is usually done in addition to your ongoing therapy. Let's say your therapist helps you to identify that you are invisible or hostile in relationships. Solving that problem in a group environment can help you to feel better.

FAMILY OR COUPLES THERAPY can be helpful when relationships are causing issues in your life and you feel you need professional help to sort them out and to teach you new ways to interact. It is not helpful when you are totally furious at everybody in your life and want to get them in a room and tell them off for an hour until they apologize. (They usually won't.)

EXERCISE—no, it's not officially therapy, but it is a powerful depression treatment. It increases the levels of mood-enhancing **neurotransmitters** (chemical messengers) in your brain, boosts feel-good **endorphins**, releases tension in your muscles, helps you to sleep better, and reduces the stress hormone **cortisol**. It also increases body temperature, which may have a calming effect. All of these changes together may account for exercise being one important part of keeping your mind healthy.

LIGHT THERAPY is the use of a light box. It's basically a bright light that simulates sunlight, and you spend time sitting in front of it. It is used for seasonal affective disorder, which is a form of depression triggered in the wintertime by limited exposure to sunlight. Light therapy may be helpful for the treatment and prevention of other forms of depression, as part of a complete treatment regimen.

RELAXATION THERAPIES AND TECHNIQUES, such as meditation, involve learning structured exercises for relaxing both your body and your mind. These can be used as helpful therapy (or preventive therapy) along with other methods for treating depression. The same goes for acupuncture, massage therapy, and yoga. These are great ways to cope with life's day-to-day stressors to minimize depression and stay mentally healthy.

HERBAL TREATMENTS can be helpful for some people. When treating my brain, I like to know that I have a reliable source of quality medicine with consistent dosing. If you have a reliable herbalist who can treat you with herbs, you may find some benefit.

But please—don't take any medicine on your own, whether it's from a natural foods store or a pharmacy. A drug made from a plant is still a drug, it still has interactions with other drugs, and it still can cause side effects. *Natural* does not mean *safe*.

Over-the-counter drugs are far more controlled, but you should still tell your doctor that you use them. There are countless bad interactions between medicines and over-the-counter drugs. For example, if your doctor prescribes a pain medication and you think it would be harmless to add some acetaminophen on top of that, you could give yourself a serious **liver** problem if the prescribed pain medication also contains acetaminophen.

SUPPORT GROUPS are not the same as group therapy; in support groups, you meet regularly with a group of people who have a common problem and support each other. Be careful about this. Support groups can be wonderful places where the feeling of connecting with others helps you to move on with your future.

Some support groups, unfortunately, become stuck in a rut with the wrong leader. Your therapist may be able to recommend support groups, or you can research them locally. Many people find that support groups are a godsend in the early days of recovery but become less important as they become stronger.

ONLINE SUPPORT GROUPS can be good for commiseration and moral support, but again, be careful! Online support groups are notorious for giving bad medical advice. Don't take any action without calling your doctor first. Use these groups for support, not medical treatment.

Some online groups are a practical tool. For example, stay-at-home moms can live in a lonely place with few neighbors. Depression often follows. You may expect yourself to be perfect, like you think your parents are, and you may hate housework. (Surprise! Your parents do, too.)

Try www.Flylady.com for help—it has practical advice on strategies (not cleaning tips), whether you are at home or not, plus an online community that is not crazy. They are also very good at talking you out of some of the crazy things moms do—like when we organize a bake sale, bake brownies for it, then go to the school and buy them back. (Just write a check!)

One method they recommend is good for all aspects of your life: buy a timer, and when you are trying to do a job that feels too big, set it for fifteen minutes. Breaking the job down into fifteen-minute "shifts" can help you with any big or unpleasant challenge at work or at home.

NOTE TO SELF

Find a support group that is positive for you. Do you leave feeling that you have learned something about yourself—something that you want to work on? That's a good group. Did you all complain for an hour about the same subjects every week? Not good.

Why Me?

Depression affects twice as many women as men. Married women are more likely to be depressed than single women; married men are less likely to be depressed than single men. Why? Nobody knows for sure.

It's easy to say that a new mother with **postpartum depression**, sleep deprivation, **hemorrhoids**, and an intrusive mother-in-law is going to be a tad more depressed than her husband, who is over-the-moon happy with a beautiful new baby. Many women work harder at work and harder at home than men do. Hmm, pretty depressing. Our hormones are a bigger roller coaster—depressing. So, although no scientist knows for sure, many women feel there's a simple answer to "Why me?" It's everyday life!

Do You Ask, Why Bother?

When you are depressed, it can be extremely difficult to take action. You just plain don't feel like it. But it's important that you do act. Depression is a bumpy road that can lead to a downward spiral, and it is treatable. You don't need to suffer.

Let's start with the symptoms. Depression needs treatment if it lasts for more than two weeks, if it interferes with your work or family life, or if you find it hard to carry on daily tasks and to enjoy activities that you used to like. You may have a decreased appetite and lose weight, or you may find you eat too much and gain weight. You may sleep too much or too little, sleep restlessly, or have insomnia. You may feel useless or joyless. You may have no energy, or you may be agitated and jumpy. You may cry often. You may think or talk about suicide or even attempt it. To be diagnosed with depression, you don't need to have all of these symptoms, just some of them, and they can range in intensity from mild to severe.

Depression often runs in families. It can be caused by changes in your brain chemistry. People taking certain medications for **cancer**, **arthritis**, heart problems, and high blood pressure may be more susceptible to depression. Hormonal changes can trigger depression, as can medical conditions like **stroke** or Parkinson's disease, a complicated and serious brain disorder that gets worse over time.

Teenagers and Young Women and Depression

Before adolescence, the rate of depression in boys and girls is about the same. Between the ages of eleven and thirteen, depression rates rise for girls, and by age fifteen, major depressive episodes are twice as common in young women as in young men. Young women have significantly higher rates of disorders, including depression, anxiety, and eating disorders. Young men don't escape the hormone wildfire: male students have higher rates of disruptive behavior disorders.

Women molested as children, abused at any time, or sexually assaulted are more likely to have clinical depression at some time in their lives than those with no history. So are women who experience other forms of abuse, such as physical abuse and sexual harassment on the job. Abuse may lead to depression by fostering low self-esteem, a sense of helplessness, self-blame, and social isolation.

Does this sound familiar to you? If it does, you deserve help. Addressing the pain in your life may sound like the biggest burden you can imagine, and you may be right. Being treated for these issues is very difficult, but it can and will change your life. It won't change the past, but it will mean a different path for you. For proof, see if you can talk to older women who sought help and those who didn't. You'll see a difference, and you have the right to that better future for yourself.

You can start with your doctor and then seek help with a good talk therapist. You may find that medication will help. Just, please, start now. I see many women who carry your pain, and I know how deeply you will benefit from treatment.

Treating Depression with Medication

The good news: Many people with depression can be treated successfully with medication, therapy, or a combination of both, which can be better than either treatment alone. Be sure to discuss all of the options with your doctor.

The bad news: Nobody can tell you for certain which antidepressant is going to work well for you, antidepressants can take a few weeks to work, and they may work for a while and then stop. If you start taking antidepressants, try to have a little patience. It may take some time to find the perfect treatment for you, or it may take time to adjust to the side effects of each drug.

I could give you a detailed history of antidepressants and a chemical analysis of each one and why we think it works. The truth is that none of that information may be true

REAL LIFE FACT: Symptoms of Depression

- **A sad, anxious, or "empty" mood that lasts longer than two weeks**
- **Loss of interest in activities you like**
- **Feelings of worthlessness, helplessness, hopelessness, or pessimism**
- **Suicide attempts**
- **Sleeping too much or too little**
- **Restlessness, irritability, or excessive crying**
- **Decreased energy, fatigue, or feeling slowed down**
- **Frequent thoughts of death or suicide or imagining means of suicide**
- **Appetite increase or decrease**
- **Difficulty concentrating, remembering, or making decisions**
- **Persistent physical symptoms that do not respond to treatment, such as headaches, digestive disorders, or chronic pain**

REAL LIFE FACT: Types of Depression

Major depression (clinical depression) includes some or all of the symptoms we've listed in the box on page 44 for at least two weeks—but frequently for several months or longer.

Dysthymia involves symptoms that are milder but also longer lasting—at least two years. Daily life is joyless and marked by fatigue.

Manic depression (bipolar disorder) has cycles of depression that alternate with mania. During manic episodes, people may become overly active, talkative, euphoric, and irritable; spend money irresponsibly; and get involved in sexual misadventures.

tomorrow. That's why I normally recommend seeing a psychopharmacologist—a doctor who prescribes these drugs—in addition to mental health therapy. This field is changing constantly, and you need someone whose job is to follow it. Please approach your treatment carefully. Take the doses as prescribed. Never change the dose on your own. Never stop taking the drug without talking with your psychopharm, as we call them. Pay close attention to your symptoms and keep a record of how you are feeling. If you are feeling worse, call your psychopharm immediately.

Tell the complete truth to your psychopharm. If you smoke, say so. Take drugs? Say so. Have bulimia or anorexia? Please, say so.

What Does It Feel Like to Take an Antidepressant?

When you first start taking an antidepressant, you'll notice nothing. It can take a few weeks before you feel any positive difference. These are not happy pills that will have you waking up singing tomorrow morning. You may start to see some improvement in energy level or sleep before you feel any change in mood.

Side effects often come before relief! The most common side effects are nausea and sexual dysfunction. Many women have less interest in sex and may even have difficulty having orgasms. However, because many women who are depressed have lost interest in activities that used to give them pleasure, including sex, the side effect may be worth it or even unnoticeable. This side effect does go away when the medication is stopped. After you have stabilized on a medication, you and your partner may want to try, as some couples do, taking a weekend break from medication under the guidance of the psychopharm.

Other possible side effects include headaches, diarrhea, nervousness, tremors, and insomnia. Often the side effects improve and even go away entirely after a few weeks. If not, you may want to try a different medicine.

As the medication begins to work, you'll feel a decrease in emotional pain. Some patients describe this as being like seeing that they have a bruise but they can't feel it; or like seeing that there is pain on the other side of the door but they don't feel like they have to open it. The pain may be in a fog that they can't quite see.

You will not feel "high." You will feel a gradual but steady improvement in your outlook. If that doesn't start to happen in a few weeks, report in to your psychopharm. As you begin medications, you will see this doctor as often as weekly, but eventually you will be on a more occasional schedule.

What happens next? You may need a short-term treatment, or you may take antidepressants for years. Everyone is different. Just be sure your psychopharm is paying attention to your symptoms, and if you are not satisfied with the results, ask your primary care doctor for another referral.

Chemistry 101: What We Think about Depression

Why do you feel depressed when you think you have no reason to? You have billions of nerve cells in your brain. They are constantly texting each other whenever you react to something, think, or feel anything. They communicate using neurotransmitters, such as **dopamine**, **norepinephrine**, and **serotonin**.

There may be countless neurotransmitters that we don't know about yet, just as you might use Facebook, MySpace, or Twitter today but will discover some new way of connecting tomorrow. Depression happens when your level of one of these molecules is down. The best-known of the molecules is serotonin. A nerve cell sends the serotonin molecule out with a message and then reabsorbs it. If you are reabsorbing too quickly, you don't get enough serotonin floating around, which we think causes some forms of depression. If we block the reabsorption—or "reuptake"—a bit, you'll have more serotonin and will feel better. The drugs that do this are called **selective serotonin reuptake inhibitors (SSRIs)**.

These drugs are often as effective as the enthusiastic commercials claim, but remember that the manufacturers also have gigantic marketing budgets. There are many other good options. Keep an open mind when you see the psychopharm. An SSRI means absolutely nothing to your brain if it has a different problem—despite the sunshine and rainbows of the TV commercials.

Anxiety

Everyone has some anxiety. If you can put your worries aside and focus on daily living, your anxiety is normal. If you can't, you may have an anxiety disorder, which can be harmful to your body's health and to your life.

Anxiety is your body's way of warning you that some kind of active response is needed in the face of danger. It's a legacy from our ancestors' lives in the wild, when predators might be hiding in the next tree. So anxiety can be a helpful tool. It can motivate you to prepare for a presentation, write a paper, or avoid a dangerous situation.

However, anxiety *disorder* doesn't help you. It can make you skip a presentation that makes you nervous, get writer's block because you are afraid the finished product won't be good enough, or stay at home because you fear unknown dangers.

We don't know what causes anxiety disorders. They can run in families, and they can be triggered by a traumatic or stressful event. People with anxiety problems often worry about the same things as everyone else, including money, health, families, relationships, and jobs. But people with anxiety disorders worry excessively and constantly. They wake up feeling anxious, and the feeling never seems to go away throughout the day.

Alleviating Anxiety

Start with a physical exam to make sure you are healthy. Consider whether you have any sister problems, such as depression.

Treatment of anxiety generally includes counseling, medication, or a combination. No one treatment works best for everyone, so you, your doctor, and/or your therapist will strive to find the best treatment for you. Behavioral therapy is an effective treatment for many people with anxiety disorders. This trains you in relaxation and coping skills. Talk therapy is also effective in helping you resolve and cope with troubles or stresses. Medication can be used successfully to control your symptoms while you are working on the other treatments.

To support your efforts, stop or reduce your intake of caffeine (coffee, tea, caffeine sodas, and . . . chocolate). Review with your doctor any over-the-counter medicines that you take, including herbal remedies. Many, many medications have the side effect of creating or increasing anxiety. Exercise daily and eat a healthy, balanced diet. (Please see chapter 17, Your Diet.) Practice good sleep hygiene. Seek counseling and support after a traumatic or disturbing experience.

REAL LIFE FACT: Symptoms of Anxiety Disorder

- **Change in appetite**
- **Difficulty breathing**
- **Difficulty concentrating**
- **Fatigue**
- **Feeling panicked**
- **Frequent need to use the bathroom**
- **Headaches**
- **Light-headedness**
- **Lump in the throat or difficulty swallowing**
- **Muscle tension**
- **Nausea**
- **Panic attacks**
- **Restlessness**
- **Sleeplessness**
- **Startled easily**
- **Sweating or hot flashes**
- **Trembling**

Premenstrual Syndrome and Premenstrual Dysphoric Disorder

Oh, the jokes. PMS stands for Pass My Shotgun. Or Provide Me Sweets. Those two lines have obviously been written by women and are actually funny. Online there are 750,000 other PMS jokes that are just plain bad.

Every woman feels premenstrual syndrome (PMS) differently. For some, it is hardly noticeable, while for others, it can be a monthly ordeal. It can start soon after **ovulation** and usually peaks in the few days before your period starts. Bloating, breast tenderness, fatigue, food cravings, anxiety, depression, irritability, and mood swings are typical problems. Premenstrual syndrome is often worse for women in their thirties. It could be that at this age women have increasing stresses, such as balancing careers with motherhood, that make underlying health problems worse. We just don't know exactly why our hormones cause PMS.

It's important to figure out if your symptoms are caused by PMS or by some other mental or physical problem. Start by keeping a simple PMS journal. Write down when your symptoms happen and how severe they are, so that your doctor can look for a pattern in your symptoms. You'll find a diary format to copy in the appendix, Tools to Use. The key to knowing whether your symptoms are caused by PMS is that you should be symptom free in the early part of your menstrual cycle. If you have the symptoms throughout the month, it's not PMS.

Premenstrual dysphoric disorder (PMDD) is a more severe form of PMS that affects perhaps one in twenty women. The physical symptoms for PMS and PMDD are exactly the same; however, in PMDD the emotional symptoms are significantly more serious and go far beyond what are considered manageable or normal premenstrual symptoms. It's like the difference between a mild headache and a migraine. PMDD is an official psychiatric diagnosis. Like PMS, PMDD occurs the week before the onset of menstruation and disappears a few days after.

With PMDD, significant depression and hopelessness may occur. In severe cases, women may feel suicidal. PMDD is characterized by severe moodiness, irritability, depression, and anxiety.

Diagnosis: PMS or PMDD?

Women with a history of depression are at increased risk for PMDD, and women who have had PMDD are at increased risk for depression after **menopause**.

To figure out if you have PMS or PMDD, first, keep a diary! List the dates of your period and which symptoms you have (and their severity) on the ten days before and after your period. After tracking your symptoms for at least two cycles, bring this symptom diary to review with your physician, along with a list

REAL LIFE FACT: Progesterone—Poor Choice

Progesterone was once thought to be helpful for the treatment of PMS and was commonly prescribed. Now we know that it doesn't work. Ignore any publicity or marketing hype about this treatment: it won't help you.

of all medications you are taking (including prescriptions, over-the-counter medications, herbs, vitamins, and supplements). Your doctor will take a complete history and give you a physical exam to rule out other possibilities, as no specific physical findings or tests can confirm the diagnosis of PMS or PMDD.

Why bother with seeing your doctor first? Because the psychopharm doctors don't do physicals. You could go for years being treated with antidepressants when you're actually suffering from constipation.

Treatment Strategies

PMS can be treated in a few different ways. The first line of treatment is in lifestyle and diet. With mild PMS, exercise and calcium, which are good for you anyway, are a good initial treatment, either on their own or with medication. A daily 1,000 mg calcium supplement has been shown to be helpful in several studies.

Exercise and relaxation help to ease the bothersome symptoms of PMS. Cutting your salt intake may decrease bloating and swelling, a very common PMS-related complaint. And some women may find relief from the physical symptoms of PMS—bloating and breast tenderness—through using oral contraceptives. The decision to take oral contraceptives must be made with your doctor because of well-known risks. The newer oral contraceptives (Yaz, Yasmine, Ocella) may also ease the moodiness as well.

Many women with PMS have been helped by complementary therapies such as biofeedback, relaxation techniques, acupuncture, and massage. For many patients, simple stress-reduction techniques such as taking long hot baths or meditating are also helpful. Multiple studies have now confirmed that SSRI antidepressants can treat both PMS and PMDD. Serotonin problems may be a cause of PMS, just as they are linked to depression. Remember to take SSRIs with your doctor's guidance and follow the instructions carefully. SSRIs are not addictive, but if they are stopped suddenly, some people may experience unpleasant withdrawal effects.

NOTE TO SELF

There are highly effective treatments available for PMS and PMDD.

Can Someone My Age Have a Stroke?

It's rare, but it happens. And even if it never happens to you, you should learn the warning signs (below and top right) as recommended by the National Stroke Association. You may save someone's life.

What is a **stroke**? It happens when your brain does not get enough oxygen because a blood vessel is blocked or bleeding. Strokes can be mild or devastating, causing paralysis or even death. Although strokes are less common in your age group, everyone should know the warning signs of a stroke. Your parents and other older people, who are at greater risk, should know the signs too.

Eating Disorders: It's Not About Food

It might seem strange to see a section on eating disorders in a chapter on your head. But eating disorders are one of the best examples of a problem that involves the body *and* the brain.

Eating disorders are mental health issues. Some women have a false idea that controlling food can make their lives wonderful or improve self-esteem. Some women starve to keep their bodies in a childlike state for reasons we don't fully understand. Both are skewed, painful, and harmful views of life and the world. Women suffer from these beliefs, but luckily they can be helped.

WHAT ARE THE SYMPTOMS OF A STROKE?	
Sudden numbness or weakness of face, arm, or leg—especially on one side of the body	
Sudden confusion, trouble speaking or understanding	
Sudden trouble seeing in one or both eyes	
Sudden trouble walking, dizziness, or loss of balance or coordination	
Sudden severe headache with no known cause	
ACT F.A.S.T.	
FACE	Ask the person to smile. Does one side of the face droop?
ARMS	Ask the person to raise both arms. Does one arm drift downward?
SPEECH	Ask the person to repeat a simple sentence. Are the words slurred? Can he or she repeat the sentence correctly?
TIME	If the person shows any of these symptoms, time is important. Call 911 or get to the hospital fast. Brain cells are dying.
Source: National Stroke Association, www.stroke.org	

More than 90 percent of people with eating disorders are women between the ages of twelve and twenty-five. However, we are seeing more older women and men who qualify too.

Eating disorders can be mild or life-threatening. At the mild end, athletes who diet to meet performance goals can become obsessive about food and exercise to a harmful degree. At the dangerous end, **anorexia nervosa** is an extremely restrictive eating behavior involving a distorted body image in which an emaciated woman sees herself as overweight. People with anorexia are unable to maintain a body weight that is at least 85 percent of normal for their height and build, and may also have **amenorrhea** (no periods).

A woman with **bulimia nervosa** has regular (at least twice a week) episodes of binge eating, with a sense of loss of control over eating during these episodes. People with bulimia purge regularly (at least twice a week), with self-induced vomiting, abuse of laxatives or diuretics, fasting, excessive exercise, or any combination of the above.

Generally, a woman with an eating disorder puts an abnormal emphasis on body image or shape in her self-evaluation. The earlier these disorders are diagnosed and treated, the better the chance of full recovery.

Disordered Eating

Disordered eating is a term used for eating habits or behaviors that resemble anorexia nervosa or bulimia nervosa but are not as serious. Disordered eating can mean changes in eating patterns that happen after a stressful event or an illness, or in preparation for athletic competition. Although disordered eating can be troublesome, it rarely requires in-depth professional attention or causes serious health problems. It can, though, develop into an eating disorder. Please, if this sounds like you, tell your doctor.

NOTE TO SELF

Like it or not, eating disorders are really not about food—they are mental health problems.

Medical Problems Caused by Eating Disorders

When weight drops far below normal, your nails grow brittle and your hair thins and even falls out. Your skin may dry out, become yellow, and develop a covering of soft hair called lanugo. Swollen **joints**, reduced muscle mass, and light-headedness are common results. Fatigue can be overwhelming from the caloric restriction. Severe cases of anorexia can lead to brittle bones that break easily because of calcium loss. Extreme anorexia leads to organ failure and even death.

Women with bulimia, who stimulate vomiting, bowel movements, or urination, are at high risk for heart failure. Irregular heart rhythms and death can happen from imbalances in **electrolytes** such as sodium and potassium. Acid in vomit can wear down the outer layer of the teeth, inflame and damage the **esophagus**, and enlarge the parotid

glands near the cheeks (giving the appearance of swollen cheeks). Damage to the digestive system can also occur from frequent vomiting, including stomach **ulcers** and long-term constipation.

How Do I Know If I Have an Eating Disorder?

You feel obsessed with your weight. You think people are lying when they call you thin. You get incredibly upset at gaining even a pound. You feel angry with yourself if you overeat. You have lost a lot of weight recently; now people are telling you that you are too thin. You purge when you feel full. You live on the scale or in front of the mirror. You hate your body and punish yourself by starving. You feel that you can't control anything else in your life except food, so you figure you'll show everybody else by controlling it to extremes.

Getting Help

People who don't know what it's like to have anorexia or bulimia find it very difficult to understand. Don't be surprised if even people who love you just tell you to go and eat something. If you suffer from an eating disorder, you really have to get professional help, usually from a combination of a therapist and a nutritionist, though sometimes hospitalization is necessary.

You watch the news; you know that these are serious problems that can make your life miserable or even kill you. If resources are scarce in your area, visit the Aware Foundation website at www.awarefoundation.org and click Eating Disorders. This will take you to a good list of places to turn to for help, including hotlines.

Migraines and Misery

Migraines attack about thirty million people in the United States. They may happen to you at any age, but they usually start between adolescence and age forty and begin to go away after age fifty. Some people have migraines a few times a month, others have them a few times a year, and still others have only a few migraines in a lifetime.

About 75 percent of migraine sufferers are women. Some women have migraines just before or during their periods. These headaches, which are called menstrual migraines, may be related to hormonal changes. Other women develop migraines for the first time during pregnancy or after menopause.

The cause of migraines is unknown, but they do seem to run in families. Migraine sufferers may inherit a sensitivity to triggers that produce **inflammation** in the blood vessels and nerves around the brain, causing pain.

What Can Bring on a Migraine?

Some common migraine triggers include alcohol, environmental factors such as weather and barometric pressure changes, perfume and other odors, bright lights, loud noises, foods, hormonal changes, sleep deprivation, hunger, dehydration, and stress.

NOTE TO SELF

Think the migraine is a modern problem? The word dates back to 1373.

Migraine Types and Auras

Migraines are classified based on the symptoms they produce. The two most common types are migraine with aura and migraine without aura.

Migraine with **aura** starts with a strange brain event (aura) ten to thirty minutes before the headache. Most auras are visual. They may appear as bright shimmering lights around objects or at the edges of your vision (called **scintillating scotomas**). They may be zigzag lines, wavy images, or hallucinations. Some people experience temporary vision loss. Nonvisual auras include weakness, speech or language abnormalities, dizziness, **vertigo**, and tingling or numbness of the face, tongue, or arms and legs. Some of these symptoms may also resemble the symptoms of stroke (see page 50), a serious neurological problem that requires immediate medical intervention. So if you are unsure, call your doctor or go to the emergency room. Don't hang around wherever you are discussing it to death. Go.

Migraine without aura is the most common type; it may happen on one or both sides of your head. You may have tiredness or mood changes the day before the headache. Nausea, vomiting, and sensitivity to light or sound often go along with migraine without aura.

Migraine pain is throbbing and usually begins in a specific area on one side of your head. Once it begins, the headache spreads and builds in intensity over several hours, then gradually goes away. Migraines can last up to twenty-four hours and, in some cases, several days. Your hands and feet may feel cold and sweaty, and odors may be intolerable to you. Migraines are made worse by any physical activity, coughing, straining, or lowering your

REAL LIFE FACT: Migraine Magnifiers

- Chocolate
- Dehydration
- Glare
- Hormonal changes
- Hunger
- Medications
- Monosodium glutamate (MSG)
- Nitrates (in hot dogs and other processed foods)
- Perfume
- Red wine
- Sleep deprivation
- Stress
- Time zone changes

REAL LIFE FACT: Tips for Easing Your Headaches

- **Drink fluids.**
- **Keep your head cool with an ice pack.**
- **Lie down in a quiet, dark room and slightly elevate your head.**
- **Keep your body warm with covers.**

head. The headache can be so bad that it interferes with daily activities. It can even wake you up. People with migraines often feel tired and weak once the headache has passed.

Migraine without aura appears to pose little risk to your health, despite the pain, suffering, and lost time from work and your personal life. For people with migraine with aura, there is a small future risk of stroke. This risk is very small and should not limit your activities in any way. It should not limit your contraceptive choices either, unless you find that hormonal birth control makes your headaches worse. For some women, hormonal contraception actually improves migraines, especially those that come with their period.

Migraine Treatment

Most people who suffer from migraines know what triggers them. Keep track of these triggers and do your best to avoid the most common ones: stress, skipping or delaying meals, poor sleep, chocolate consumption, or alcohol intake. Other triggers, such as menstruation or weather fluctuations with rapid changes in air pressure, are unavoidable.

There are many effective medications to treat migraines. Medication works better if you take it early in the attack. Even the right medicine won't work if taken too late. For mild attacks, over-the-counter pain relievers usually work if you take the right dose, discussed with your doctor. Oddly, caffeine is sometimes a good addition, either added to the medications or in a beverage. Caffeine helps in treating migraines by causing some narrowing of the dilated (widened) blood vessels in the brain that cause the pain.

Moderate to severe migraine attacks usually require prescription medications. Discuss them carefully with your doctor. One group, called **triptans**, works on those neurotransmitters or messengers in your brain. They come in different forms: oral tablets and wafers, nasal sprays, and injections.

Prescription pain relievers containing codeine and a **barbiturate** can be effective treatments for moderate to severe attacks, but your doctor needs to monitor your use carefully, because they can be habit-forming.

If you have frequent and severe migraines, a preventive medication may be taken daily to reduce them.

Why Should I Bother with All of This Mind-Body Stuff?

If this is a book about your body, why am I telling you all of this stuff about your mind and your life? It's easy: you'll feel great when you pay attention to all of it together. You'll feel great as a young woman and as an old one. If all of this sounds like too much, remember that you'll be breaking these new habits into small pieces and making change in your life a little bit at a time.

Start with a good night's sleep. Let the *whole you* take a break. Tomorrow, your brain and your body will start talking to each other again.

Now we'll move to a big issue for young women—stress—with some tips, both traditional and new, for dealing with it.

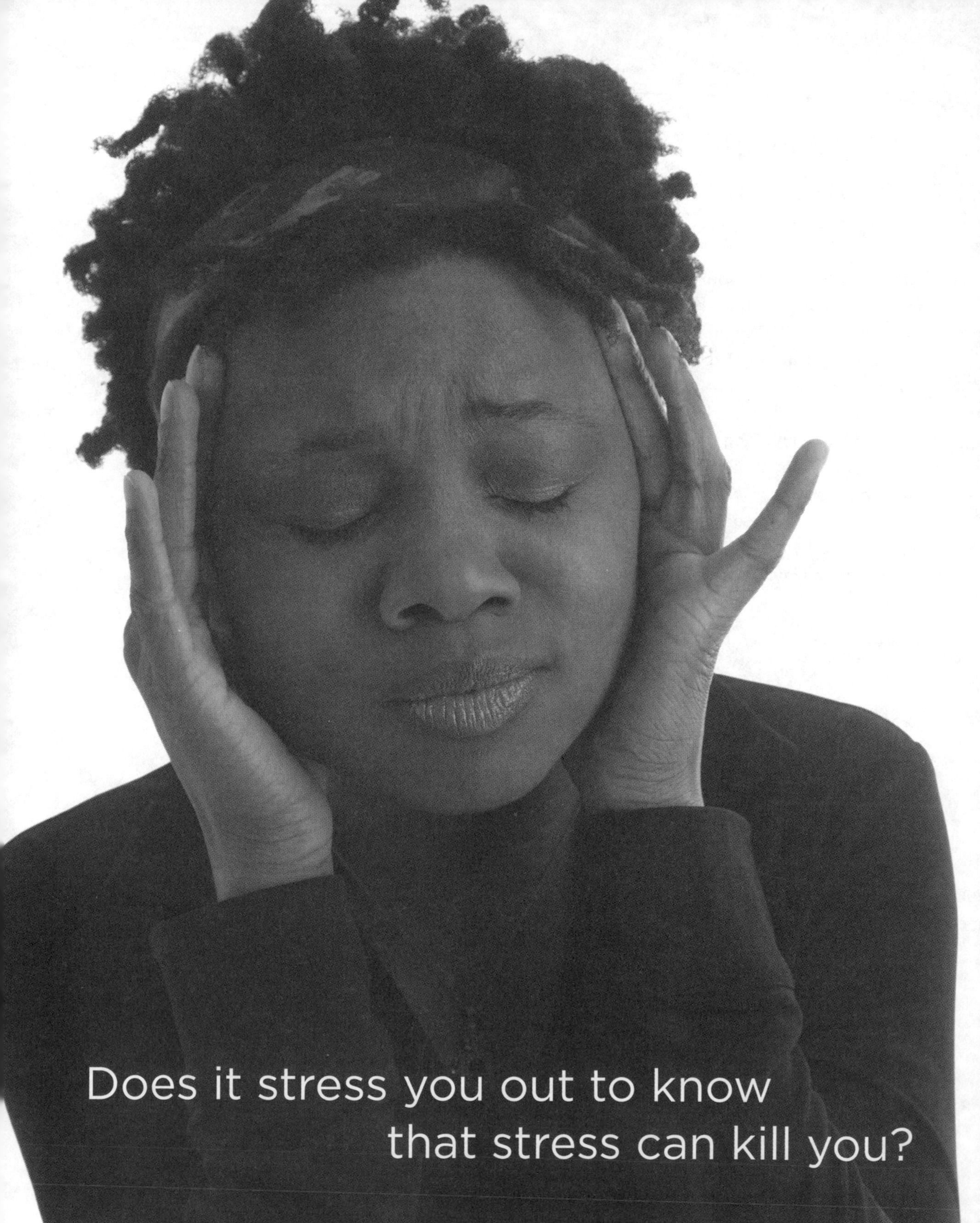
Does it stress you out to know
that stress can kill you?

stress and your body

You know the feeling. You have ten important things to do but time to do only one. Then one more thing gets added—meeting the boyfriend's family, going on a business trip when you hate flying, losing your wedding ring. Stress.

Life is stressful. Sometimes even good things—a new partner, a new job, a vacation—can trigger stress. Of course, bad things—a failed test, the end of a relationship, losing a job—can worsen stress. So can wearing tight shoes all day.

Too much stress can increase your risk for heart attacks, **strokes**, high blood pressure, **ulcers**, colds, and **PMS**, just for starters. Even if it doesn't kill you, stress can definitely cause physical problems like headaches, upset stomach, diarrhea, back and neck pain, fatigue, and insomnia. Stress can also cause you to feel depressed, angry, and anxious, and it can affect relationships at home and at work.

Believe it or not, a little stress is good for us. It keeps us striving and energetic. Studies show we are more motivated, more productive, and even happier when slightly stressed. But too much stress is not good, so let's take a look at what the biggest causes of stress are and review some tips on how to manage stress better.

Before we start, remember that we're talking about lots of individual women here. Even if your particular stressors are different from my list, the tips for reducing stress and the damage it can do to you can work no matter what pushes your stress buttons.

What's Stressing You Out?

So what are the biggest causes of stress for women age twenty-one to thirty-five? For some women, it's career building. For others, it's starting a family. For many, it's not having enough time, being overextended, and not having a good work-life balance. However, the biggest stressor for women in this age group is relationships.

Sound like an odd topic for a body book? Not when we're looking at your whole body. If relationships, good or bad, are causing you stress, there's a classic mind-body connection that's important to pay attention to. We know the impact that stress has on you and your organs!

Stress and Other People

Your family, friends, and partners create a core of happiness in your life. Every good relationship you have helps you relieve a ton of stress. But at some dark point in your life, you—like everyone else—are going to think "I hate people. I hate every single one of them."

Since relationships are a major part of your life—and often your stress—we're going to look at some typical situations and the problems that other people sometimes cause. We're looking for stressors that you can change. And if you can't change them, we're looking for ways to stop the stress from damaging your health.

Love, Lust, and Stress

You have many relationships in your life, but I'm going to start with the one you're probably thinking about right now. Your boyfriend, your girlfriend—or whatever you call your partner—s/he brings joy and stress into your life just as you do his or hers!

Here's your doctor's view. Today's world is complex, and relationships change all the time. We tend to settle down with a long-term partner a lot later in life than our parents did, so most of us are likely to be exposed to more than one sex partner. And that partner has probably been with someone other than just you. Not always, but usually.

So as your doctor, I'm going to remind you to be aware of protection from disease and pregnancy, and to be certain you're in a safe environment. I strongly recommended serial monogamy—one partner at a time. Ideally, before you have sex with a new partner, you should know that both of you have been checked for sexually transmitted infections, including **HIV**. At the very least, use **condoms** until you do. (And remember to pack your own.)

As your whole body doctor, however, I want to know if your lifestyle makes you happy, miserable, or depressed—in other words, stressed! I've seen all three. There's the woman who wanted to have sex with many partners before settling down but became miserable when her biological clock began ticking and her party girl ways hadn't found her a partner. I have a happy patient who had an uncountable number of sex partners, chosen "only by their sexiness, not their character," and then married a great guy and never looked at another man. Another woman feels desperately sad and guilty about sex, especially early in relationships, because her sex partners rarely call after sex. Relationships can unfold in lots of ways, but they all have the potential to cause stress.

Most healthy relationships don't start with sex; however. They start with friendships—at work, through friends, and through family, community, or houses of worship. Even online dating services have become a popular way to meet partners for real relationships. They're worth considering, and I've been seeing more and more people form lasting relationships this way. Just remember: Play it safe. If you're going on a date with a stranger, meet for lunch first. Get there and leave there on your own. Don't give out your address or any other personal information until you know the person better.

Are you more interested in relationships with women than men? The same rules apply. Protect yourself. The only risk you don't have to worry about is pregnancy. Every sexually transmitted infection can be transmitted from woman to woman.

Are you already an "old married lady"? Because this book is written for women from age twenty-one through thirty-five, we're addressing the needs of a wide age group. At thirty-five, you may be in a long-term relationship, if not a marriage. You may have children. You are settling into the years of life when you may be happily married or not.

If you are happily married—which one of my patients defines as "I didn't kill him today . . . "—there are still going to be stressors. You are not yet an expert at relationships, and neither is your partner. The moments of stress when you feel crazy that you ever married this galumpf, are shared by both of you (which you just cannot believe, and neither can your partner!).

If your dating and sex life is filling you with misery and guilt, it's time to kick it to the curb. It's time to set standards for yourself that rule out sex until you know a person, and to limit alcohol consumption too. It's time for a plan that works for you. Any place or source that gives you a supportive, constructive way to live your life and your relationships is a good stress reducer.

Books? Retreats? Role-model couples? The secret to having a mostly happy long-term relationship or marriage is still a mystery to most of us, but if you refer often to the tips listed on the next page, you'll have a good chance of moving in the right direction.

Relationships can be your rockiest source of stress. Worrying about meeting the right person, deciding to get married or not, hoping for or avoiding pregnancy, worrying whether you married the right person, trying to get along, learning to grow with another human being, questioning your sexuality, dealing with sexual relationships for the first time, and feeling pressure about sex all take a toll. Every woman shows different signs of stress. Many of us feel it first in the bowels, don't we? Constipation and diarrhea can both be warning signs that stress is building up.

Close your eyes and pay attention to all of your muscles for a moment. How many of them are tensed up? Start at your shoulders and work your way down, including your butt. Many people tense the butt first when stressed. Review all of the symptoms of stress we're going to describe here. If more than one applies to you, it's time to de-stress yourself.

My job as your doctor is not to counsel you about your relationships, but to reduce your stress, which you will feel whether your relationship is a fairy tale or a nightmare. Check back in with this chapter whenever you have relationship difficulties. Those hard times will come and go, and it's your job to reduce your stress so that it doesn't weaken your body.

The Abusive Partner

You know by now if your partner is abusive, controlling, or violent. For many women, an abusive relationship starts with a partner who is excessively attentive. S/he sends flowers more than once a day after one date, starts planning the future immediately, or begins to edge your friends out of the picture. The romance of it all can sweep you off your feet, like in a movie, until you realize that your pedestal is really a cage.

You need help. Don't try to handle this on your own. Talk to your friends and family first, and listen carefully. See what they can do

REAL LIFE FACT: Tips for Good Relationships

Make sure that:

- **You respect your partner's character and s/he respects yours.**
- **You care about your partner's well-being and s/he care about yours.**
- **You are both monogamous.**
- **You know each other well.**
- **You listen to each other.**
- **You both remember that you can make mistakes.**
- **You both know what buttons you can push to upset your partner, and you don't push them.**
- **You feel comfortable that you have similar goals for the future.**
- **You have some balance in your life.**
- **You have some time to have fun.**
- **You both like to laugh.**

to help. For example, if you have decided that this partner cannot or will not change, you will need a place to stay, perhaps, or legal advice, or help with children, or even help from the police department.

If your partner is violent, you're going to need special help to keep yourself and your children safe. A violent person very often is enraged by a restraining order, for example, so you've got to know how to stay safe after you get one. This is why you need a little team in place—lawyer, family, friends, police—because unfortunately you, like many thousands and thousands of women before you, wound up with the wrong partner.

You'll notice that every time you go to a doctor's appointment or hospital, somebody or some sign will ask you if you are safe at home. I hope this is a good reminder that your health care provider or hospital is also a good place to turn to if you do not feel safe. Hospital social workers can help you to find the resources you need to get the help you deserve. Don't worry—the hospital social worker is not going to charge you for these services.

The one thing you need to know? You have to do something. Few situations are more stressful than being with an abusive partner, so it's important to get this relationship fixed or ended. The person who yells a lot because that's how his or her parents resolved their differences may have the potential for change. The person who hits a lot probably does not. But you are much safer working in a team. And please be sure you have some professionals involved.

The In-Law Stressor

If you have already found and married your partner, then you are probably very familiar with the stress of dealing with your partner's parents. We all need a "Beginner's Guide to In-Laws," don't we? Maybe your new family is filled with angels and you fit in like a dream. Maybe you burst into the family acting like the new big sister. Or maybe you nervously avoid the control-freak bossy bosses that they are. Regardless of the situation, there are two essential steps you can take to make it work.

Understand your partner's mother. She cares about her child's happiness. Make your partner look happy before you see your in-laws, and you're all set. You can worship rocks, eat the dog's breakfast, wreck the family car, and ask Grandma if she's heard of bikini waxing. . . . If your partner looks happy, acts happy, and you make him or her call Mom more often than usual without ever taking credit, you will be loved. If your partner looks unhappy, there is nothing you can do. Those parents will not like you. Guess which way of life is better?

Understand your partner's siblings. They've known your partner forever, and they don't want to break up the family team. You represent separation. The best you can do? Go in from the beginning knowing that you are in second place. Don't try to overwhelm everybody with your accomplishments and your talents. Just ask questions to show your curiosity about your partner's family. If they want to play a game, play a game. If it's a game you really can't play—like football, maybe, not cards—then you can stand by and cheer. Otherwise, play.

Oh, and learn everybody's names before you meet them.

Did you already get off to a bad start? It's never too late to try the ideas above. Eventually the family will notice that you're making a new effort. You can also try the direct approach and invite your in-laws to talk about it. If all of your efforts fail, you're stuck with a stressful problem, which means you'll need to focus not on fixing the relationship, but on reducing the impact of the stress on you and your partner.

Your Parents: The Joys and Stresses of Leaving Home

When you leave home to live on your own for the first time, your first and most important relationships change. Your parents—who may have adored you, nurtured you, abused you, taught you, been great role models, been terrible ones—are starting to be in the distance a little bit more. Back in grade school, when you got a good report card, your parents were the first people who saw it. What about now, when you have a bit of nice news, or bad? Chances are you're not calling home unless nobody else is around.

Are you thrilled to be independent? What a feeling! Each generation of women seems to have its own symbol of the free, single woman in the city. Thanks to cable television, you can still see Mary Tyler Moore throw her past, in the form of a beret, into the sky.

Well, even this great feeling has its stresses. And by the way, have you ever wondered if your parents are as happy as you are? Maybe they're not. Maybe they miss you—a lot. Maybe they start asking you when you'll call next or when you'll be home next. All you want to say is "When I feel like it, you'll see me." You manage to say "I love you." You say you'll try to be home for Thanksgiving, but you don't want to go.

Your parents may start to feel like they are losing you. And guess what? This is going to push all kinds of stress buttons for them. Let's say you want to go skiing with a girlfriend when they had invited you home for the weekend. Let's say Mom was poor as a young woman and couldn't afford much. (By the way, apparently all parents were poor when they were young.) Now it gets really complicated. Mom is remembering all the times she went out on dates wearing handmade dresses and sporting hairstyles that her sister cut for her. She starts to see you as a person who lives in a different world—a ski weekend world, a world with money. She wants that for you, but she is deeply hurt that you are turning your back on her. This is especially true if you're the first child in your family to have a professional-level job or the first to go to college.

You, of course, know absolutely nothing about any of this. This makes Mom think you're insensitive. Now she's getting mad: *I cleaned up 1.8 acres of vomit from that child, and now she's too good for me.* You are two steps away from having a relationship with One-Word Mom. You know her: "How are you,

Mom?" "Fine." "How's Dad?" "Fine." "How's the weather today?" "Fine." Now you get completely irritated, and the phone call turns silent. Before you hang up, you'll sigh, which she will hear, and that will send her right into orbit with anger. Does any of this sound familiar?

Many young women see therapists to help with separation from their parents. That may be very helpful for you, and if the issues are overwhelming, it's a good idea. But whatever you do, choose to put the brakes on these kinds of downhill slides you have with your parents.

The best way to do that? Information. Let's assume for the moment that you have had a pretty normal childhood with sane parents. Tell your folks about your plans in advance and talk to them often, at least once a week. If you live some distance away, make sure that four times a year you do something with just your family. If you live nearby, do it more often. If you get resentful over giving up your prime dinnertime, suggest lunch. When Mom suggests that the two of you could bond by cooking together every night, remind her that you really enjoy your lunches where the two of you get to sit down and relax.

Keep your parents informed with little bits of information about your life. You got a raise. You colored your hair. You don't have to tell them everything. Just give them a steady stream of information and they will be much happier. A parent without information is like a dehydrated camel. Moms especially need enough information to tell their friends something specific about you. Give her a little information, and she can last a long time on that.

On the subject of sex and romance, keep it to yourself. While you love to joke about the horrors of imagining your parents having sex, believe me on this: it is a whole lot worse for your parents to imagine you having sex! Give your folks information about dating and understand that this is your bag of gold. Make it clear that you want to be able to talk about your partners without being judged and without everybody thinking you're engaged. Then be a little open about your life. It won't kill you, and it will make your parents very happy.

When Parents Become Grandparents

Are you a mom? Congratulations! Well, you didn't only give birth to a baby; you gave birth to a grandchild. Four people, sometimes more or fewer, just got very, very excited. In a perfect world, the grandparents all live next door to each other. Holidays are one big happy event, with dessert held at the other house each year. For most people, that's not the way things turn out. You live far away from both sets of parents. There are four words of advice I'm going to give you to handle every problem this stressor creates: It's up to you.

Do you have an aggressive mother who insists that everybody be at her table on Sunday night, but you don't want to go? It's up to you to tell her that you'll come once a month. You have a mother-in-law who insists that Christmas Day be at her house every year?

It's up to you. Do yourself a favor and say, "No thanks." People who are that insistent about Christmas rarely host a good one. Come up with lots of creative ways to spend times with your in-laws the way you, as a couple with a new family, want to do it, knowing that sometimes there will be occasions you must attend (funerals and weddings).

The point is that you need to guide these relationships or they can be never-ending sources of stress. If you think it's bad now, wait until your fourteen-year-old comes to Grandma's with piercings.

While you wait for that day, you will be disagreeing with your parents (and even your parent's parents) on a thousand topics, from the best way to potty train to whether a boy should have a baby doll. The best way to handle this is to give your parents and in-laws the respect they deserve, but do what you believe to be right. It's not always easy, especially when you clash over co-sleeping, thumb sucking, learning how to swim—you name it, you'll disagree.

Grandparents can often be a fabulous part of your life and your kids' lives. They are wonderful teachers, cohorts, spoilers, kissers, huggers, and playful babysitters. Just remember that managing the relationship is always up to you. If your mother-in-law would never insist on anything, don't let your aggressive mother get every special occasion with you.

The Abusive Parent

I have no tips and tricks for separating from the abusive parent. I'll be the last person to recommend staying in touch. And don't let anybody else tell you to call home when they can't possibly know what you experienced. I recommend a good therapist who is experienced with this process. I don't suggest it because you need fixing, but because you will need support as you continue to separate from this very difficult situation.

The wider your world grows and the more you see how other people grew up, you may feel intense and understandable rage about your own childhood. You don't have to go home for Thanksgiving, or for any other reason, to be with abusive people. Do you have siblings who don't believe that you were abused and who try to make you visit Mom and Dad? Skip that, too. The way you were treated can infect so many parts of your life, from your health to your own relationships; you don't owe them anything.

Brothers and Sisters

Unless you're an only child, your connection with a sibling is your first relationship with an "equal." Siblings can be a wonderful and enriching part of your life. However, if you had an abusive sibling, take a break from that relationship. There's no rule that says you have to continue relationships with any abusive person, including those in your family.

Even in adult life, that older sister who beat you up and the brother who tickled you beyond mercy are going to make you uncomfortable. And believe it or not, some siblings never get over competing for Mom and Dad's attention. No matter what you do, they will try to do it better. Whatever your children do, your siblings will claim that their children are brighter, cuter, more talented, and Grandma's favorites.

Do yourself (and your partner and children, if applicable) a favor and get off that sibling roller coaster. Stick with siblings you love and who are good for you. Work on on relationships that are worth having. The rest you can see once a year during the holidays. You can get through one day with them, right? Just take a few deep breaths and try to avoid the mind games.

Your Coworkers

If you have a choice, pick your job based on the best possible people you could ever meet. It will take years of stress off your life. If, on the other hand, you find yourself in a toxic place, where half the people spend their time in the lunchroom gossiping about the other half, you've got to find a way out. Don't join that lunchroom crowd, no matter what!

You can try being a positive example, but let's face it, bad people hate positive examples. They won't learn from you, usually. They'll make fun of you, sure. One patient of mine tried making everybody feel good by bringing muffins to work once a week and sitting together socially for a minute. Turns out the people thought she was sabotaging their diets. With mean people, it's pretty hard to win.

If you have to stay at your job—and before you make that decision, please examine whether or not that's really true—you're going to need all of the antistress methods we'll talk about below. Lots of deep breathing (but don't do that while on the phone with a client).

Your Relationship with the World

Have road rage? Want to kill the person standing next to you on the bus? Ready to start kicking the seat of the person sitting in front of you on a plane? Cool it down. If you pay close attention to how your body feels when you are getting mad at the slowpoke in front of you on the highway, you will see the physical effects of stress. Notice that your muscles are tensed. Bad sign. Notice that your pulse rate is up. Not good. Your face is red. You're starting to sweat. I bet your blood pressure is inching up, too, but you can't feel that silent killer.

Before you head out in the morning, stop for a two-minute stress buster. Take some deep breaths or use a method that works well for you. Look over your schedule for the day and get prepared for it; allow yourself some extra time to get to work when you have a meeting that's making you nervous. Picture yourself handling everything well. So when that idiot in front of you doesn't see the light turn green, maybe you'll be mad, but your body won't be. Breathe again. You are the Zen driver.

Stress and Time Management

Time is today's most valuable commodity. We all juggle choices, anxious to please family, colleagues, and friends, whether they want us to or not!

If you are time stressed, change is up to you. This sounds harsh, but you can't complain about time stress if you are letting everyone else decide your priorities. What are your own priorities? What goals do you want to achieve—and what's most important to you? Keep your important goals in the very front of your mind. They are your decision-making tools.

Let's say you feel it's extremely important to be involved at your child's school. What does this mean? Does it mean what the PTO or PTA says it means, or what you believe in? Maybe you want to run bake sales. Fine. Or maybe you want to work in the classroom or be a community service mentor. Just don't do all three. The crazy people who take on ten projects? Stay away. Remember, they are crazy. You are not, so you choose a few priorities.

True, this will mean that you are not in the PTO or PTA inner circle—but that will save you even more time! Focus on the teachers, the administration, and the families of your child's friends, and you'll be doing your job as a mom.

It's more difficult at work, where you may be the boss or not, but you still feel that everyone else takes up your time. Again, take a good hard look at your day. Write down how you spend your time as the day goes by. What unimportant things did you spend time on? Maybe it's important to you to have an open office in which people feel motivated to own their jobs and feel respected. Great! Unfortunately, the office whiner thinks that means your time is his. If you are the boss, remember you're the boss! Interrupt him. Ask him for his ideas on helpful solutions or tell him to go off and think of some. If you are a colleague or a subordinate, look at your watch and say something like "My time isn't mine—let's talk over coffee when I take a break."

Tackle Your Stress One Little Piece at a Time

If stress is overwhelming you, there are two ways to make it better: The first is to reduce the stress in your life so it never has a chance to affect your body. The second is to reduce the damage that stress can do to you if there's no immediate or easy way to get rid of it completely. Here's an example of how this works.

Let's say you have an aggravating coworker. She socializes with people all day long and gossips about everyone, including you. She has a high-pitched voice and a frequent sniff. And she never gets caught. Not only that, her parents pay all of her living expenses (you know this because you've had no choice but to overhear her talking all about it). She's really beginning to stress you out; so what can you do?

Start with what you can do to reduce or get rid of your stress. Can you tell her you have trouble hearing your clients on the phone because she has a powerful voice and ask her to pipe down a little? Can you tell her that you love to talk with her but that you don't want to talk about other people? Can you move to a different location? Would your boss let you wear headphones while at work to drown out your coworker's voice?

If none of these are viable options, then you need to look at how you can reduce the damage that this woman's loud gossiping is doing to your body.

First, don't board the gossip train. Seriously, spreading the bad word about your coworker isn't going to improve the situation, and it will likely increase your own stress. Next, practice some relaxation techniques: take a quick walk around the office or outside, stand up and do some simple stretches, or take a couple of long, deep breaths.

Now, set some boundaries: tell her you've got a deadline and you have to get to work. Change the way you think about the situation by reminding yourself that often you can learn important lessons from awful people—like how destructive gossip is. By the end of your career, awful people will have taught you almost as much about life as your wonderful mentors have. And remember that it's always better to talk with the problem person early on. If you were to talk to this coworker on her first few days of work, you'd handle it differently from the way you erupt at her a year later.

Despite the anxiety they may cause, minor stressful situations happen pretty often. But what if something major happens, like your mom being diagnosed with **cancer**? These bigger stressors require a different approach.

Let's say that you've just found out your mom is going to be in treatment for a long time. You won't be able to spend as much time with her as you would like. Not only that, but your relationship with your parents is complicated and your awful sister still lives at home and doesn't help.

To reduce this kind of major stress, start by breaking the problem into smaller pieces. Your worry about your mother is one piece, your concern about your father is another, and thoughts about yourself or your sister are another. Deal with one thing at a time, and each piece will become easier.

This sounds simplistic—and it is. My point is that we all need to learn how to reduce big problems into manageable ones and then learn how to keep stress from getting under our skin.

Stress Busters

The best way to cope with stress is to do things that are good for you and that make you feel good, like exercising, laughing, napping, pampering yourself, or listening to music. Be on the lookout for common unhealthy responses to stress so you can avoid them. These include drinking alcohol, denying the problem, using drugs, overeating, and smoking.

Many people turn to behaviors that are not only ineffective but also unhealthy to cope with their stress. The stress busters described above offer some positive ways to manage your stress. Try one, try them all—just do something to bring some calm back to your life. Your body will thank you for it.

There is definitely not a one-size-fits-all answer when it comes to stress. But it's worth reviewing some of the most common and effective stress reduction techniques because some may work for you.

Dr. Alice Domar, an expert on stress, calls this the mind-body buffet. Once you find approaches that work for you, if you work them into your life you will be amazed by how much better you feel both physically and psychologically.

The approaches that tend to work for most people are relaxation techniques such as progressive muscle relaxation (PMR) or meditation, stress management strategies such as cognitive restructuring (challenging your automatically recurring negative thoughts) or journaling, lifestyle changes including exercise and nutrition, and social support.

Practicing Progressive Muscle Relaxation

If you can work progressive muscle relaxation (PMR) into your schedule at least once a day, you'll feel relaxed and de-stressed. With PMR, you tense muscle groups one at a time as you inhale and then release them as you exhale.

Start by sitting in a quiet room wearing comfortable clothes and no shoes. Some people recommend that you sit in a chair so you don't fall asleep, but this is also a wonderful way to relax before you fall asleep at night.

Close your eyes and take a deep breath. Tense each muscle group for five to ten seconds, then release and exhale. You'll work with the muscle groups in order, starting at

REAL LIFE FACT: Stress Busters

- **Practice good sleep hygiene (see page 33).**
- **Break the stressor into small parts and tackle one at a time.**
- **Exercise regularly.**
- **Try doing progressive muscle relaxation (see above).**
- **Do some mental health therapy, including cognitive restructuring.**
- **Have a massage.**
- **Get a manicure or pedicure (a sanitary one; see page 397).**
- **Listen to music—or write your own!**
- **Take a cat nap.**
- **Read.**
- **Try a new relaxation technique (meditation, deep breathing, yoga, or self-hypnosis.**
- **Slip into a warm bath and soak.**
- **Laugh.**
- **Spend time with a good friend—go to lunch, go shopping!**
- **Eat a healthy diet and allow yourself an occasional treat.**
- **Bring calm to your space with aromatherapy.**

the feet and working up or starting at the face and working down. Regardless of where you start, be sure to include all of the groups listed below. And don't tense any muscles that hurt. This is supposed to feel good!

MUSCLE GROUPS

- One foot
- One foot and lower leg
- One whole leg
- The other foot
- The other foot and lower leg
- The other whole leg
- Buttocks
- One hand, in a fist
- One hand and forearm
- One whole arm
- The other hand, in a fist
- The other hand and forearm
- The other whole arm
- Abdomen
- Chest and shoulders
- Face

Cognitive Restructuring

Cognitive restructuring is best learned with a pro, who is usually a mental health therapist. It's a very practical approach to reducing stress because you examine negative thoughts and find practical ways to deal with them. It isn't about your childhood or other issues, which are better addressed in talk therapy.

If you want to try cognitive restructuring, find a therapist that is trained in it (to know, you just have to ask). If you can't find a specialist in your area, there are some online tools you can try. Go to www.mindtools.com and search for "cognitive restructuring." This won't replace having sessions with an expert, but it can be very useful.

Meet Your Own Needs

I've noticed that women have a hard time meeting their own basic needs, and in fact, men do a better job of this. When they are hungry, they eat. When they are tired, they sleep. I think most women need to add their own needs to their daily to-do lists as more of a priority. Self-care is not selfish—you are better able to care for those around you if you care for yourself. Remember the airplane emergency procedure: put on your own oxygen mask before attending to others who may need help. The same thing goes for meeting your own needs in general.

Set Priorities

Sometimes when you have a to-do list in your mind it can feel overwhelming. Once the list is on paper, it may feel a lot more manageable.

Make a list with two columns. In column one write down the highest priority tasks for that day or week. In the second column note the lower priority tasks. Include phone numbers, addresses, or other information you need to complete the task so all the details are in one place. Then tackle each task one at a time. The most important step: What can you cross off your list?

Develop Relationships

Don't go it alone. Humans are social beings, and sometimes just describing your problems out loud to trusted family members or friends can make a huge difference. Share your worries—talk with friends, counselors, therapists, support groups, or family members about what is bothering you. Take note of warmth and love from others and reciprocate. Make eye contact and say hello to colleagues at work. Listen more and talk less. Ask lots of questions to be sure that you have understood correctly and to show your interest in others. Try to be less self-absorbed. And remember the wisdom of this great bumper sticker I saw recently: Wag More, Bark Less.

Relax

Don't say you don't have time to relax. Take time for things you love to do. Slow down when you can, and recognize when you are being a workaholic. Learn to meditate or use structured relaxation and breathing techniques to reduce your stress load. You can do this in a minute, while driving or sitting at your desk at work. You'll be amazed how well it works. Try yoga or your favorite exercise.

"Fall Down Six Times, Get Up Seven."

This is an old saying, and it has a lot to do with stress. Life is filled with mistakes and accidents. You probably know people who are truly handicapped by a "failure" that they just can't get over, like being fired from a job.

Most of the time, life's burdens are smaller than that, but they add up to a big bundle of stress and anxiety that you carry around. Monique says that the best advice she ever found was on the back of a shampoo bottle: "Lather. Rinse. Repeat." You get it: Try something. If you fail, rinse it off. Now try again. It takes practice, and the sooner you start, the better you will be at managing stress. Try applying shampoo advice to daily tangles: Say the project you proposed was rejected. Maybe the recommendation you made was innovative but wrong. You've got to gather yourself and move on.

For one patient, "lather, rinse, repeat" meant gathering up all of the rebate forms and receipts that she had never mailed in. She collected all of the expired rebates she had never followed up on and shredded them, vowing never to make a purchase based on a rebate price ever again. She said she used to think of that pile when she lay awake at night.

Don't Strive for Perfection

You may have things to "shred" too. Let go of the anger over the small fight you had with your partner. Be the one who apologizes sometimes. Only save coupons for things you already use or stores you already shop at. Only give the kids nonstaining snacks for the backseat of your car—no grape drinks.

Remember, you and many other people are in the same boat and feel exactly the same way. There's something positive about knowing you have company that relaxes your body. Are you furious that you just bought a computer and two weeks later a new version came out? "Join the club," your IT director says. "Ahh," you think. I'm not alone. Doesn't that feel better? Perfect is the enemy of good. Most of the time, good enough really is enough.

In chapter 4, we'll talk about another issue that's universal: skin problems. That's where we're headed next.

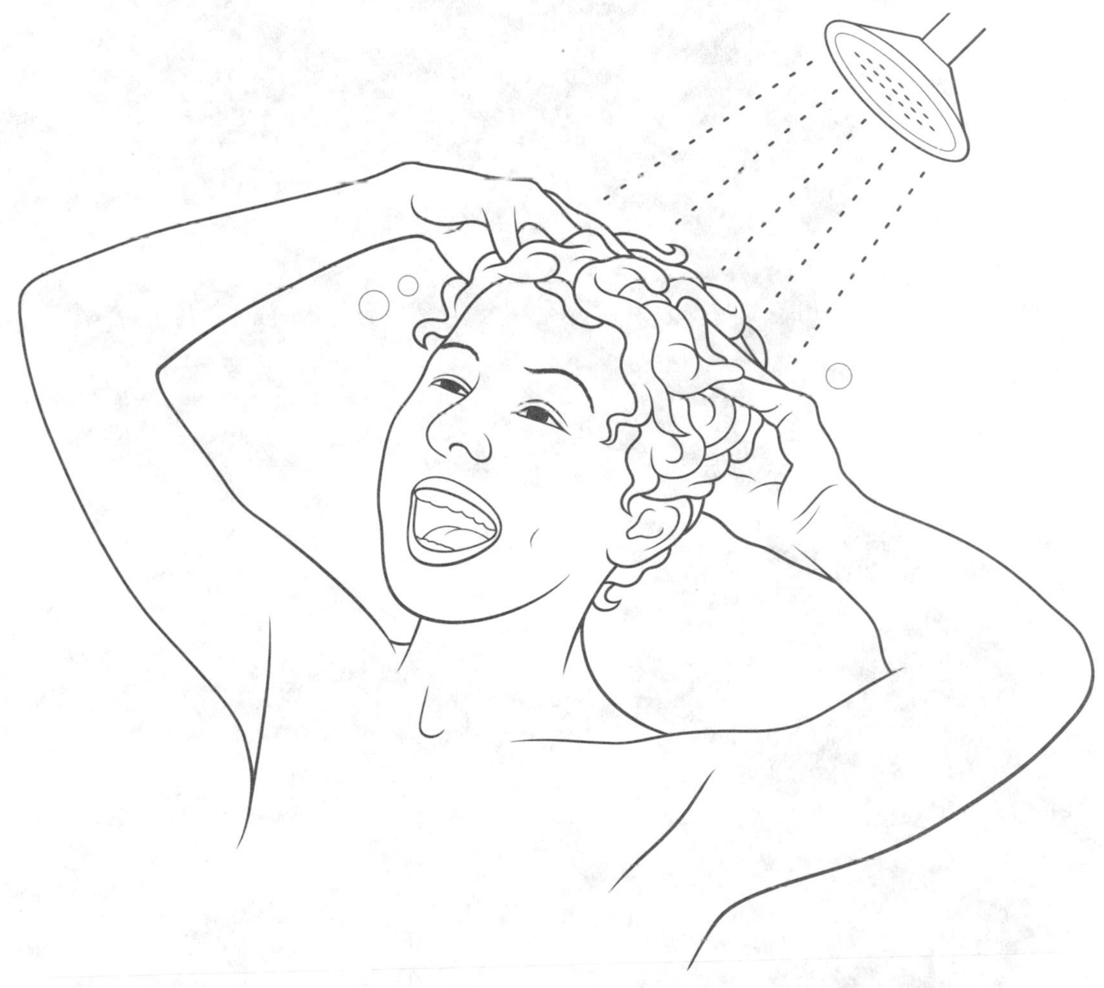

Lather. Rinse. Repeat.

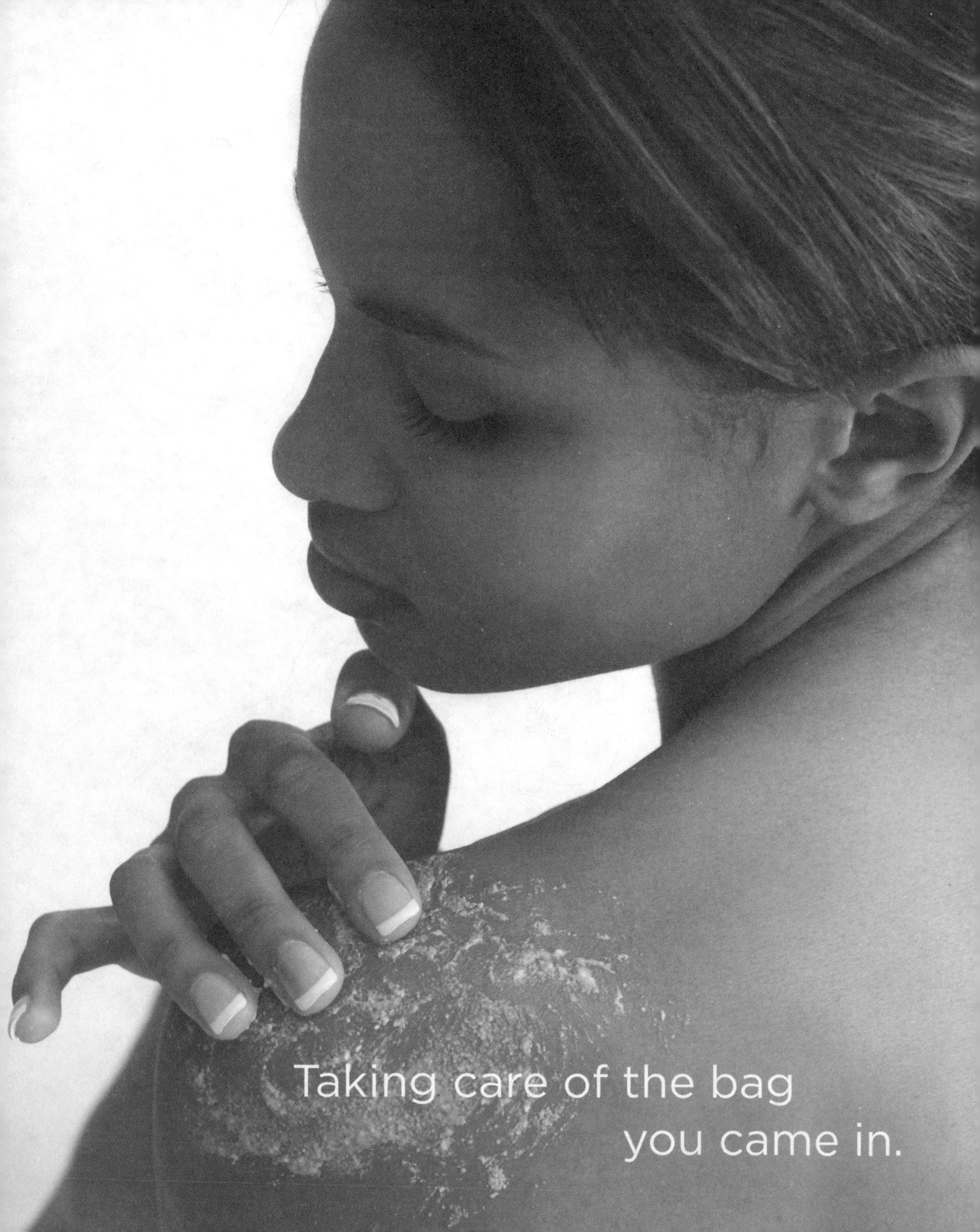
Taking care of the bag
you came in.

your skin

Maybe this has happened to you: You have a favorite moisturizer. It's a

department store brand, and it's your only splurge. You buy a jar twice a year, plus your aunt gives you a jar for your birthday. You both wait until the store is giving out a free gift with purchase before you buy.

At the cosmetics counter, the saleswoman smiles when you ask for your moisturizer. Then she frowns. "Hmm." She looks closely at your skin, then *hmms* again. "When was your last personalized beauty strategy exam? Let's see, your personalized profile says it was a year ago! I bet you never pamper yourself, do you? Well, sit down, because I'm going to pamper you until you feel fabulous. You deserve some "me time." Don't worry, this is entirely complimentary."

Your entirely complimentary makeover turns out to be moisturizer plus makeup. It will cost you $200, because that's how much makeup the saleslady will convince you that you need. You'll walk out of the store feeling so fabulous, looking so fabulous. Then you'll get in the car, quickly flip down the mirror, and see yourself in real daylight. Hmm. You look a little like a clown, true, and a somewhat slutty one. And guess what? You forgot to get the moisturizer. Live and learn: you won't do that again, at least not too often.

What's wrong with leaving your skin care in the hands of department store clerks? Your skin is the container you came in, and it's a living organ, like your lungs, **kidneys**, and **liver**. It's the largest organ you have, not just a blank canvas to be painted. Its job is to protect you from the outside world—dehydration, heat, cold, infection, and pollution—in much the same way that some moms dress their kids in rubber from hat to boots just in case it rains.

The appearance of your skin is often a sign of your body's health. So it is important to learn the basics of pampering your skin now, because many of the preventive and protective measures I'm recommending will keep the rest of your body healthy, too. It's a good idea to take care of this big organ just as carefully as you take care of the others.

Also, your skin is a great big giveaway about your lifestyle. Think nobody knows you stayed out all night? Your skin advertises what kind of life you lead. If you've had too much junk food, too much alcohol, and too little sleep, no amount of makeup will hide that shade of gray. Poor nutrition, neglect, and too much sun can damage not just how you look, but also the vital protective mechanisms of your skin.

We women spend zillions of dollars—and hours—on skin care. I'm pretty sure that part of that time and money is wasted, but which part? Well, what's important? What's harmful? And what is skin, anyway? Let's look under the surface of your skin and learn how to keep it looking great no matter how old or young you are. We'll even make a scary trip through your under-the-sink shoebox of disaster makeup.

Anatomy of Your Skin

Your skin is made of two major layers: the dermis and epidermis. The epidermis is the thin outer layer of your skin, the one you can see. The epidermis contains cells called melanocytes, which make the pigment that gives your skin its color. The pigment comes from a substance called melanin, which determines the shade of your skin and also makes freckles.

The dermis is the thick inner layer of skin. It contains sweat **glands**, oil glands, hair **follicles**, fat, nerves, arterioles, and **veins**, as you can see in the illustration on page 75. The glands produce the sweat and oil that make it to the skin surface. Sweat and oil make you want to wash your face as soon as you can, but they are actually designed to protect your skin. (Don't worry, we're not going to tell you to stop washing your skin just because sweat and oil have a useful purpose.)

The dermis is where new cells are made to replace the old ones. When you wash or exfoliate or scratch your skin, old cells flake off. You need new ones to form the new surface, which are made in a 24-7 factory down in the dermis. The dermis also contains connective tissue. This is a stretchy net, made of collagen and elastin, that gives structure and resilience to your skin. This net makes you look young.

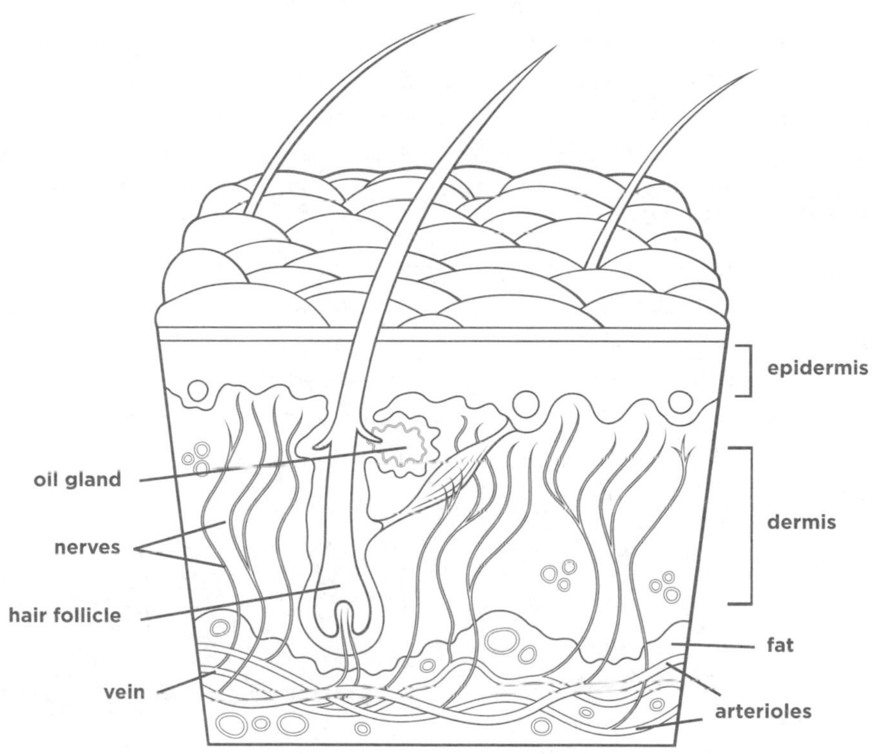

Anatomy of your skin: Your skin is made of two major layers: the dermis and epidermis. The epidermis is the thin outer layer of skin, the one you can see. The dermis is the thick inner layer of skin. It contains oil glands, hair follicles, fat, nerves, arterioles, and veins. The glands produce the sweat and oil that make it to the skin surface.

Acne: It's Number One

Acne, pimples, breakouts, zits—it's the biggest skin problem for many people. Twenty percent of visits to the skin doctor are about acne. It could follow you through your teenage years and stop—or it might come back as your faithful companion during pregnancy or **menopause**.

Young women are especially troubled by acne. They get more of it than anyone else because of the hormone tornado raging inside of them. Acne usually pops up on the face and shoulders, but it can also thrive on your arms, legs, trunk, and even your booty. The worse your acne is, the more you may be bothered by it. Many people find acne embarrassing, and some people have it so severely that they end up with scars. Let's get to the bottom of this common skin condition.

What Is Making You Break Out?

Start with great news: It's not chocolate! There is no link between chocolate and acne. And there is no evidence that any food causes acne. The myths of chocolate, sweets, pizza, oil, and milk as causes should be put to rest. A healthy diet will help your skin, of course, but none of these individual foods will trigger acne. So what does cause it?

Acne Activators

How and why do zits happen? Step one begins with **bacteria** on your skin. You have normal bacteria on your skin, as you do everywhere in and on your body. On your skin, the little harmless germs are supposed to live on the surface, but when they get trapped *beneath* the skin, they can cause trouble.

In step two, your hormones rev up your skin's oil glands, which are called sebaceous glands. Normally, the oil glands help keep the skin lubricated and help remove old skin cells. During your teen years and early twenties, hormonal changes make these glands work overtime. Too much oil can clog pores, especially when old skin cells are added to the mix. You might also be adding oil from lotions and makeup.

Your natural oil, or sebum, is collecting in your hair follicles. Look closely at the hair on your body. Each hair is growing in a little tube called a follicle. When your glands make the right amount of oil, your face looks moisturized. When they make too much, your skin looks and feels greasy.

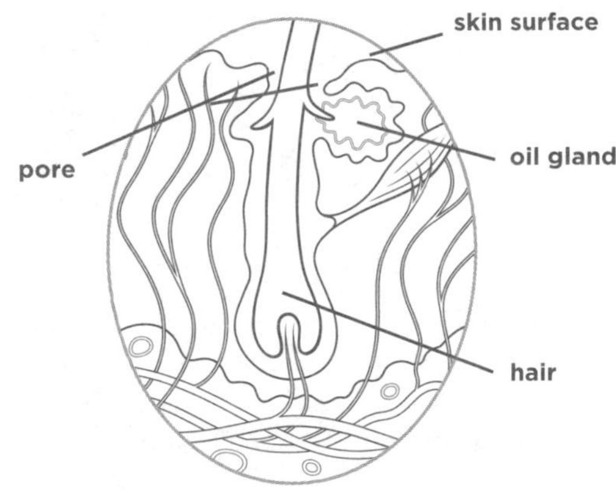

Close-up view of a hair follicle and oil gland.

REAL LIFE FACT: How Acne Happens

Oil glands in your skin produce too much oil, or you add oil with makeup and lotions. Old skin cells get stuck in your pores. Bacteria gets trapped under the skin's surface. When it joins the mix, a mini infection grows, with redness, swelling, and pus.

REAL LIFE FACT: When to Throw Makeup Out

We're heading for the bathroom cabinet, including under the sink. That's where you have the shoebox of disaster makeup that looks terrible on you but is too expensive to throw away. Here's a helpful life secret: If you can satisfy your conscience, it won't bother you to toss it. Tell yourself that all of that stuff has an expiration date. It could be bad for you.

You still can't toss it? Well, ditch anything that could be contaminated: mascara, eyeliner, lipstick, and anything with a brush that you touch to your face and then put back into the bottle. Your conscience can be clear. See? It doesn't matter what you spent on the purple mascara; it has to be thrown out now.

Those gorgeous eye shadows and foundations that would be perfect on any color skin but yours? The peach blush and brown lipstick? That's what nieces are for. She'll be grateful, or at least appear to be, before she realizes that nobody, not anybody, can wear that blush.

In step three, the bacteria and the oils combine. The bacteria trapped below the skin surface combine with the oils in your skin, causing a chemical reaction. The oils break down into free fatty acids. Free fatty acids irritate your skin. Next stop: redness, swelling, tenderness, and warmth. Acne.

If a pore gets clogged at the surface of your skin, step four is a whitehead. If a pore gets clogged beneath the skin but remains open at the skin surface, the clog inside darkens when exposed to the air, and the result is a blackhead. The black tip is not dirt stuck there, but the oily contents reacting with oxygen at the surface of the skin.

If the wall of the clogged pore breaks open underneath the surface of your skin, pimples come next. Oil, bacteria, and dead skin cells leak out under the skin, causing tiny eruptions, which are pimples. (If the eruption is deep under your skin, the pimples may grow to form cysts. Cystic acne is described in more detail below.) **White blood cells**, which eat bacteria, multiply in the clogged pore. They cause bigger bumps and pus pockets beneath the surface of the skin. Ugh.

Together, this oil and dead skin blockage is known in medical terminology as a comedo; in a group it is called comedones. Because this word looks so much like *condoms*, I'll just add a detail that it is pronounced *com-ee-DOHNZ*. *Comedo* is pronounced *com-EE-doh*. When you buy any product for your skin, make sure that it is noncomedogenic. This means it doesn't clog pores.

Biggest Acne Triggers

Your family history plays a part in whether you get acne. You can inherit a tendency for acne, hormone levels, skin thickness, and oil production that can cause you problems. Yet another gift from Uncle Harry, the man with acne scars and red back hair.

However, this isn't cast in stone! Plenty of acne-plagued parents have children with clear skin.You may not inherit this tendency. Plus, there are many products available today that your parents didn't have. Remember, these are people who fashioned their makeup on TV shows like *Dynasty*.

Besides your genetics, acne can be triggered by:

- Sweating
- Your menstrual cycle
- Pregnancy
- Birth control pills (which can also be used to relieve acne!)
- Cosmetics, lotions, and hair products
- Tight clothing, hats, or tightly-strapped backpacks

Cystic Acne

Cystic acne happens when pimples grow to become large oil-filled chambers beneath the skin surface. Acne in this form begins like all acne lesions and has the same factors involved—bacteria, too much sebaceous oil, and plugging of the follicles with oil and dead skin.

In cystic acne, however, you have a mini atmosphere with no oxygen, called an anaerobic environment because it is cut off from the oxygen at the skin surface. This environment is a perfect place for bacteria to grow. So next come the white blood cells to fight the bacteria. They use **enzymes** that break down the oils into free fatty acids. Cysts begin to form under the skin. If the opening to the cyst is totally blocked, surgical drainage may be necessary, along with **antibiotics** to help eliminate the bacterial infection.

Hormone Hurricanes

Do you ever notice that your skin tends to break out right before and during your period? Your hormone levels rise and fall during your menstrual cycle, and your skin is very sensitive to these changes. From the teens through the early twenties, hormones are in an especially powerful cycle of change. How does it work?

We all have both female and male hormones in our bodies. The female hormones, especially **estrogen**, tend to prevent acne; male hormones, such as **testosterone** and **androstenedione**, stimulate the oil glands in your skin, which can lead to breakouts.

When your estrogen level is high, this powerful female hormone acts to reduce or prevent acne. It neutralizes male hormone activity. It helps your body to produce a substance that will bind with the male hormones and slow them down. The "free" testosterone that hasn't been bound by this **protein** is the active form, which causes acne or makes it worse. So the more estrogen you have circulating, the less male hormone activity there is to affect your skin.

At the beginning of your menstrual cycle (right after your period ends), your ovaries produce large amounts of estrogen to prepare for **ovulation** (release of an egg). After ovulation, another female hormone, **progesterone**, goes to work. It creates a nourishing environment in your **uterus**, getting it ready for the arrival of a fertilized egg. These female hormones keep the acne-causing male hormones in check.

As your body moves through your monthly menstrual cycle and your uterus prepares to shed its lining during your period, the levels of your female hormones drop. This is what those male hormones have been waiting for. Free at last, they spring into action, stimulating your oil glands to become active—and causing acne breakouts. This is why you may notice breakouts right before and during your period. Then the cycle starts again.

Later in the chapter we'll see how birth control pills can help to ease acne by increasing the levels of female hormones and suppressing the acne-causing activities of male hormones.

Acne Attackers

If acne is a problem for you, take action. First, gently wash your face only twice per day, morning and evening. Too much washing can irritate your skin. Ideally, use only your hands and a gentle cleanser to avoid irritating your skin. You can use a washcloth to remove makeup or lotions, but use it gently. Washing by itself does not clear breakouts, as dirt does not cause acne, so there is absolutely no need to scrub.

NOTE TO SELF

Make sure your washing machine's rinse cycle leaves your washcloths free of harsh detergents. To check, put the cloth in water after you wash it and see if you can work up some suds. If you can, do two rinse cycles.

Now, on to good treatment options that may help clear up your skin.

To Pop or Not to Pop

"Never pop!" is the advice you get from your friends, your doctors, and your mother. But it can be okay to pop a zit . . . under the right circumstances (a pimple almost ready to pop on its own that can be removed with very gentle pressure). But please don't beat up on your face. If you pop too much, you will make a bad problem worse and do more harm than good.

What are the rules? The key to productive popping is to choose the right zits to zap. Only pop zits that are close to the surface of your skin and have come to a raised head. You'll know a zit is poppable because you can see the white pus lurking just under the surface of your skin. Wash the area and then use a clean washcloth to press gently (gently!) on each side of the zit. Don't use your bare hands to apply pressure; this can traumatize your skin.

The oily contents should squeeze out pretty easily. Wipe this off gently and apply an antibiotic ointment from the drugstore (such as Neosporin or Bacitracin) to prevent more bacteria growth.

If a zit doesn't pop easily, it probably isn't ready to be popped. You can try the next step, gently and carefully, which may draw the pimple to the surface so it becomes poppable in a few days. Take a warm, wet washcloth. Press lightly on the zit to bring it to a head. Hold the cloth on the spot for a few minutes, and repeat this warm compress a couple of times a day to coax the oily material to the skin surface. Don't use hot water or you'll burn your skin and end up with more bright red blemishes than you started with.

Remember, less is better when it comes to popping zits. (Don't do any of this the day of the prom. Your skin needs a few days to recover!)

NOTE TO SELF

Popping pimples is not prohibited! The key is choosing the right pimples to pop and doing it the right way.

A few more emergency pimple popping tips:

- Wash your face with a washcloth to remove all lotion and makeup.
- Steam your face before you pop zits. Steam will open your pores and soften your skin surface. Sit in front of a bowl of hot water with your skin near the water—but not touching it! Make a tent over your head with a towel to trap the steam. Some people take a hot shower to do this, but many will just get irritated skin this way.
- Wash your hands thoroughly to prevent infecting the pimple with bacteria from your hands.
- Sterilize a needle or pin by holding it in a flame or wiping it with alcohol so you don't introduce bacteria with the procedure.
- Prick the surface (and only the surface) of the pimple with the needle.
- Using a washcloth or gauze, apply gentle pressure to the sides of the pimple to coax out the pus. Do not press hard!
- Apply antibiotic ointment to the area.

Over-the-Counter and Prescription Medications for Acne

These are two of the most popular and effective acne medications that you can buy at your local drugstore:

- Benzoyl peroxide is a topical (skin) treatment that comes in liquid, bar, lotion, cream, and gel forms. Whatever form you choose, *topical* means that you apply it to your skin. It helps by killing acne-causing bacteria, but it may take four to six weeks before you see the effects.
- Salicylic acid is applied as a topical cream or face wash. It helps to slow down shedding of the cells inside the follicles, preventing clogging. Salicylic acid also helps break down blackheads and whiteheads.

If the over-the-counter options don't work, ask your skin doctor (dermatologist) about these prescription medications for acne:

- Adapalene (trade name Differin) is a topical gel. It slows down the accumulation of skin cells inside the follicle that plugs the pores.
- Azelaic acid (trade name Azelex) is a natural acid found in whole-grain cereals and animal products. This topical cream is thought to help the skin to renew itself more quickly and prevent the buildup of cells that can plug pores, thereby reducing pimple and blackhead formation. It also helps to kill *Propionibacterium acnes*, the bacteria that causes acne.
- Clindamycin and erythromycin are antibiotics used topically and orally for treatment of acne. They work by killing the bacteria that cause acne. They may be used alone or in combination with other treatments, and it may take up to twelve weeks for the full effects to be seen.
- Isotretinoin (trade name Accutane) is a kind of vitamin A that is taken in pill form for fifteen to twenty weeks. It is prescribed for severe acne that does not respond to other treatments. It reduces the amount of oil produced by the oil glands. A single course of fifteen to twenty weeks has been shown to result in complete clearing and long-term remission of acne in up to 85 percent of people. No other acne medicine works as well for severe acne.

But wait: as powerful as isotretinoin can be in improving your skin (and your life), its negative effects can be just as powerful. Isotretinoin must be used with caution. It is known to cause miscarriages and severe birth defects. In rare cases, patients develop serious problems affecting the liver, **intestines**, eyes, ears, and skeletal system. Some patients taking isotretinoin have developed serious psychiatric problems, including depression. More rarely, patients have developed suicidal behavior. Because of the miscarriage and birth defect risks, it is essential to use a reliable birth control method while taking this medication.

Birth Control Pills Do Double Duty

Birth control pills are another option for acne treatment. They are well proven for treating acne in women ages fifteen or older. Studies show that nine out of ten women who take birth control pills show significant improvements in their skin. Some formulations of the birth control pill are better than others for acne control, but all types help to some degree.

Birth control pills contain the hormones estrogen and **progestin**. (Progesterone and progestins are cousins. Progestins are synthetic hormones and mimic the action of natural progesterone.) In all pills that contain estrogen, the estrogen component helps to minimize acne by decreasing the level of **androgens** (male hormones) that contribute to the development of acne. Estrogen in the pill helps prevent acne by increasing **sex hormone binding globulin (SHGB)**, which binds more of the free (acne-causing) testosterone in your body. Bound testosterone is not active, and with lower levels of free testosterone in your body, the severity of your acne decreases.

Birth control pills today contain low doses of the hormone estrogen, and almost all contain the same (or a similar) form of estrogen. Some pills are lower dose than others.

The real difference from one pill to another is in the progestin component. Some of these progestins work together with the estrogen component to make the pill a good treatment for acne. The progestin component is originally created in the laboratory based on androgens: scientists start with androgens and alter them to turn them into progestins. Progestins that are the least androgenic (the least like testosterone) are the best for your skin. Pills that are good choices for acne treatment are those that contain so-called third-generation progestins. These newer and less androgenic progestins include desogestrel and norgestimate (found in the drugs marketed as Mircette, Desogen, Ortho-Cept and Ortho-Cyclen). Oral contraceptive pills containing these progestins have been shown to reduce and even resolve acne.

Even newer and probably even better for your skin is a new progestin not based on androgens at all, called drospirenone. Drospirenone (found in the pills marketed as Yasmin and Yaz) is a unique progestin. These pills start with a different hormone building block called **spironolactone**. When made naturally in your body, the hormone spironolactone helps to balance salt and water and prevents water retention. When you take a birth control pill that contains a progestin made from spironolactone, there can be a weak diuretic (increased urination) effect when you first start it. Studies suggest these spironolactone-containing birth control pills, because of their lack of male hormone effect, are very good in helping to clear up or prevent acne.

NOTE TO SELF

Pimples are not caused by dirt on your skin, and pores do not get blocked on top of your skin. Your pores get blocked deep inside where you can't reach. No amount of washing prevents this, and too much washing is actually irritating to your skin.

The Truth about Your Skin

There are people who seem to have perfect skin for a lifetime. The color is even, there are no zits, the pores are invisible, and the wrinkles are only the most charming smile lines. In real life, these people are statues in museums, because no real person actually looks that way. Some of us have dry skin, some oily;

thick skin or thin; giant pores or tiny; or sensitive skin or tough. And some of us are one color from head to toe, while others are covered with freckles and moles.

It's too bad you can't pick your own genes from perfect-skinned parents. Instead, you must take steps now to have the healthiest, most attractive skin you can have. These steps are proven, evidence-based practices. I know that every magazine tells you about "the one trick you need for beautiful skin" and it turns out to be making facials from recycled tires and oatmeal or something. Skip the tricks. Try to practice all of the guidelines below. They work better than any cosmetic you can buy, and they work now, later, and much later:

- Live a healthy lifestyle, eating healthy foods that keep your body working at its best. If your body has to struggle to get what it needs to be healthy, everything suffers, including your skin.
- Quit tanning . . . on the beach, at the salon, everywhere. Take a look at elderly women who come from cultures that kept women out of the sun. Their skin looks good at eighty. I'm not promoting their lifestyles, just pointing out that they prove the damage that sun does to beautiful skin.

  The tanning bed is just as bad as the sun, and we now know that tanning beds cause melanoma, the most serious kind of skin cancer. Your dermatologist has probably been telling you to quit for years. Now the International Agency for Research on Cancer (IARC) puts tanning beds up there with arsenic. They are as bad as smoking and asbestos. Please, stop using the tanning bed. It's urgent!
- Wash your face and body once a day with a gentle cleanser. Don't cleanse too often—once a day is usually plenty unless you sweat heavily or live in a highly polluted area. If you wear makeup, remove it before bedtime.
- Moisturize. A daily moisturizer just after cleansing the skin is good for everyone. Choose a product for oily, dry, or normal skin; let your skin be your guide. If your skin still feels oily ten minutes after applying your moisturizer, you're using too much or the wrong kind. If your skin is often scaly, you need more. Change with the seasons—in cold climates, winter is very tough on dry skin. Keep hydrated inside and out.
- Use sunscreen every day. Many moisturizers contain sunscreen, so this can be a great way to get a double benefit from your moisturizer. If you have dry skin and like to use a moisturizer at night, use one without sunscreen then to minimize applying extra chemicals to your skin.

Does your sunscreen burn your eyes? You are probably applying it too closely. Lotions all move around a bit and will work their way toward the eye. Leave a small margin, perhaps a quarter of an inch, around each eye. Be sure to wash your hands thoroughly before you touch your eyes. Most of that sunscreen "eye burn" is caused by your fingers!

- Exfoliate. You've got to get rid of those old cells for your moisturizer to do its job. Many experts believe in once-a-week microdermabrasion to remove the top layer of dead skin cells from the face. Use a gentle scrub with small grains, as larger ones can traumatize your skin. If you have sensitive skin, though, don't do this more often than once a week or it might do more harm than good.
- Facial masks, like exfoliation, can be beneficial, as long as you don't overdo it. If you have dry skin, they can help hydrate it.

  You'll notice a big difference between results from exfoliation at home and those from having a scrub at a salon. The salon worker spends minutes gently circling each inch of your skin, but at home most of us squirt some exfoliant out and do a quick rub around the face. If that sounds like you, you might benefit from the exfoliating kits that use a battery-operated pad to do the work for you.

  Remember that if you're having an acne breakout, scrubbing is too tough for your skin.
- Read the label. When you buy makeup and skin care products, buy water-based or oil-free products if you have oily skin or are prone to breakouts. Even if you have dry skin, buy products that are labeled noncomedogenic.

Topical Tricks

Creams and lotions can play an important role in the care and maintenance of your skin. However, no serum or cream works for everyone. And no serum or cream works as well as it does in "before and after" pictures. But there are ingredients that you may find helpful. The first two have been proven to have a helpful effect on aging skin:

- As you age, the circulation in your skin decreases, resulting in a decreased supply of vitamin C, which is needed for collagen production. Vitamin C can be incorporated into creams that penetrate deep into your skin, where it works to enhance collagen production.
- Topical use of antioxidant vitamin A creams, such as tretinoin (trade name Retin-A), also help to produce collagen. Tretinoin can lessen the shallow wrinkles around the eyes. However, the improvement lasts only as long as you keep using it, and the wrinkles come back when you stop. The vitamin A creams can be irritating to some skin types. Remember that a little wrinkling is going to happen no matter how well you treat your skin. (Retinol is the non-prescription-strength version of tretinoin.)
- Glycolic acids, alpha hydroxy acids (AHAs), and lactic acids exfoliate the skin without scrubbing. They can be tough on sensitive skin, but if you can

tolerate them, they will make your skin feel and look smoother.

- Antioxidants are designed to address **free radicals** (see page 87). They include vitamins A, B, C, and E, alpha-lipoic acid, chamomile, grape seed, papaya, some evergreens, wine extracts, green tea, rose hips, coenzyme Q10, and other new compounds discovered every day.
- Peptides are an old ingredient that's part of a new craze, a trend to focus on aging at the cellular level. This approach tries to speed up the production of new cells so that the surface of the skin will appear younger.
- Dimethylaminoethanol (DMAE) is a hotly debated ingredient claimed to firm skin. It is a known organic compound that is studied for antiaging impacts on the brain. Nobody knows whether putting it on your skin will slow aging. I have a few problems with DMAE. It is a cheap ingredient that's easy to get, but the creams that contain it cost a fortune. This ingredient, like many cosmetic and herbal ingredients, has not been proven to be safe.
- Collagen, elastin, and hyaluronic acid are among the most marketed ingredients. These are all part of that stretchy net that keeps your face firm. The truth: Applied topically, they can't penetrate the skin, so they will not replace that aging net. However, they hold an amount of water many times their own weight and can be part of a great moisturizer.

REAL LIFE FACT: Money-Saving Advice

If you are planning to spend hundreds of dollars on antiaging cosmetics, you are better off seeing a dermatologist. Dermatologists can prescribe products such as Retin-A and do procedures such as chemical peels that are many times more powerful than what you'll find in over-the-counter jars. These approaches, however, can be rough on the skin. Many people find them to be too abrasive. But if you see a reputable dermatologist, you may get good advice tailored to your own skin.

What about having facials at the salon? If you love having a facial, go ahead. Just allow a few days between your facial and a big event because you are likely to have some redness in spots, especially if your facialist really works at those clogged pores. As a young woman, you may not have discovered that there are different types of facialists. This is going to sound like a stereotype, and it is, but eastern European facialists tend to be rigorous on those pores. You either like that sensation or you don't, but your skin will recover.

If you're doing your own facials, remember to read labels and look for basic ingredients that address your needs.

You can spend many hundreds of dollars for a single ounce of specialty skin care products. Many celebrities do, because they can and because we all know that a new jar of cream is fun to try. Just remember that when you see the most beautiful woman in the world in a magazine, she has been airbrushed to perfection. You know, because you've seen it, that two weeks later a tabloid will snap a photo of her without makeup, studio lighting, her stylist, her big sunglasses, and airbrushing. She actually looks a whole lot older than you do, doesn't she?

Keep that in mind before you go into debt for any cosmetic. Also beware of the expression "clinically proven." Cosmetic companies can legally use that phrase if just one woman said she liked the product! I'm not exaggerating here. In medicine, "clinically proven" refers only to peer-reviewed, highly structured testing that is published for other scientists to review. In cosmetics, it can mean "my neighbor liked it."

For the best moisturizing, read the label. The first ingredient will be water. Next, be sure to look for noncomedogenic ingredients. Two of the most effective moisturizing ingredients—glycerin and petroleum jelly (Vaseline)—can clog pores. So can mineral oils and lanolin. You'll find them listed as ingredients on the label, and they may be perfectly fine if you have dry skin.

Apply these products to damp, clean skin before bedtime for an overnight mois-

REAL LIFE FACT: Holistic Skin Care Secrets that Manufacturers Don't Want You to Know

Because the baby boomer generation is aging, we're seeing an explosion of antiaging products in magazines and on TV. These ads mostly show a thirty-year-old woman using an antiwrinkle serum, even though she doesn't have any wrinkles yet.

The truth is, when you are eighty you will probably look twenty years younger than any baby boomer you know now. When they were your age, baby boomers didn't use sunscreen, didn't eat for health, and didn't have the most basic information about healthy skin. Now they are targeted by every cream and lotion manufacturer, and some of these products do help a little. On TV, however, manufacturers show results that really can only be had through plastic surgery or Botox injections. Studio lighting can make a wrinkle look deeper than it is—and then make it "disappear."

The "miracle" treatments work on the surface, but that's not where your skin future is happening. Real miracle treatments don't come in a jar when you are fifty. They start for you right now, at *your* age.

ture facial. If you have oily skin or acne, avoid these; you should look for an oil-free moisturizer that may come as a gel.

Your Best Skin for Life

So you've started taking care of your skin and yourself. What are the critical steps you can take to keep your skin looking great? You already know the basics: Quit tanning. (You can use self-tanning products, but give up the tanning bed forever.) Use gentle cleansers. Moisturize. Limit the amount of alcohol you drink. But let's look a little more closely at three more steps.

Feed Your Skin: A Pound of Prevention

Nourishing your skin from the inside maintains healthy skin that ages slowly. We'll need to go back to high school chemistry to explain.

A great deal of skin damage is caused by free radicals. Free radicals are real, even though your parents may have never heard of them. They are molecules that are unstable because they contain unpaired electrons. In your body, they are produced when your cells interact with oxygen. Free radical production is an unavoidable part of life. They are produced every time we breathe oxygen or are exposed to sunlight. They are also caused by toxins: cigarette smoke, alcohol, and air pollution.

Free radicals are part of normal body functions, such as killing bacteria in your body, but they have many negative side effects. Scientists are studying the connections between free radicals and premature aging, wrinkles, and even some of the devastating illnesses of age, such as Alzheimer's disease, **heart disease**, and osteoarthritis.

Your body can stabilize free radicals and prevent them from causing damage by counteracting them with the body's antioxidant system, which slows the damage from free radicals. If you squeeze a lemon—an antioxidant containing vitamin C—onto a cut apple, it will keep it from turning brown. The apple turns brown because of the exposure to oxygen and the resulting free radicals. Vitamins C and E and other antioxidants found in the diet donate electrons to unstable molecules and prevent them from damaging our tissues, like the lemon juice on the apple. A diet rich in the antioxidants contained in fruits and vegetables will prevent oxidative damage not only in your skin, but in your whole body too.

Nourishing your skin from within is good for the whole body. Eat natural, whole foods, such as whole grains, vegetables, fruits, nuts, and seeds. Your diet can supply antioxidants. Look for highly colored foods, which are typically rich in antioxidants: cantaloupe, spinach, berries, and cruciferous vegetables (broccoli, cauliflower, cabbage, and brussels sprouts). These foods, along with green tea, also have other beneficial phytochemicals (**nutrients** from plants) to help protect against oxidative damage and free radical attack on skin and other cells in the body.

Omega-3 fatty acids can help the skin stay healthy and keep it more supple, smooth, and soft. Fish, flaxseed, walnuts, and canola oil provide omega-3 fatty acids.

Cigarettes and Skin

Cigarette smoking is second only to the sun as your skin's worst enemy, yet young women are the fastest-growing group of smokers. The skin of smokers ages much more quickly than the skin of nonsmokers, and the combination of smoking and sun exposure compounds the problem. Women who smoke often have a grayish skin tone, circles under their eyes, loose skin, and more wrinkles, especially around their eyes and mouth. Nicotine in cigarettes affects blood circulation, so smokers have poor nutrient delivery to their skin. Cigarettes and their many toxic ingredients also increase oxidative damage to the skin from free radicals.

Compared with the skin of nonsmokers, smokers' skin does not replenish itself as well, is less hydrated, and lacks important nutrients that keep it healthy, including the antioxidant vitamins. Smoking also lowers estrogen production by the ovaries, which normally helps to maintain the skin's structural proteins, elastin and collagen.

It's so easy for nonsmokers to tell you to quit smoking. In fact, it can irritate you and make you reach for a cigarette. Quitting smoking will be one of the hardest, most challenging, and most important things you can do for your health and your skin.

We know a lot more about getting off cigarettes than we did when Grandma quit cold turkey, which she did every day and then started up again, adding a martini. We know about medications that can help and relaxation techniques that will take the place of that nicotine pleasure. Please see your doctor about it, even if you have been pretending to be a nonsmoker. Your doctor may have done the same. You may have had the experience of

REAL LIFE FACT: Priming the Canvas

If you are bothered by the look of large pores, use the makeup artist's trick: apply a primer to your skin and let it set before applying makeup. A primer, which usually contains silicone (often called dimethicone on labels), settles into the pores and seems to reflect light away from them. They're not gone, but they look a lot smaller. Apply makeup a tiny bit at a time, and your pores will look smaller. Spackle your face with a thick layer of makeup, and your skin will look like the surface of the moon. When you are finished with the makeup, dust with a layer of very fine clear powder and the look will last for hours.

REAL LIFE FACT: Seven Steps to Lifelong Skin Health

- **Protect your skin from sunlight.**
- **Moisturize regularly.**
- **Avoid harsh soaps.**
- **If you drink alcohol, make it a little, not a lot.**
- **Feed your skin well.**
- **Get enough sleep and minimize stress.**
- **Quit smoking.**

going out at night with people from your non-smoking office, only to discover that everyone smokes "just when I drink." See your doctor, get help, and make this your highest priority. Your young body may not feel the effects of smoking yet, but it will soon. You won't like how it feels.

Why are young women the fastest-growing group of smokers? Look carefully at the movies and TV shows you watch. If someone is smoking on screen, chances are they are being paid to smoke by a tobacco company. The company decides that you are a good target, picks the actors and actresses you like, and pays them to smoke on film. Seriously.

Sleep Well, Limit Stress

Stress takes a big toll on your body. When you are stressed—by a job interview, a problem at work, an exam, a crying baby, a noisy neighborhood, a conflict with someone, an unhappy relationship—your body has a standard reaction. It goes into motion as the human body has for thousands of years when we were stressed. It produces chemicals to make you react, to punch, to run.

The problem: We are made to respond to one-minute stresses like saber-toothed tigers, not continuing stresses like finding a job. Our stress responders work overtime because they can't tell the difference. You are left with a great big overdose of stress responders, and they affect everything from your stomach to your period. Worst of all, stress affects your sleep. Lack of sleep makes you more vulnerable to stress, which makes you have more trouble sleeping. If you already read chapter 3, Stress and Your Body, you know what I'm talking about. We modern humans have to convince our bodies to relax, so that the flood of chemicals we produce under stress can slow way down. For now, learn to take a few deep, slow breaths. Tell your body that this stress is the threat of a possible layoff, not a volcano erupting.

The Knife and the Needle

I seethe when I see a woman defend a decision to have major surgery in order to look younger. "If it makes you feel better about yourself, I say go ahead!" This is the grown-up version of anorexia. Mine is not a popular opinion, but I feel it strongly.

Young women are tortured by the body image war around them, in magazines, videos, movies, and television. As they age, they also see that, for women, body image issues extend far into the sixties and maybe longer. The older star on the entertainment news show who jokes about her Botox shots or her liposuction is no different from the young actress whose breast implants are her identity or who starves to stay picture-perfect.

Yes, every woman wants to look her best. I do too. By all means, take care of your skin and do everything you can for it. But if it involves needles or knives, stop. Unless there is a health reason to undergo anything invasive—say, reducing extremely large breasts to ease your back pain—then your decision about surgery is really about body image.

If you have body image issues, see a therapist first, not a surgeon. Yes, you may feel elated with your new breasts or tummy for a little while. You may say it's the best thing you've ever done for yourself. You may feel angry that I seem to be judging you. But it's not *you* who I'm judging, it's the money-making system that makes older women feel just as bad about themselves as teenagers do. I wonder why we let that happen. If you are a patient in my office with butt implants and breast implants and a facelift, I'm not going to judge you, but I am going to wonder why you were that unhappy.

Some women consider Botox and surgery to be in the same category as using cosmetics. Perhaps this is true at some level, but Botox and surgery are miles apart from cosmetics in their severity, risks, and irreversibility. I'm just saying this: if you think plastic surgery is going to make you happy, make yourself happy first. Then decide if you still need the surgeon. (And always see a therapist before you see a surgeon.)

None of this advice applies to you if you have an uncomfortable or disfiguring problem that a surgeon or a dentist could fix. Go ahead.

Here Comes the Sun—So Watch Out!

Unlike the baby boomers—who, back in the 1950s and '60s, would apply a mixture of iodine and baby oil and lie in the sun—today's young women have heard it a thousand times: too much sun is bad for your skin. If you don't believe it yet, try leaving a newspaper or a piece of colorful cotton out in the sun. It is hard to understand that a sun ninety million miles away can hurt the paper, the cloth, or you, but it does, and in many ways. Before we go any further, remember that a *little* sun is good for your health (think vitamin D) and your spirits. But as a species, we were not made to lie down in the sun to color our skin.

Why is too much sun bad for your skin? Sunlight generates those damaging inflammatory compounds called free radicals (described earlier) in your skin. This is how it happens: the sun gives off ultraviolet (UV) radiation. As far as we know today, three bands of UV radiation affect the skin: UVA, UVB, and UVC. UVA rays make up 90 percent or more of the sun's radiation that reaches the earth, and these cause most of the skin damage. The earth's ozone layer filters out the UVC and many of the UVB rays, but damage to the ozone layer now allows more of these rays to get through. UVB, which is most intense in the two hours before and after noon, can cause sunburns and skin cancer.

Free radicals in your skin damage its structural scaffolding proteins—collagen and elastin. These flexible yet sturdy proteins give your skin its firm tone and fullness and allow it to stretch and contract. Damaged collagen molecules break down and then repair themselves in a process known as cross-linking. Cross-linking causes the normally flexible and elastic collagen to become stiff and less mobile, resulting in skin with less tone and resilience. Besides skin tone loss, sun damage causes wrinkles, sagging, uneven pigmentation, brown spots, and a leathery appearance. Aged skin that has been protected from the

REAL LIFE QUESTION: Are tanning salons safe?

No. No. No.

According to the Skin Cancer Foundation, thirty minutes in a tanning bed is like eight hours of sunbathing. And according to the International Agency for Research on Cancer (IARC), tanning bed time is carcinogenic: it causes cancer in humans.

It's not just your skin that's in danger in the tanning salon. There is evidence that the level of ultraviolet exposure in tanning beds is so strong that it may cause damage to the eyes and even cause ocular melanoma, or cancer of the eye. Don't listen to claims that the tanning salon uses harmless UVA rays, because UVA rays also cause skin damage, although more slowly than UVB rays. The problem is that they go deeper into the skin than UVB rays, and so can be even worse.

What about spray-on tanning? Self-tanning creams with the active agent dihydroxyacetone (DHA)—not to be confused with the other DHA, an omega-3 fatty acid called docosahexaenoic acid—is probably safe. They work by creating a temporary staining of the skin. One thing we know for sure: if you foster the idea that a tan is beautiful by spraying it on, it remains difficult to convince young women to quit tanning in the sun or in tanning salons.

sun is thin and may have some reduced elasticity, but it is otherwise smooth and unblemished.

If you still haven't quit tanning, compare your body parts that rarely, if ever, see the sun with those that do. This is why your bottom has no wrinkles.

Skin Cancer: What to Look For

You can prevent most types of skin cancer. Exposure to ultraviolet radiation from sunlight is the major cause of skin cancer, so protecting your skin is the first line of defense in preventing it.

Tanning in a salon is just as dangerous as burning in the sun. There is no such thing as getting protection from a "base tan." Even when you don't tan or burn, exposure to the sun's UV rays may still increase skin cancer risk by weakening the immune response in skin cells. And don't rely on cloud cover for sun protection. Even on cloudy days, 60 to 80 percent of the sun's rays can get through. The same is true for swimming—the water filters out only a small amount of the sun's rays.

You don't have to stay indoors to protect your skin from the sun. Sunscreen can minimize the damaging effects of sunlight on your skin. Make a habit of using it anytime you will be outside. Choose a sunscreen with a sun protection factor (SPF) of at least 15. Make sure it has both UVA and UVB protection. Another application may be needed after exercise, swimming, or sweating. Whenever possible, stay in the shade for outdoor activities, and wear a hat that shades your face and neck. Avoid sun exposure between 10:00 a.m. and 2:00 p.m., when the sun's rays are strongest.

NOTE TO SELF

This is worth repeating: there is no such thing as getting protection from a "base tan." Even when you don't tan or burn, exposure to the sun's UV rays may still increase skin cancer risk by weakening the immune response in skin cells.

Examine Yourself for Dangerous Moles

There are three main types of skin cancer: basal cell carcinoma, squamous cell carcinoma, and melanoma. Basal and squamous cell carcinomas grow on areas of the body that have been repeatedly exposed to the sun. They tend to pop up when you are older, years after tanning—especially on your face, neck, or hands. (More motivation to avoid tanning: if you tan when you are young, you get those awful-looking brown spots when you age.) Basal and squamous cell carcinomas grow slowly and rarely cause death because they usually don't spread. These cancers are easily removed by minor surgery, but if left untreated they can look terrible.

Melanoma is a different and scarier skin cancer. Thankfully, it makes up only 1 or 2 per-

SKIN CATEGORIES	SKIN COLOR IN UNEXPOSED AREA	TANNING HISTORY	SKIN SENSITIVITY VALUE
Never tans, always burns	Pale or milky white	Red sunburn, painful swelling, skin peels	4–10
Sometimes tans, usually burns	Very little brown, sometimes freckles	Usually burns, pink or red coloring appears, can gradually develop a light brown tan	10–12
Usually tans, sometimes burns	Light tan, brown, or olive, distinctly pigmented	Rarely burns, moderately rapid tanning response	11–14
Source: Classification developed by the U.S. Environmental Protection Agency			

cent of all skin cancers, but it can be very serious, and sometimes deadly. It tends to happen at a younger age and is not just limited to sun-exposed areas of your body. It can develop on almost any part of the body, and it can spread quickly. Sun and especially bad sunburns are risk factors for developing melanoma. Some people are more vulnerable to the damaging effects of UV radiation. Do you have fair skin? Freckles? Blue eyes? Fair hair? If you do, you're at greater risk.

The U.S. Environmental Protection Agency has a system for grading skin sensitivity to damage from the sun. Everyone is at risk, but some skin types are at higher risk than others. (Please see the table above for details; the lower your number, the more sensitive your skin is.) Some medications can also affect your skin's sensitivity to sun damage. If you have not quit tanning yet, be sure your doctor knows that before you start taking any medication.

How Can I Tell If My Mole Is Normal?

You can't judge a mole by yourself, but it's very important to examine your skin and become aware of your moles. This way, you'll notice changes, because a change in the appearance of a mole or the development of a new mole may be abnormal. Let your doctor know if you notice any of the following:

- Dark or discolored patches or spots in a mole
- Bleeding or crusting over a mole
- Change in the color, size, or shape of a mole
- Persistent itchiness in a mole

The majority of **benign** (normal) moles appear on your skin by age thirty. A normal mole is tan or brown colored with smooth and well-defined margins. It's usually smaller

REAL LIFE FACT: The Cotton Swab Problem

Have your read the fine print on a box of cotton swabs? It tells you not to use them to clean your ears. Seriously. It tells you not to use the ear cleaners you just bought—to clean your ears with—to clean your ears.

So now, because you're not one of the people who have damaged their ears with a cotton swab, you think every warning is just fine print—an overblown scare tactic. You're reading our message about food and your skin, or the sun, or fiber, and you're thinking it's all just fine-print stuff that you don't really have to do.

If you were sitting in my office and we were talking face-to-face, I hope you would believe me. There is nothing in this book that isn't important for your health. What you eat, what you smoke, how much you move, how much you sleep, how much stress you carry—every single thing will affect how your skin looks now and how it looks when somebody calls you Grandma. It's not fine print. It's real, evidence-based science to help your body live well and look good for a lifetime.

than ¼ inch in diameter (smaller than a pencil eraser) and has a round or oval shape. The edges are regular and the shape is symmetric (the same on one side as the other). It should be flat or only slightly raised.

It's common for moles to darken from hormonal influences, such as during adolescence or pregnancy or when taking birth control pills. If a mole appears after age thirty, have your doctor examine it. Other changes in moles to report to your doctor include bleeding, rapid growth, crusting, a nonhealing sore, or itchiness.

If you have a family history of melanoma, many doctors recommend that you see a dermatologist once a year for a full body skin exam. Even a great **gynecologist** is not as experienced at skin cancer as a dermatologist is.

A Word about Vitamin D

Now that I have you totally worried about skin cancer and sun, here is some good news: sunlight is not all bad. When the sun penetrates the atmosphere, the UVB in sunlight reacts with **cholesterol** in the skin to produce vitamin D. Our bodies can produce up to 20,000 international units (IU) in the skin after one small exposure—that is, until the skin just begins to turn pink. In certain parts of the world, particularly at higher latitudes, vitamin D production in the skin is usually not sufficient, especially in the winter, so vitamin D deficiencies are common. To help prevent deficiencies, milk is fortified with vitamin D, usually about 100 IU per glass. The RDA (recommended daily allowance) for vitamin D is

200 IU, and some nutrition scientists are recommending this amount be increased.

Many of us do not get enough vitamin D. A severe deficiency of vitamin D leads to rickets in children and osteomalacia—a softening of the bones—in adults. Recent medical studies also associate vitamin D deficiency with most cancers, heart disease, depression, **diabetes**, **hypertension**, **autoimmune disorders**, gum disease, and obesity. A small amount of sunlight is one good way to obtain vitamin D, but don't overdo it. Limit unprotected exposure, without sunscreen, to thirty minutes daily. Vitamin D is being recognized as increasingly important for health, but getting it in supplement form rather than too much sun is your best bet.

Check out www.vitamindhealth.org for some groundbreaking information about vitamin D.

When to See the Doctor about That Rash

We all get rashes, which are mostly harmless. If you have a fever with your rash, call the doctor today, especially if you were not vaccinated against the major diseases that cause rashes, such as chicken pox. These illnesses can be very uncomfortable for adults; even if your doctor can't offer a cure, you'll learn the measures you need to take to be more comfortable.

An itchy rash may happen often if you have sensitive skin. A new sweater, a new detergent, new sheets, new body lotion, new cleanser, new hair color, a new boyfriend's detergent, new anything can cause a rash. Investigate anything new that you've been doing and eliminate the new "foreigner." Strangely, sometimes you can develop an allergic rash after you've been exposed to the same thing more than a hundred times, so even if it's not new, it can be a new offender. Either way, if the rash doesn't clear up, it's time to call the doctor for an appointment.

Some rashes are itchy patches that won't go away. Your doctor may have creams to eliminate these or s/he may just ask you to use moisturizer. Many people learn to recognize these patches and know how to treat them, but until you are experienced, have your doctor check them out before you self-medicate. And always call your doctor if the rash doesn't go away after two weeks.

Many skin conditions can be diagnosed and treated by your general physician. However, if you are not getting relief, ask for a referral to a dermatologist.

Tats, Rooks, Tragus Piercings, and Scrumpers

Body art, such as piercings and tattoos, has really jumped in popularity. I'm not your mother, so what I tell you is based on science, not on society's views. But one of my goals as a doctor is to help you make personal decisions armed with the medical facts.

Personally, I think there's something beautiful, interesting, rebellious, creative, and exotic about all of this skin decoration. Patients who have tattoos and piercings tell me that they feel sexy or different in a good way.

So is it possible to make these very permanent changes to our bodies in a healthy and smart way? Yes! Safety depends on a few things: the tattoo or piercing artist, the part of the body you are adorning, and the cleanliness of the whole process. Luckily, there are medical facts that we can rely on to help us make the right choices.

Tattoos

About a quarter of young American adults aged eighteen to thirty—at least half of them being women—have tattoos. Age twenty seems to be the most common age for getting a first tattoo, as this is when young women want to express their uniqueness and identity.

Tattoos were once worn only by sailors, pirates, and criminals among men, and by "loose" women. Grandma still sees them that way. And you thought your mom did, too—until the day she and her friends had hearts and butterflies tattooed on their behinds. (She swears the tattoo stopped her hot flashes.) Tattoos are even showing up at PTA meetings (but they are probably hidden under clothes.)

Some religious groups have strong opinions about tattoos. In Islam and Judaism, tattooing is usually forbidden, especially among the most orthodox believers. In Christianity, it varies widely, with many fundamentalists strongly opposed. Other faiths, such as Hinduism and Buddhism, take a more liberal view.

Most women are happiest with tattoos in the long term when their decision to get one was deliberate and they placed it in a discreet location. In other words, don't have a few drinks with your friends and make a spontaneous decision that you will later regret. As tattoos have gotten more popular, dermatologists have increasingly heard stories of regret and received requests for tattoo removal. About 20 percent of women change their minds and wish they hadn't tattooed, even when they made a careful decision about getting the tattoo. Usually this change of heart is really a desire to move away from their past or to change their self-identity; most women seeking tattoo removal do so because of embarrassment, negative comments, or problems with tattoos showing underneath their clothes.

Before you decide to get a tattoo, talk with people working in your chosen career field because even today there's some discrimination against body art in certain industries. If you are an artist, a tattoo might be acceptable. If you want to be an accountant, you might want to get the tattoo in a location that you can hide with clothes all year round. For instance, your back might be a good spot, unless you're a lifeguard or a ballroom dancer who wears backless dresses. (If you don't have a chosen field yet, be especially thoughtful about your body art decision. And keep in mind that you may well change fields several times in your lifetime.)

What If You Change Your Mind?

Removal of tattoos is expensive and painful, so be sure to give your tattoo plan some clear and rational thought before you go ahead with it. We all change our minds from time to time, however, so here is what you need to know about removal.

Laser therapy is used for most tattoo removal. It's not a perfect method, but it *can* be done and improvements in technology have made it better. Depending on your skin type and your tendency to form scars (which varies from person to person), there can be some scarring or skin texture changes, and some pigmentation may be left behind. Usually you'll have one or more of these side effects even in the best hands. Because treatment with lasers is painful, a local injection with a topical skin numbing cream can be used before treatment. As laser techonogy gets more advanced, laser tattoo removal will likely continue to improve.

Piercings

As a gynecologist, I get a unique view of all the latest piercing trends. I'm also asked to treat the problems they create, like pain and infections. Piercings, especially body piercings in places other than the earlobes, have become more and more common. I find jewelry in the tongue, lips, upper ear, nipples, belly button, and genitals.

Are piercings harmful? They can be, but usually they aren't. Occasionally I see minor scarring. (Some people are genetically predisposed to overgrown scars called keloids.) And rarely, I see piercing-related infections, which generally resolve pretty easily with topical cleansers or oral antibiotics. If these methods don't work, you have to remove the jewelry immediately. By the way, these problems happen with earlobes, too. We don't know yet if the genitals will be more or less prone to problems because these piercings are a much newer trend.

Ask most doctors about piercings or tattoos and they will tell you eighty-seven horror stories about the tragic deaths of young people. Some are true; many are not. Here are the facts.

Medical Risks of Tattoos

Tattoos are made with needles and dye. Dye is inserted into the skin with repeated needle sticks, like a sewing machine needle going in and out, inserting more dye with each skin prick. Large tattoos can take several hours. They are painful, just like a shot is painful, except there are a lot more needle sticks with tattoos. If you have a needle phobia, don't even consider it!

There are a few medical risks to be aware of with tattoos, some of them serious, others minor. A small number of people get allergic reactions to the ingredients in the dye, which can lead to pain, rash, or even scarring. Tattoos on the lower back create a worry for anesthesiologists, because this is the place an epidural or spinal is inserted for pain relief during childbirth or surgery. This is a controversial concern, however, because it is not clear that this a problem. Until we know for sure, most anesthesiologists try to avoid putting needles through tattoos.

The most serious issue is infection, which can be caused by unsterilized needles. Be sure you go to a reputable place where proper sterile techniques are used. If you don't, you put yourself at risk for hepatitis B, hepatitis C, and **HIV** infections

Medical Risks of Piercings

Allergic reaction is one of the most common problems related to piercings. Most good-quality jewelry is made of gold or silver, and allergic reactions to them are uncommon. However, you get what you pay for, and to keep prices lower, nickel is often mixed into cheaper jewelry sold as gold or silver. Nickel is usually the culprit when I see allergies. And buyer beware: Sometimes high-quality earrings are paired with cheap earring backings! If you are allergic to nickel, you'll notice redness, swelling, and tenderness in the area. This usually disappears within a day or two if you remove the jewelry.

If you take blood thinners or corticosteroids, or if you have diabetes, you are more likely to have infections or bleeding. And if you have congenital heart disease (you were born with a heart defect), there are some rare but very serious reports of infections in the heart after having tattoos or piercings. People who have heart defects usually know it. Is this you? Before going to the dentist, for example, do you take antibiotics to prevent bacteria from the mouth from entering the **bloodstream** and seeding abnormal areas of the heart, especially the heart valves? This same seeding of bacteria into the heart is also possible with piercings and tattoos. So if you have congenital heart disease, avoid tattoos or piercings. If you feel you must adorn, talk to your cardiologist (heart doctor) first.

One doctor who is completely opposed to tongue piercings? Your dentist! Your teeth have a long and important road to travel over the duration of your life, and banging a piece of metal against them is a bad idea.

For most people, piercings are usually safe. If you have problems, they will likely disappear when you remove the jewelry for good. If you have an infection, be sure to call your doctor. Warning: Genital piercings can damage condoms and **diaphragms**! Take the jewelry out before sex, especially if yours has any sharp edges.

REAL LIFE FACT: Skin-Saving Vitamin C

Vitamin C does more than inhibit skin-damaging free radical activity. Remember the net of collagen in your skin that gives it structure and resilience? Without that net, your skin wrinkles and sags. Vitamin C is needed for the body to make collagen, but aging skin makes less and less collagen. So the bottom line is, what you put inside your body can make your skin healthier.

A Healthy Body Equals Healthy Skin

To have healthy skin, you need to take good care of your body. So, in a way, taking good care of your skin also gives you the bonus of a healthier body. It's a win-win situation!

In the chapters to come, you'll learn more about which lifestyle and diet changes—like eating more whole grains, fruits, and vegetables—will help you to create both beautiful skin and a healthy body. Are you starting to see how all of this stuff is connected? Keep reading for more.

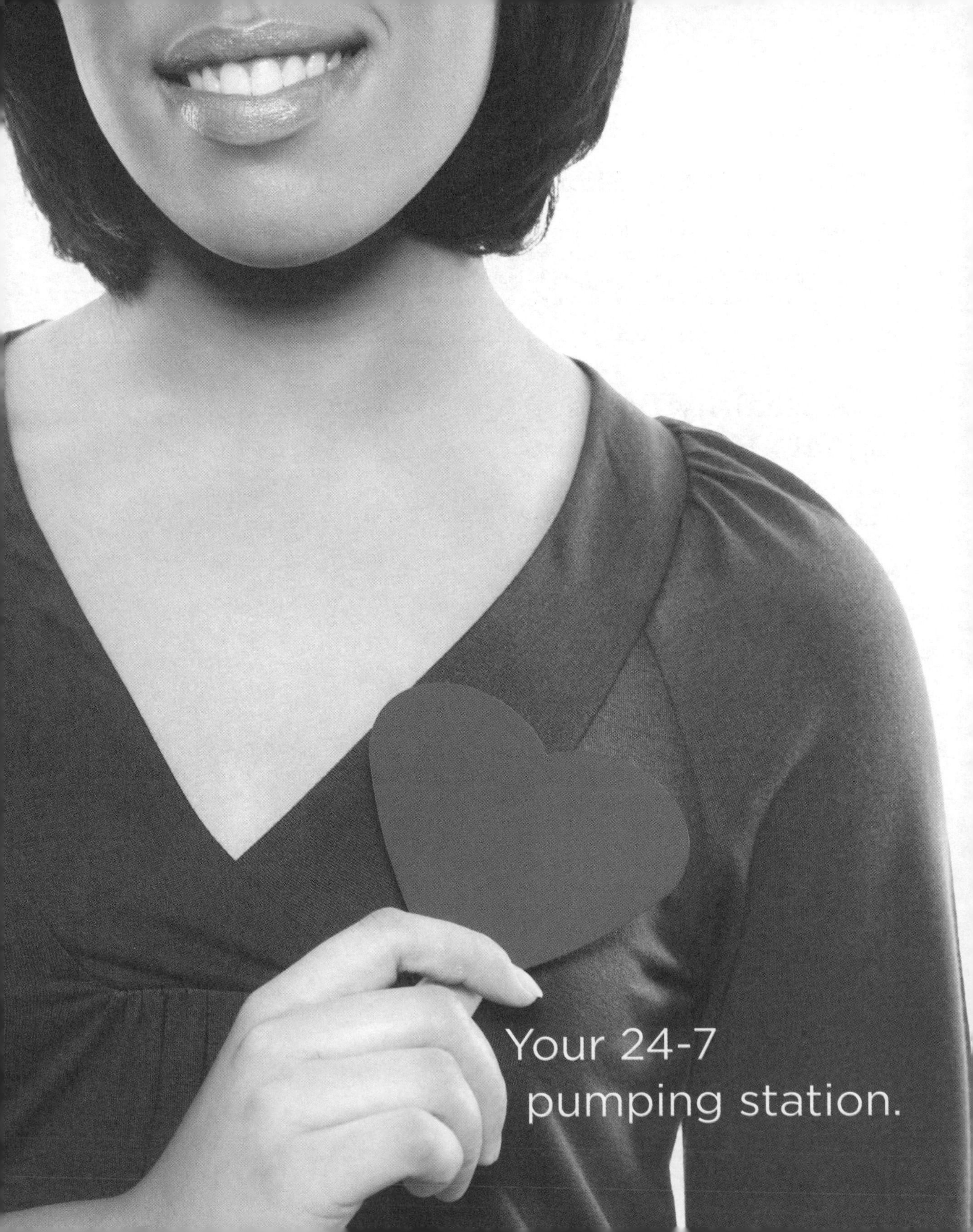
Your 24-7
pumping station.

your heart

What's a heart? Silly question, maybe. But it runs your body, and without it, well, your body would stop. Your heart is pumping blood all day, all night, even when you're asleep. So let's take a quick look at it, and then go on to see what can go wrong and how to keep it healthy.

The heart is an organ, which means a part of the body that has a function you can't live without. I always imagined it to be a giant thing, given how important it is, but it's only about the size of your fist. Its job is to circulate blood through the body and lungs, in two trips. You can tell it's working because it beats, which you can feel in your pulse points. During one hour that you spend reading this book, your heart will beat almost five thousand times.

Take a look at the illustration on page 102 and follow the two blood trips. Even if you have a perfect ticker—and chances are that you do—this will help you in those family conversations with Grandma about hers. First, the heart has four chambers. They appear on *Jeopardy* so often that we all ought to know them, but many people don't.

The four chambers are two **atria** (which is the plural of *atrium*) and two **ventricles**. The atria collect blood, and then push it through to the ventricles. Ventricles pump. So your blood goes into

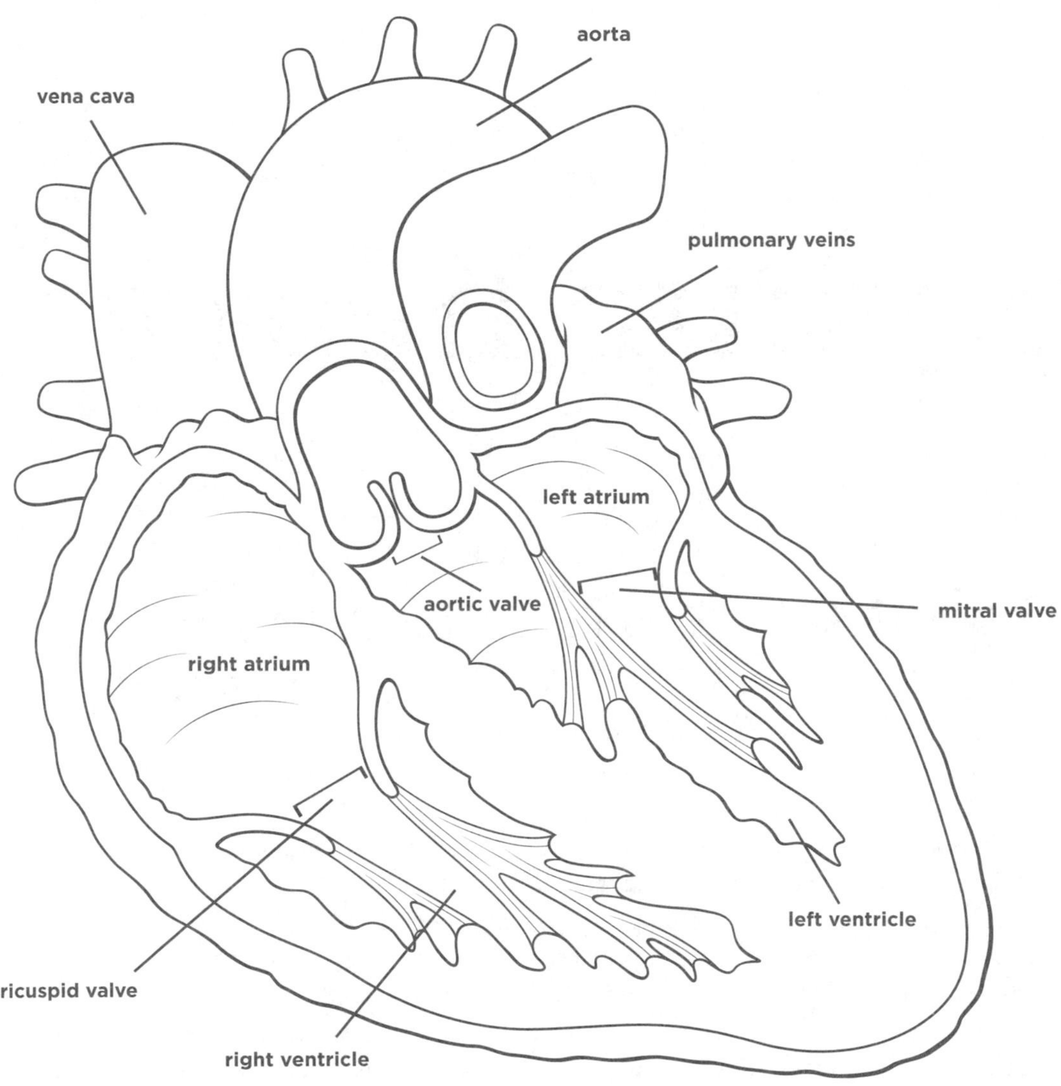

Anatomy of the heart: The heart has four chambers—two atria and two ventricles. The atria collect blood, then push it through to the ventricles. Ventricles pump blood to your lungs and the rest of your body.

the atria, collects there, then gets pumped to the ventricles, and from there gets pumped out to the body.

It's headed for your blood vessels—an incredibly complex network of **veins** and **arteries**. Your arteries take your blood from the heart to the body's tissues, and from there, the veins carry it back to the heart.

Your heart also has four valves, which do the same job that the valves in your car do: they stop backflow or backwash (like when a friend takes a sip of your drink with a mouthful of pretzels and you end up with icky half-chewed pretzels in your glass).

Let's start in the right ventricle. The ventricle pumps blood through the pulmonary valve, which is connected to the pulmonary arteries, which are the doorway to the lungs. Here the blood picks up oxygen. Now that the blood is **oxygenated**, it heads back to the heart through the pulmonary veins. Next stop is the left atrium, which is blood's waiting room. The left atrium sends the blood through the **mitral valve** into the left ventricle, where it is pumped into the **aorta**. From there it gets sent all over your body. Now it's time for trip number two: the veins pick up the blood and take it back to the heart, through the vena cava, to the right atrium. And we're back to the beginning, where the right ventricle pumps blood through the pulmonary valve.

All together, this is called your **cardiovascular system**. And during the time it took you to read this section, your blood started and finished its two trips!

NOTE TO SELF

Heart disease is the leading killer of women worldwide. It claims more women's lives than all forms of cancer, including breast cancer, put together.

The Business of the Heart: What Can Go Wrong?

Do you have to worry about cardiovascular disease? You may think that just because you're young, you don't need to be concerned about heart health. **Heart disease** happens to old people and to men, right? Nope.

It's true that heart disease in women is more common after **menopause**. Still, it can affect women of all ages. Despite the widespread belief that heart disease is a man's problem, it is also a devastating health problem for women. Many women mistakenly believe that **cancer** is more of a threat, when in fact heart disease is our number one killer. Why do I keep repeating this? Because you see so many reminders to take care of your breasts and so few to take care of your heart. That's changing, and more red ribbons are showing up to remind you about heart disease in women. But still, you are more than ten times as likely to die of cardiovascular disease as breast cancer.

According to the American Heart Association, 10 percent of women ages forty-five through sixty-four have heart disease, 25 percent of women age sixty-five and over have heart disease, and 13 percent of women over age forty-five have had a heart attack. Over 40 percent of women do not survive their first heart attack.

Why should you care? Because that could be your future! The only way to travel on a different road is to choose yours now, as early as possible. So it's time to readjust your thinking. Make heart disease prevention a priority in your life, and love your heart. I'll talk more about risk factors and what you can do to prevent heart disease later in the chapter. But first . . .

What Is Heart Disease?

Heart disease is caused by the narrowing of the coronary arteries, which carry oxygen-rich blood to your heart. Your heart is a muscular organ that works hard 24-7. To stay healthy and work effectively, it needs oxygen and **nutrients** to keep it going. The coronary arteries carry blood to supply your heart with these essential elements.

The three big villains of heart disease are:

- **Cholesterol**
- **Hypertension** (high blood pressure)
- Smoking (no big surprise)

First, let's talk about cholesterol and high blood pressure. (You will hear plenty about smoking later in this chapter.) Cholesterol leaves leftovers in your coronary arteries. Eventually, the cholesterol buildup will narrow the arteries—a process called **atherosclerosis**—and not enough blood will be supplied to your heart. The result can be a heart attack. It takes years for cholesterol deposits to build up in your coronary arteries, and often a heart attack is triggered by an abrupt clog when a blood clot sticks in a cholesterol deposit that narrows an artery.

Cholesterol Conundrum

You probably think of cholesterol as a type of bad fat. While that's true, cholesterol is also an essential ingredient that your body uses in its normal functioning. Cholesterol serves as the basis of cell walls, certain hormones and vitamins, and **bile** acids. However, it takes only a small amount of cholesterol to meet these needs, and the leftovers are deposited in your arteries, where they can cause narrow passages that lead to heart disease and circulation problems.

Can you blame your parents if you end up with heart disease? Well, a tendency to have a high cholesterol level can be inherited. However, you can try to stay in a healthy range by minimizing **saturated fat** and **trans fats** in your diet and increasing the amount you exercise.

Alphabet Adipose

You've probably heard of **HDL** and **LDL** cholesterol. What are these alphabet fats?

Fats (called lipids) don't mix with water, and since your body is full of water, fats need

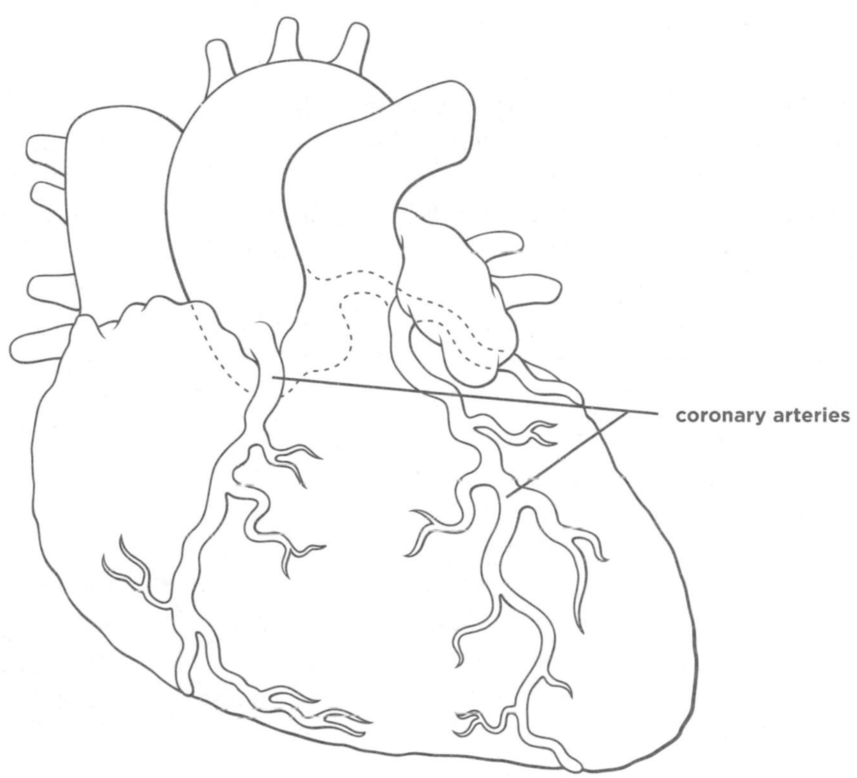

Heart disease is caused by the narrowing of the coronary arteries, which carry oxygen-rich blood to your heart.

CHOLESTEROL TABLES

Total Cholesterol Levels		HDL Cholesterol Levels		LDL Cholesterol Levels	
Less than 200 mg/dL	Desirable	Less than 40 mg/dL	Major risk factor	Less than 100 mg/dL	Optimal
200–239 mg/dL	Borderline high	40–59 mg/dL	Better	100–129 mg/dL	Near or above optimal
240 mg/dL and above	High	60 mg/dL and above	Protective	130–159 mg/dL	Borderline high
				160–189 mg/dL	High
				190 mg/dL and above	Very high
Source: Adapted from the American Heart Association					

special treatment during digestion so your body can handle them. After they leave your stomach, for example, fats are carried through your blood in little bags called lipid-protein complexes. This tiny luggage takes fat to the **liver** or to adipose tissue (*adipose tissue* is the medical term for your stored fat).

There are two types of cholesterol: high-density **lipoproteins** (HDL) and low-density lipoproteins (LDL). The levels of these substances affect your risk of heart disease. High levels of HDL indicate a lower risk of heart disease and high levels of LDL mean a higher risk of heart disease. That's why we call HDL the "good cholesterol" and LDL the "bad cholesterol." (To remember which is which, I think of H for high and L for low—the desired levels, that is.) When your doctor checks your risk of heart disease, tests should include both an HDL level and a total cholesterol level.

Your weight and diet can affect your HDL and LDL cholesterol levels. Being overweight tends to increase your LDL ("bad") cholesterol level; weight loss helps lower LDL cholesterol and raise HDL ("good") cholesterol levels. Exercise can improve your lipid profile by helping to lower the LDL cholesterol level and raise the HDL cholesterol level.

Saturated fat and cholesterol in your diet have a negative effect on your lipids and raise your LDL cholesterol level more than any other factor. If you can reduce the amount of saturated fat and cholesterol you eat, you'll have taken a very important step in reducing your cholesterol and LDL levels. (The section "Preventing Heart Disease," beginning on page 111, will give you more ideas about how to increase HDL cholesterol and lower LDL cholesterol.)

High Blood Pressure

So, what is blood pressure anyway? *Pressure* means "force." As your blood makes its two trips around your body, it puts pressure, or force, against the walls of your arteries. Measuring your blood pressure is very important because the reading can warn you about serious health problems, including heart attack risk.

You've probably had your blood pressure taken. It looks a bit like magic, but it's pretty simple. When your heart pumps, or beats, your blood pressure is at its highest point, called the systolic pressure. When it is at rest—that tiny pause it takes between heartbeats—your blood pressure drops to its lowest point, or diastolic pressure.

We take your blood pressure using a sphygmomanometer (pronounced *SVIG-mo-man-ah-mitter*, or *thingie*). We wrap your upper arm with a cuff and then inflate it to measure the pressure in your brachial artery. We put a stethoscope on your arm under the cuff and then listen for two important sounds. The first sound is a repetitive beat, like a heartbeat. As soon as we hear that beat, we look at a dial on the machine to get a reading of your systolic pressure, the higher number. A few seconds later, the beats stop. We look at the dial for your diastolic pressure, the lowest number. We write the two measurements like a fraction, with the systolic on top. If your blood pressure is 120/80, we say it's "120 over 80." You can search www.youtube.com for a video that includes the sounds we hear.

Many new devices have been designed to speed up the process, like a cuff that inflates automatically and a digital screen. The automatic cuff learns your typical blood pressure and only inflates the cuff to about that level, which is much more comfortable for you than a full inflation. The digital screen then gives your blood pressure all at once. While all of this is going on, the nurse also has time to take your temperature and pulse (heart rate).

Your blood pressure changes throughout the day. It's at its lowest when you sleep and at its highest when you are really anxious. As you learned in chapter 1, some people get "white coat hypertension," a brief upswing in blood pressure that goes away as soon as the doctor does.

Your "Real" Blood Pressure

Picture a woman running late for her doctor's appointment. She is anxious and is wearing high heels that hurt. She races into the elevator but drops her bag, which spills her cell phone out through the door just as it closes. That can cause temporary high blood pressure. The high blood pressure reading that we worry about is not temporary.

Your whole body takes a beating from high blood pressure. It increases your heart's workload. As your heart pumps blood through your body's arteries, your nervous system regulates how dilated (relaxed) these blood vessels are. But sometimes this system goes a little nuts and the vessels stay narrowed, which we call constricted. This results in high blood pressure, which means your heart has to work harder to pump blood through these constricted blood vessels. Blood vessels can get damaged from this wear and tear.

When it is not treated, high blood pressure can result in heart disease, heart attack, **stroke**, and even **kidney** failure. Now, what if you add in obesity, smoking, high cholesterol, or **diabetes**? Those conditions also damage blood vessels.

Yikes! Is there any good news? High blood pressure is treatable, so see your doctor regularly to make certain your blood pressure is well controlled. You may be able to control it to a degree with your diet, although often medication is still needed. A diet called DASH (Dietary Approaches to Stop Hypertension), which includes lots of fruits and vegetables and less salt, has been shown to lower blood pressure in some people, especially when their diets also contain healthy fats.

Studies using the DASH diet show that cutting back on salt decreases blood pressure to a small degree in people who are salt sensitive. If you have normal blood pressure, we think it is okay to salt your food in moderation. Keep in mind that very little of the salt in your diet comes from the saltshaker. The vast majority of it comes from processed foods like canned goods and fast food.

Often, salt is hidden in these processed foods, even when they don't seem salty. Check it out by reading the labels—you'll find salt listed on almost anything in a can or box made in the United States. The nutritional information will show you the sodium content in a serving. You should always compare how many servings the manufacturer thinks are in the package (twenty servings of potato chips, for example) to how many servings *you* plan to get from it (one serving).

Be sure to read chapter 17, Your Diet, and remember this basic habit: When grocery shopping, stick to the outside aisles of the store. That's where you'll find the fresh and lower salt foods: produce, dairy, fish, and lean meats.

Eating fresh, whole foods, rather than processed foods, is the best way to minimize salt in your diet. You can then prepare fresh vegetables with a bit of salt to enhance their flavor. Explore spices from around the world and you'll miss salt less and less.

Later in the chapter you'll find more suggestions for decreasing your cholesterol, blood pressure, and risk of heart attack.

Deadly Gender Differences

Heart disease is different in women than in men. Although women and men are equally likely to have heart attacks, women are more likely to die after their first heart attack than men. About 38 percent of women versus 25 percent of men will die within one year of a heart attack.

It is not clear what accounts for this deadly difference. Some scientists have theorized that it's because the symptoms of heart attack are different in women, or because women tend to be older when they have their first heart attack. Men's symptoms are often more dramatic; they usually have strong—even crushing—chest pain during a heart attack. Women have more vague symptoms such as chest tightening, indigestion, shortness of breath, nausea, and fatigue. Reread those lists of symptoms for women and men, so someday you may be able to help a friend or a parent—or yourself—by responding quickly to an emergency.

Diagnosis Dilemmas

Heart disease in women can easily be mistaken for indigestion, **gallbladder** disease, or even anxiety. The likelihood of misdiagnosing a heart attack in women is also increased by the fact that women tend to have heart attacks when they are older, and therefore they often have other diseases, such as **arthritis** or diabetes, which can confuse the picture. Prevention is the best medicine! If symptoms that cause suspicion of heart attack do occur, you will need thoughtful evaluation, and potentially different tests than what men receive. You still call 911 without hesitating! The thoughtful part is up to the doctors. Your job is to get to the hospital quickly.

Second-Rate Treatment?

Several studies suggest that not only is heart disease different in women, but women may also receive second-rate treatment. Women suffering a heart attack are given fewer tests and are less likely to be prescribed medication for the prevention of another heart attack compared to men. Medical treatment with cholesterol-lowering drugs is also more commonly prescribed to men, despite scientific evidence showing that men and women benefit equally from the drugs. Finally, women are less likely to be referred for surgery than men. Besides gender, race also influences treatment recommendations. A study that used actors as patients found that black males were about half as likely to be referred for heart surgery as white males.

I admit that's a mystery to me. While I have met doctors who are sexist and racist, I've never known one who intentionally made a medical decision that would harm a patient. Still, I have to advise you to be on your guard. You're a woman. You're going to have to advocate for yourself and sometimes get second opinions. You already know, in your heart, when you are meeting a sexist or a racist, don't you? When you are not comfortable with what is recommended, protect yourself and get second opinions! And keep your doctor on his or her toes. Good doctors want you to be an equal partner in your health care.

I suppose all men get second-rate treatment if they find a lump in their chest. Maybe their doctor has seen male breast cancer so rarely that s/he explores all other options first. By the way, if a male loved one or friend ever gets male breast cancer, remind him that the most famous male breast cancer patient was Richard Roundtree. Shaft, the original. There is nobody tougher or more manly than Shaft, is there?

How Do You Know If You Have a Great Heart Doctor?

You'd like to think you've got a great doctor, right? Well, the first sign of a good doctor is a willingness to listen to a second opinion.

REAL LIFE QUESTION: How can I be sure that my doctor knows the gender differences in heart attack symptoms?

You can ask your doctor to tell you the gender differences in heart attack symptoms. This is relatively new information. Ask what the differences are, and if your doctor gives you a blank stare, switch doctors.

Seriously. I've never met a good doctor who would object to your getting one. If s/he does, you just learned something: your doctor is not in the "great" category.

Second Opinions

If you decide to seek a second opinion, first call your insurance company for permission to get a second opinion, and then get one. Most insurance companies will cover second opinions for you.

Next, find a doctor for your second opinion. How? Ask everyone you know who has been treated for heart disease, had a heart attack, or had heart surgery. Eventually, a small list of names will surface. When you are dealing with your heart, remember that you've only got one. You can't fool around with it, and you can't let politeness interfere with how or where you are treated. I wish I'd never heard of patients who died at the hands of inattentive staff, but I have. Often enough to urge you to get the right care.

Seeing a Specialist

When you are trying to see a specialist like a cardiologist, delayed appointments are a big problem that's getting bigger. If the doctor tells you s/he can see you in six months, then you need to try these tips: your best bet is to have your doctor call the specialist personally to ask for an earlier appointment. Sometimes your doctor will be willing and sometimes s/he will be shyer than you are. On to plan B.

The person who scheduled your appointment was not the doctor, it was the receptionist, right? See, the actual doctor knows s/he can't say no to a patient in need. So the receptionist out front, whose job it is to say no to just about everyone, is the gatekeeper. Your objective? To get around this barrier.

Here's how: You can say "Yikes! My doctor really wants me to be seen earlier than that. Do you think you could talk to the doctor and see if there might be a slot you could put me in?"

No luck with plan B? Time for plan C. Ask to see a nurse in the office first. If the nurse finds something wrong, s/he will involve the doctor. Poof! Instant appointment.

This method does not work 100 percent of the time, but if your situation is serious, it probably will. Remember that most doctors are truly caring people who will figure out a way to see you when it's urgent.

Beating Gender Bias

Don't let gender bias affect your health! To become an equal partner in your health care, remember that no one knows your body better than you do. Trust your instincts. If you think there is a problem with your heart, press your doctor to take your symptoms seriously, and ask for more comprehensive testing if you are dissatisfied with a diagnosis. Do your research, too. The websites listed at the end of this chapter (see page 122) contain excellent information about heart health and the diagnosis of cardiovascular disease.

Heart Disease Risk Factors

How do you determine whether or not you are at risk for heart disease? Start by seeing your doctor for a thorough evaluation. Next, ask about your personal risks and ways you can lower them. Heart disease risk factors:

- Diabetes
- Hypertension (high blood pressure)
- Abnormal lipids (high cholesterol, low HDL, high LDL, high **triglycerides**)
- Obesity
- Smoking
- Family history of premature coronary heart disease (CHD; defined as a first heart attack of a male relative less than fifty-five years old or a female relative less than sixty-five years old)

You may be surprised to know that even the shape of your body might give you a clue to your heart disease risk (see page 112).

Preventing Heart Disease

Many studies have shown that the more risk factors you have for heart disease when you are young, the more likely you are to have a heart attack later. You need to stay motivated now to protect yourself later. One strong motivator might be, as you've learned, that heart attacks are deadlier for women at any age than for men.

The good news: Cardiovascular disease can often be prevented. The challenge is that this requires an ongoing commitment to a healthy lifestyle, which can be a lot more difficult than taking a pill. Important measures that you can take include controlling your weight, exercising regularly, eating a healthy diet, and quitting smoking. It's never too early to begin taking healthy steps in the right direction.

It's so easy to list these measures here and so hard to achieve them. Whenever you make a major change in your habits, remember that it takes three weeks before any new habit becomes second nature. Also remember that all change is best handled in baby steps. So imagine yourself a year from now, when those baby steps have added up to major changes that have become such a normal part of your life that you can't imagine living any other way.

NOTE TO SELF

Smoking is the single biggest risk factor for having a heart attack. And it gives you wrinkles.

Stomp Out Smoking

If you smoke, you really do have to quit! Smoking is the single biggest risk factor for heart attacks. Women who smoke are up to six times more likely to have a heart attack and

REAL LIFE FACT: Fruity Risk Factors

Two different body shapes are known as apples and pears. Men and women with an apple shape store their fat around the waist and chest, while those with a pear shape store it around the hips and thighs. Scientific evidence has shown that those who store fat around their waists have higher risks of heart disease. Doctors can assess your risk through a measurement called a waist-to-hip ratio (calculated by dividing your waist measurement by your hip measurement). Simply measuring your waist is also a pretty good indicator of this risk. Even if your weight remains stable, an expanding waistline can be a sign that you need to make some changes in your diet and exercise.

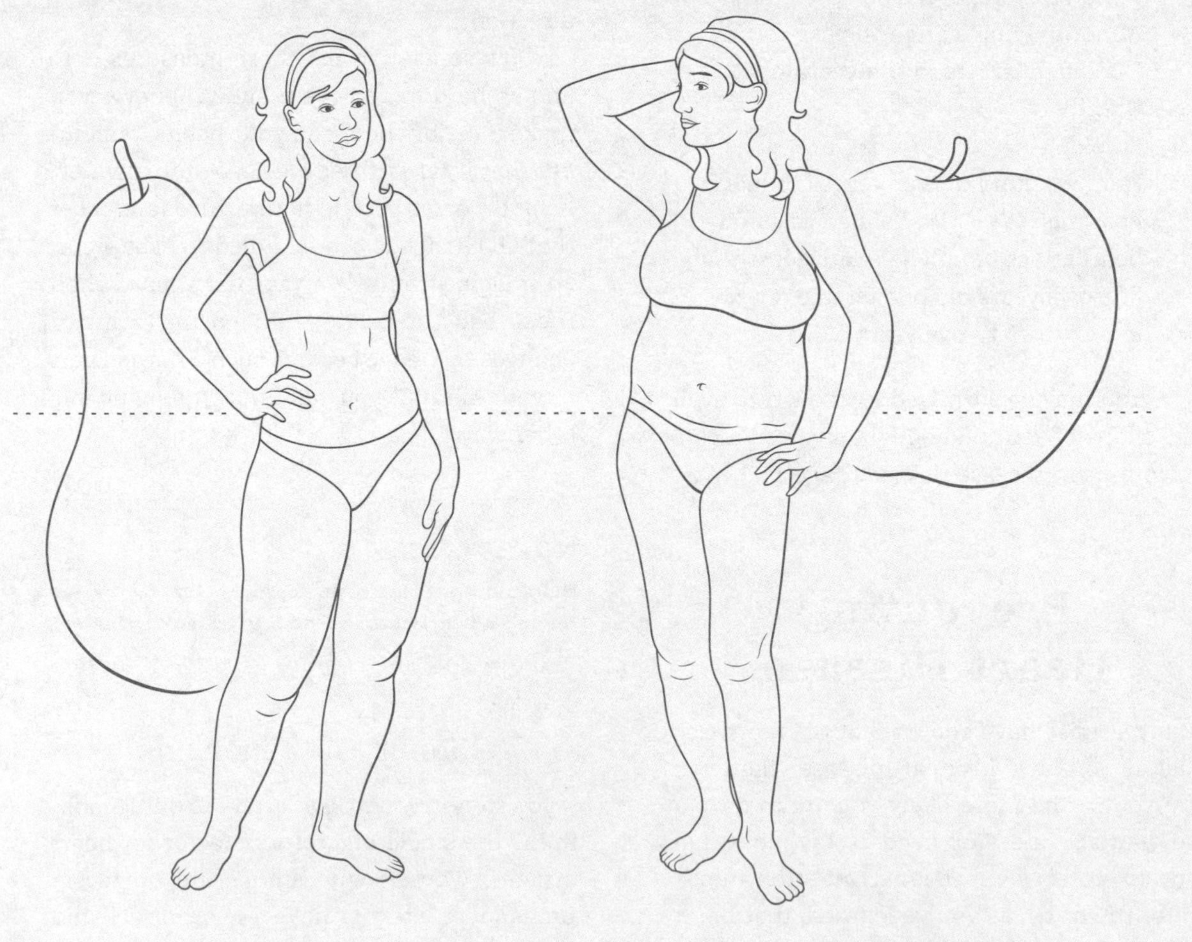

risk having it almost twenty years earlier in life than nonsmoking women. Blood vessels in the body react to the presence of nicotine in cigarette smoke by constricting. This makes the heart work harder to pump blood through narrowed blood vessels. If blood vessels are already partially blocked by cholesterol deposits, smoking further narrows them. And once an artery that supplies blood to the heart is completely blocked, a heart attack results.

The American Lung Association estimates that 18 percent of all adult American women today are smokers. According to the Department of Health and Human Services, approximately 1,500 female teenagers start smoking every day. Tobacco advertisers make promises of desirability, slimness, and independence for women who smoke, and they target women, especially young women, with their ad campaigns. Don't fall for it! Don't start! Smoking is not very cool. It makes your teeth yellow and your clothing and hair smell, and it gives you wrinkles. It is difficult to quit smoking, but it is the single most important thing you can do for your health.

How can you quit? Some people do quit cold turkey. That used to be the only way, but today there are many ways to help you quit that are more likely to be successful. Please read on for some tips on quitting smoking. There are also some useful websites on the topic listed at the end of this chapter. There are many options and programs to help that do not use the cold turkey method. Anyone who thinks it's easy to quit has either never quit or doesn't remember their own struggle. Quitting is going to take tremendous motivation on your part and constant reminders about why you want to quit.

NOTE TO SELF

If you are able to stop smoking for two weeks, you are very likely to succeed in quitting permanently!

How to Quit Smoking: Some Tips

Have a plan and don't compromise—decide that you'll go all the way. You might develop your plan as part of a quit smoking group, with a doctor, or as part of a support group in addition to taking medication.

Forget about "quitting lite." If you're like most people, you think you can cut back. Smoking even a few cigarettes a day is bad for your health. Cutting back works for a short while, but most people find that after a few weeks they go back to smoking more. And switching to low-nicotine or low-tar brands doesn't help either. Studies show that people who switch to these so-called "healthier" brands actually inhale more deeply to achieve the same level of nicotine in their bodies. Don't believe that? If you've been "smoking lite," buy a pack of the regular version of your brand. With one puff you'll find that you've been puffing pretty hard on your "reduced" cigarette, because your puff on the regular one feels incredibly harsh. The only safe choice is to have a plan to quit completely.

Write down why you want to quit.

- To be healthier?
- Improve your stamina?
- Smell fragrances again?
- Set a good example for your friends, family, and children?
- Save money?
- Live longer?
- Taste food again?
- Avoid lung cancer, which will kill you?
- Avoid emphysema, which will also kill you, just more slowly?

A person who is strongly motivated to quit smoking has a higher success rate with quitting permanently. For example, smokers who survive a heart attack or lung cancer are the most likely to quit for good—they're very motivated. Make the choice to quit smoking before you have no choice.

I mention emphysema here. Just about everyone knows that smoking causes lung cancer, but emphysema has gotten less publicity. When you see people walking around Disney World with oxygen tanks, that could be emphysema—and it could be you. With emphysema, you gradually lose the ability to breathe normally. Toward the end, your life becomes a struggle to breathe at all.

NOTE TO SELF

"It's easy to quit smoking. I've done it hundreds of times." —Mark Twain

KNOW THAT IT WILL TAKE EFFORT TO QUIT SMOKING. If you could be made unconscious until all of the nicotine in your body was gone and your addiction was broken, it would still be hard to "stay quit" when you woke up. Nicotine is highly addicting, and it can help to recognize and admit that quitting smoking will take a great deal of resolve and support to overcome. Sometimes being aware that quitting will be a struggle makes it easier to tolerate the physical symptoms of nicotine withdrawal.

It is very normal for the new ex-smoker to crave cigarettes, and moodiness is a common symptom of withdrawal from nicotine. Nicotine replacement products such as gum and patches can help diminish cravings, but it still is not easy to quit. It gets easier with time, and after a month most people find that the worst cravings go away. Like many habits, it can help to not look too far into the future when trying to stop. Just take it one day at a time, and feel good when you have made it through another day smoke free.

MILLIONS—YES, MILLIONS—OF PEOPLE WHO ONCE SMOKED HAVE QUIT. That's a reassuring and powerful statistic. There are millions of former smokers enjoying good health and happiness today as nonsmokers. Ask any one of them—anyone who is honest—what it was like. Every one of them will say, "I never thought I could do it." Those who say, "I quit cold turkey and never gave it a single thought after that," don't remember making everyone else's life a living hell for a month because they did it with no help.

HELP IS HERE. Your doctor or dentist, as well as friends and relatives who have successfully quit, are all good sources of help and support. There are many resources available to guide you in quitting—pamphlets, books, group programs, and the Internet can help you get started.

We know a lot more today about fighting nicotine addiction. Medications are available to help you with cravings or at least get them under control. For everyone, the important message of this quitting process is that you will not feel this way for the rest of your life. Things really will get better, you'll feel better, and you'll enjoy being free from cigarettes.

In the first few weeks, you'll think about every way in which you are married to cigarettes. "Why take a break when I can't smoke?" "Why bother with our vacation when I'll be craving a cigarette the whole time?"

I promise: these feelings will go away with time. You may not believe me now, but it will happen. And when you've succeeded at quitting, you'll join the millions of real heroes. They all know the struggle you've been through, and you'll know that you can accomplish anything!

SMOKELESS TOBACCO? THIS DOES NOT HELP. IT'S ANOTHER KILLER. Many young men and women alike think that chewing tobacco is a good way to quit smoking. They think "chaw" is harmless, especially because they see a constant stream of brown spit on national television during baseball season.

In fact, chaw is just as dangerous as smoking—it just destroys a different part of your body. If you could see a ballplayer who was treated for mouth cancer and lost half his face in the process, you'd never call this stuff harmless.

NOTE: These tips were adapted from the National Center for Chronic Disease Prevention and Health Promotion, www.cdc.gov/tobacco/quit_smoking/how_to_quit/quit_tips.

NOTE TO SELF

Three of the legendary Marlboro Men died of lung cancer.

You Knew It Was Coming: Weight Management

Your weight plays a role in your risk of developing heart disease. Here are some good weight indicators for assessing heart disease risk:

- How much you weigh in relation to your height. (Please see the Body Mass Index chart, opposite.)
- Your waist measurement. (Please see Fruity Risk Factors on page 112.)
- How much weight you gain after your early twenties. (Less is better.)

ADULT BODY MASS INDEX CHART

BMI	19	20	21	22	23	24	25	26	27	28	29	30	31	32	33	34	35
HEIGHT (inches)	**BODY WEIGHT (pounds)**																
58	91	96	100	105	110	115	119	124	129	134	138	143	148	153	158	162	167
59	94	99	104	109	114	119	124	128	133	138	143	148	153	158	163	168	173
60	97	102	107	112	118	123	128	133	138	143	148	153	158	163	168	174	179
61	100	106	111	116	122	127	132	137	143	148	153	158	164	169	174	180	185
62	104	109	115	120	126	131	136	142	147	153	158	164	169	175	180	186	191
63	107	113	118	124	130	135	141	146	152	158	163	169	175	180	186	191	197
64	110	116	122	128	134	140	145	151	157	163	169	174	180	186	192	197	204
65	114	120	126	132	138	144	150	156	162	168	174	180	186	192	198	204	210
66	118	124	130	136	142	148	155	161	167	173	179	186	192	198	204	210	216
67	121	127	134	140	146	153	159	166	172	178	185	191	198	204	211	217	223
68	125	131	138	144	151	158	164	171	177	184	190	197	203	210	216	223	230
69	128	135	142	149	155	162	169	176	182	189	196	203	209	216	223	230	236
70	132	139	146	153	160	167	174	181	188	195	202	209	216	222	229	236	243
71	136	143	150	157	165	172	179	186	193	200	208	215	222	229	236	243	250
72	140	147	154	162	169	177	184	191	199	206	213	221	228	235	242	250	258
73	144	151	159	166	174	182	189	197	204	212	219	227	235	242	250	257	265
74	148	155	163	171	179	186	194	202	210	218	225	233	241	249	256	264	272
75	152	160	168	176	184	192	200	208	216	224	232	240	248	256	264	272	279
76	156	164	172	180	189	197	205	213	221	230	238	246	254	263	271	279	287
	healthy						**overweight**						**obese**				

Source: Adapted from the U.S. Department of Health and Human Services

A healthy weight and a healthy heart are closely related. Being overweight or obese is associated with heart disease as well as many other diseases. If you have put on extra pounds, you are not alone. As a nation, we are getting heavier. Overweight bodies and obesity are increasing problems in the United States—and the world, as our fast-food lifestyle spreads to other countries. Even the famously skinny French are eating larger portions and gaining weight. It may surprise you to hear that 32 percent of adults in the United States are obese. The problem cuts across all ages and racial and ethnic groups, and both sexes. Among women, 23 percent of white women, 38 percent of black women, and 36 percent of Latina women are obese.

Despite the constant flood of hundreds, even thousands, of new diets and strategies for weight loss, we are losing the battle of the bulge. Now, more than ever, we need an even greater emphasis on the simple message of weight control through restrained eating, good food choices, and exercise for health. (You can read more about weight loss in chapter 17, Your Diet.

There is no magic diet, no drink, pill, or program that will make you skinny. The simple fact is that if you eat more calories than you burn, you will gain weight. Keeping your weight in the normal range is a critical part of reducing your risk of heart disease.

One good way to determine whether you are at a healthy weight is the body mass index. It's adjusted for height and accounts for the fact that taller people weigh more than shorter people. A body mass index of less than 25 is considered healthy and is associated with a lower risk of dying from heart disease. Body mass indexes of 25 to 30 are considered overweight, and those over 30 are classified as obese.

Conquer Cholesterol

Improving your cholesterol and lipid levels—lowering total cholesterol and LDL (bad) cholesterol and raising HDL (good) cholesterol—through dietary changes and exercise can significantly reduce and even prevent heart disease. Everyone can benefit from efforts to lower cholesterol. Even if you have normal cholesterol levels, you can greatly reduce your future risk of heart attacks and death due to heart disease.

So don't wait until you develop heart disease. Start to lower your total cholesterol and LDL cholesterol now by watching your weight, eating healthier fats, and increasing the amount you exercise. Start a little bit today. Do that until it is easy. Then you'll be ready for the next step. It's all about viewing life one day at a time, one hour at a time, and even one minute at a time when you have to.

Fat versus Fiction

A diet low in saturated fat, trans fats, and cholesterol is important in heart health—but remember that a heart-healthy diet does not need to be a low-fat diet. Nonhydrogenated oils such as canola, peanut, or olive oil, and

REAL LIFE QUESTION: Trans what? Saturated with what?

Here's a quick breakdown of what fats are. First, if you were to take a bit of any kind of fat and rub it on your hand, your hand would feel greasy. Whether it's olive oil or butter, you know there's fat content there. But that's where the similarity ends.

Saturated fats are mostly from animals. Many of these fats stay hard even in warm temperatures. This category includes butter, cheese, whole milk, poultry skin, palm oil, and coconut oil.

Unsaturated fats come from plants and fish and come in two major groups—polyunsaturated and monounsaturated. The mono group usually comes from plants, such as olive, canola, and soy. The polyunsaturated group includes two important groups—omega-3 fatty acids and omega-6 fatty acids.

We know that omega-3 fats are very important for good health. These are found in fatty fish, including salmon and anchovies, and in walnuts, flaxseed, and flaxseed oil.

Trans fats come from unsaturated fat that is processed into a different, unhealthy form that is more shelf stable. Food made with trans fats lasts much longer on store shelves, saving businesses money, but it's bad for your body. Put your heart health first!

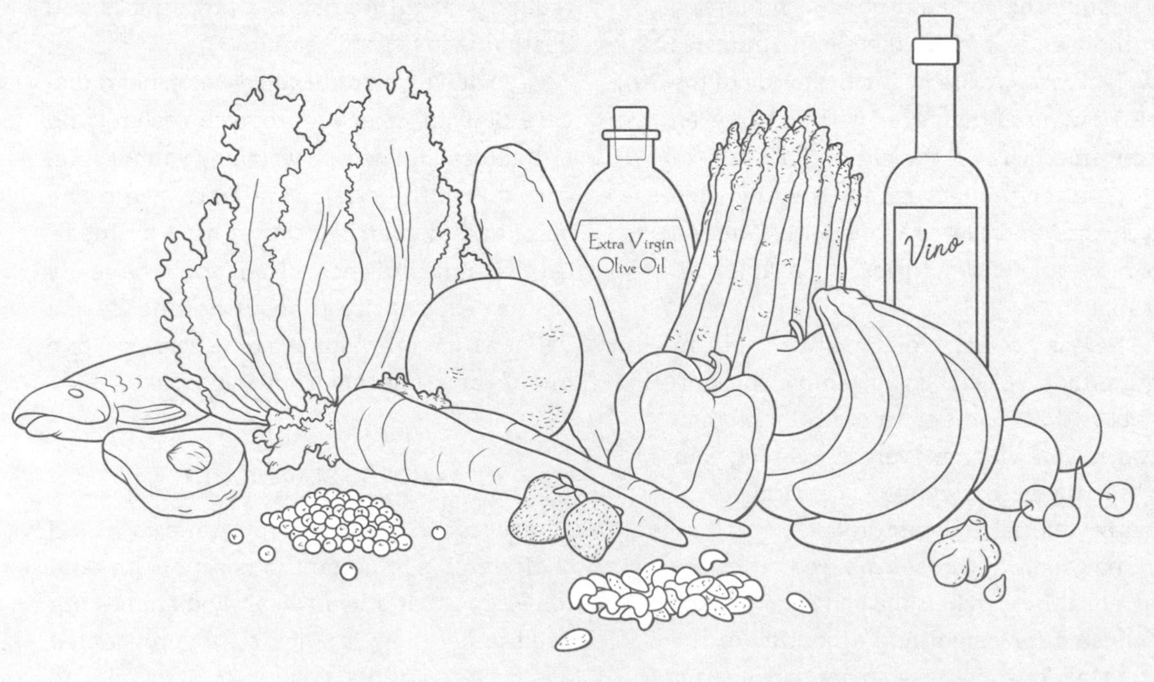

the fats found in nuts and avocados are heart healthy. Unhealthy fats that you should keep to a minimum in your diet include saturated, hydrogenated, and trans fats. Avoid processed foods made with hydrogenated and trans fats, such as french fries, doughnuts, and commercial baked goods including cookies and crackers. Foods that are high in saturated fat include butter, whole milk, cheese, beef, and the skin of poultry. Your diet and lifestyle can keep your cholesterol lower and reduce your risk of heart disease.

NOTE TO SELF

A heart-healthy diet does not need to be low in all fats. It just needs to be low in unhealthy fats, like saturated fat and trans fats, and cholesterol.

Emphasize Exercise

Did you know that your farming ancestors could eat thousands of calories a day and be thin? A huge breakfast including pork, a big lunch out in the field, a big dinner, and then sleep . . . why, oh why, can't we?

Look around your kitchen and count the laborsaving devices: the dishwasher, the stove, the canned goods, the frozen foods. Labor, of course, equals exercise. Suppose you had to catch that chicken, pluck it, do other unbelievably gross things to it, somehow get a fire going with wood you chopped, and cook a nice, high-fat meal for everybody, plus a pie. You made the pie yourself; in fact, you made the lard for the pie crust by yourself, and you planted the apple trees yourself and harvested them yourself. You milked the cow and churned the butter. You certainly didn't need more exercise. You could be eating 4,000 calories a day and be rail thin.

Now look around your whole house. The lawn mower, the washing machine, indoor plumbing (!), heat, the vacuum cleaner . . . You can keep your rugs clean without having to take them outside to whack them clean with a broom.

Okay, enough of that. It's about the exercise. Our ancestors, and most of the developing world, would not believe that we have to make a special effort to exercise. We do: lack of physical activity is a major risk factor for heart disease. According to the American Heart Association, two-thirds of Americans do not get any exercise. Worse, up to 80 percent of women spend much of their time sitting.

It's very important for you to hear my message clearly. I am not talking about weight control or exercise because I want you to be skinny or so buff that you look like Serena Williams. I only want you to begin making changes in exercise and fat consumption and diet in general so that you can live a long and healthy life.

Another good reason: Have you looked around at old people? Have you noticed the big differences among them? Some are straight-backed and healthy at ninety. Others look ancient by seventy-five. Which road do you want to take?

Regular, moderate-to-vigorous exercise for thirty to forty minutes a day can help control blood cholesterol, diabetes, and obesity, as well as help to lower blood pressure, all of which lowers your risk of cardiovascular disease and heart attack.

Physical activity also builds muscle, a key ingredient in weight control. Fat tissue in your body has much lower metabolic activity—meaning it burns fewer calories, even at rest. If you build and maintain muscle, your resting **metabolic rate** increases and your body requires more calories every day to perform its basic functions. So if you build more muscle mass, you can even burn calories in your sleep!

NOTE TO SELF

You can burn more calories while you sleep if you do strength training (use free weights or weight machines). The more muscle in your body, the higher your resting metabolic rate.

Is Alcohol Okay?

Alcohol in moderation is probably good for your heart. There is evidence that alcohol increases the amount of HDL (good) cholesterol. It also reduces the formation of blood clots that block arteries to the heart, which can cause heart attacks.

The question of what is meant by moderate alcohol consumption is tricky, especially for women. Studies show that drinking as little as one drink a day can increase the chances of developing breast and other cancers. Two drinks a day can increase breast cancer risk by 20 to 25 percent. This does not mean that 20 to 25 percent of women who have two drinks a day will get breast cancer; rather, it indicates the increase in the total lifetime risk that a woman has for developing breast cancer. For example, with a baseline risk of twelve of every one hundred women over their lifetimes, the cancer rate increases to fifteen of every one hundred women.

Most authorities, including the American Heart Association, say that one drink a day for women is okay. A drink is one 12-ounce beer, 4 ounces of wine, 1.5 ounces of 80-proof spirits, or 1 ounce of 100-proof spirits. Even as little as one drink a day may slightly increase your risk, so if you have a strong family history of breast cancer—such as a sister who's had it or a mother who developed it at a young age—you may want to limit your consumption even more.

NOTE TO SELF

Alcohol in *moderation* is good for your heart.

Not-So-Magic Markers

Having a high level of an **amino acid** called homocysteine in the blood is increasingly seen as a marker (warning sign) for cardiovascular disease, although it is controversial whether this is actually the cause of the problem or just a sign that things are not healthy on a cellular level.

Some evidence indicates that homocysteine damages the lining of the blood vessels, which promotes fatty buildup (atherosclerosis) in the vessels. A good diet may counteract this process, because folic acid and B vitamins such as B_6 and B_{12} help break down homocysteine in the body.

So far, though, studies of folic acid supplementation and heart disease risk reduction have been mixed, and more recent studies have not shown them to be helpful. It may be that the vitamins and other substances that reduce heart disease risk need to come from the whole food, and shortcuts with vitamin supplements are not enough.

Another vitamin supplement that was once thought to reduce heart disease risk is vitamin E. Although early research indicated that vitamin E might help prevent heart disease, rigorous experiments have not shown that routine use of vitamin E protects against the development of heart disease.

Based on these facts, the American Heart Association is currently not recommending the routine use of vitamin supplements to try to prevent heart disease. Instead, a balanced diet that is rich in fruits and vegetables, whole grains, and healthy fats is your best bet. Folic acid is found naturally in most vegetables, citrus fruits, and tomatoes, and also in fortified grain products. Vitamin E is found in most nuts and seeds.

A new test for **C-reactive protein** is showing some promise as an indicator that can help combat heart disease. The idea for this test comes from new evidence that **inflammation** (for example, in response to bacterial or viral infections) may be another cause of heart disease. However, at this point experts are recommending only that C-reactive protein be measured when other risk factors for heart disease are present, such as abnormal cholesterol or lipid levels.

REAL LIFE FACT: How to Love Your Heart

- **Replace saturated fat and trans fats with monounsaturated and polyunsaturated fats.**
- **Eat fruits, vegetables, and whole grains regularly.**
- **Control portion sizes.**
- **Exercise for thirty to forty minutes on most days of the week.**
- **Do not smoke, and do not let others smoke around you or your family members.**

Love Your Heart

So the truth is, there is no magic bullet to prevent or cure heart disease. The key lies in the ways in which you live your life: what you eat, how much you exercise, whether or not you smoke, and how well you control your weight. It isn't easy, but the rewards are great. If you love your heart and give it an environment in which it can flourish, it will serve you well and potentially give you the gift of a long, healthy life.

For More Information

CHOLESTEROL

http://yourtotalhealth.ivillage.com/cholesterol.html

HEART ATTACKS

http://yourtotalhealth.ivillage.com/heart-attack.html

QUITTING SMOKING

Agency for Health Care Policy and Research Clinical Practice Guidelines on Smoking Cessation

Instant fax 301-594-2800 [press 1] or call 800-358-9295 for physician materials and a "You Can Quit Smoking" consumer guide.

www.ahcpr.gov/consumer/tobacco/card.htm

American Cancer Society

800-ACS-2345

www.cancer.org/docroot/PED/content/PED_10_13X_Guide_for_Quitting_Smoking.asp

American Heart Association

800-AHA-USA1

www.americanheart.org/presenter.jhtml?identifier=3038010

American Lung Association

800-LUNG-USA

www.lungusa.org

California Smokers' Helpline

800-NO-BUTTS

www.californiasmokershelpline.org

Institute of Social and Preventive Medicine

www.stop-tabac.ch/en/welcome.html

Office on Smoking and Health

800-CDC-1311

www.cdc.gov/tobacco/index.htm

National Cancer Institute (NCI)

800-4-CANCER

www.cancer.gov/cancertopics/tobacco

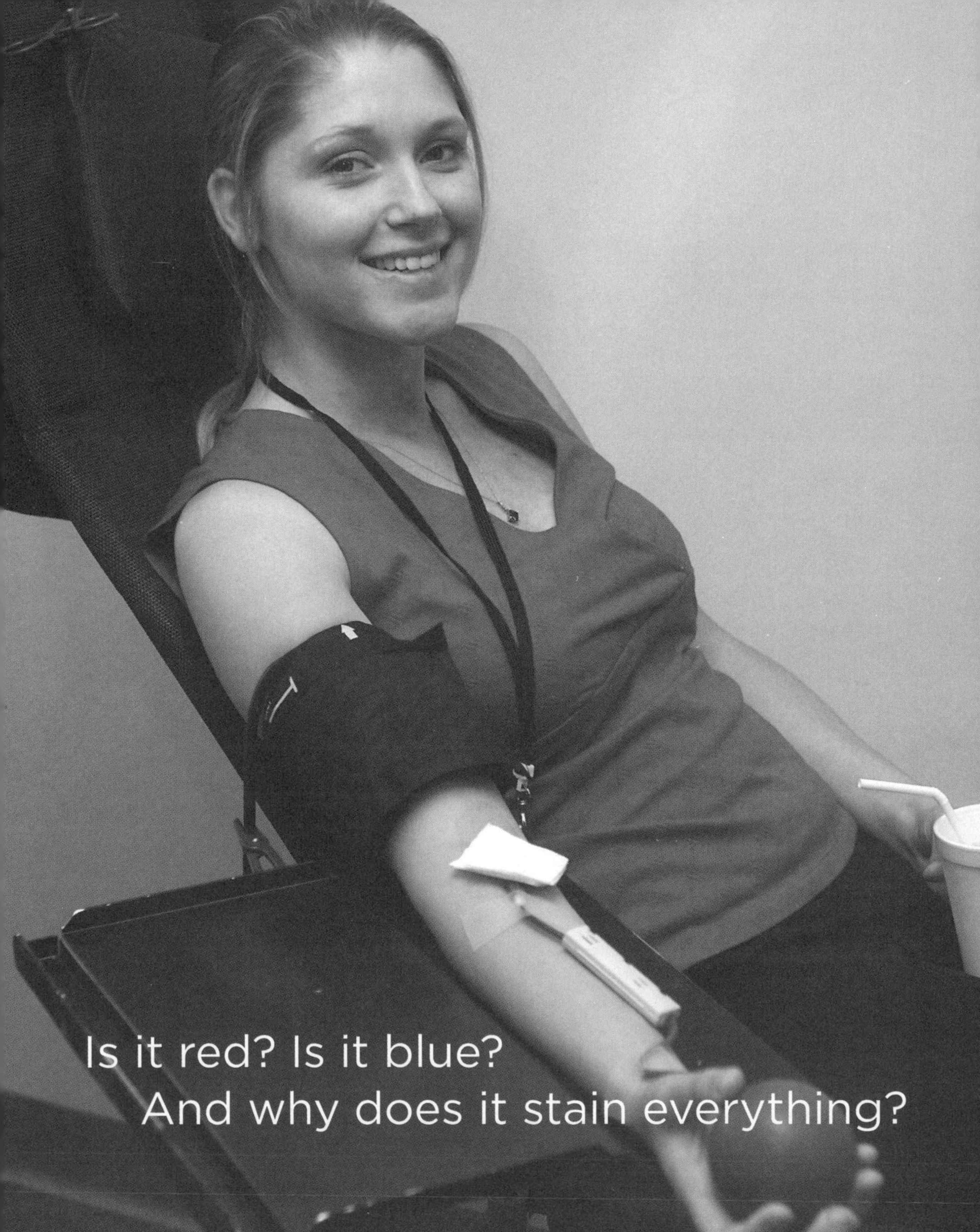
Is it red? Is it blue?
And why does it stain everything?

your blood

Your doctor wants you to have a blood test, so s/he fills out a form for you to take to the lab. She checks off about a million tests on the form, and your inner soap opera goes into full swing. You're sure that you have a terrible disease, something very, very rare—you just know it. Why else would she order so many tests? Scientists will be working around the clock to save you. Everyone will be praying, including everyone who was ever mean to you, especially people at work. On the way to the lab you copy down all of the names of the tests you are having so you can Google them later. Then you do, but they seem even more mysterious. Lord, your disease must be the rarest one on earth!

What's the reality? Your doctor has ordered the standard blood tests that we all have during a regular checkup. Chances are you are completely fine. In this chapter, we'll look at your blood in detail. And by the time we're finished, you'll know why a blood test is something that's done even when you're perfectly healthy.

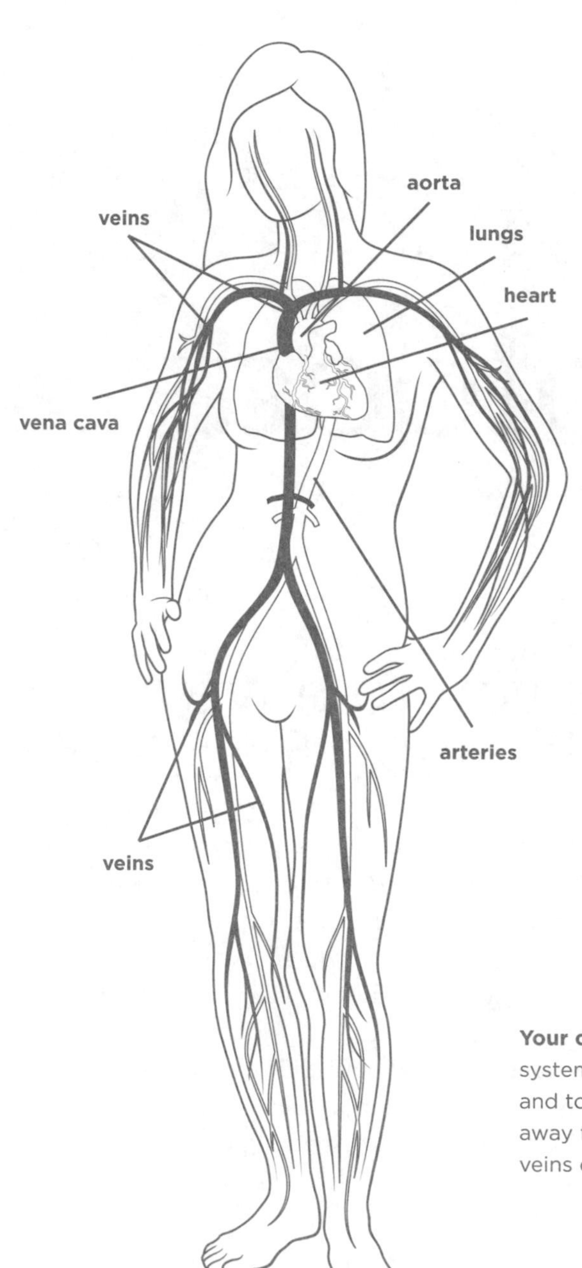

What Is Blood?

Your blood contains your body's oxygen delivery system and also helps protect against infection. It's made of three kinds of cells (red cells, white cells, and platelets) plus a lot of liquid called plasma. The cells are made in your bone marrow, which is the soft inner core of your bones. Plasma is mostly water, which your body absorbs from your **intestines** and your **kidneys**. Your body contains four to six quarts of blood, which is at least a gallon. Picture the large two-liter soda bottles: you could fill two to three of them with your blood depending on your size and how much water you drink.

Your blood travels around your body constantly. The path it takes is called the **circulatory system**. Your heart is the center of the system, pumping blood nonstop. Your blood keeps you warm, cools you off, picks up your body's waste products, and delivers **nutrients** and oxygen to your organs and tissues.

Your circulatory system: Your heart is the center of the system, pumping blood nonstop through your lungs and to your organs and tissues. The arteries carry blood away from the heart to the rest of the body and the veins carry blood back to the heart.

Blood's Four Parts

Blood part 1: **Red blood cells** are the delivery and trash service. They carry oxygen from the lungs, are pumped all the way through your system, and pick up waste products along the way. The waste you exhale as **carbon dioxide** were brought to your lungs by your red blood cells.

How do the cells travel? Through your arteries, veins, and capillaries. Your **arteries** are major outbound routes that take oxygen away from your heart and bring it everywhere in your body. Your **veins** are inbound feeder routes that deliver waste products back to the red blood cells for trash pickup. Your **capillaries** are like tiny roads that connect the arteries and veins. In a medium-sized person at rest, blood takes about a minute to work its way around the body once. That timing varies greatly, depending on so many factors that this is not a very useful number, but I think it's a fun fact to know.

Are red blood cells red? Yes, when they're carrying oxygen. That's when they're in your major arteries, deep under the skin where you can't see them. When blood cells are traveling inbound through the veins, they are carrying the trash, not oxygen. That's why your veins look blue—the blood in there is sort of bluish. Your skin makes it look light blue, but if you had X-ray vision you'd see that it's really much darker. As soon as it hits oxygen, though—like when you get a cut—blood turns bright red again immediately.

To some people this is like a "refrigerator light" puzzle. How do you know whether the light goes out when you close the door? How do you know that venous blood is blue? That blood is blue you have to take on faith (and on what you see through your skin), because there aren't any experiments you can easily do with-

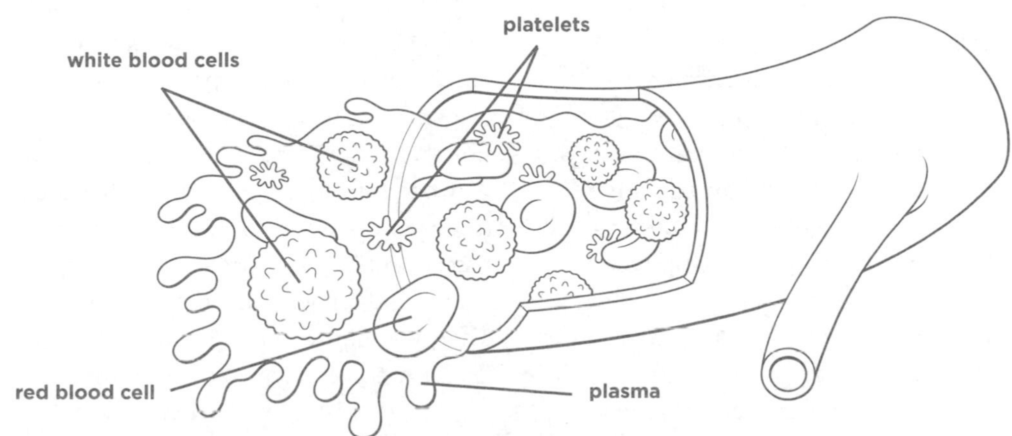

Blood's four parts: Red blood cells are delivery and trash services, white blood cells make up the army, platelets build dams, and plasma carries the cells through the circulatory system.

REAL LIFE QUESTION: Does it hurt to have blood drawn?

It's a quick prick, over in less than one second. That's it. In goes the needle (a fine needle, not a big fat one like in a cartoon), and on goes the tube to collect the blood.

You might feel some stinging when you donate blood. This is from an anticoagulant that is added to the tube to keep your blood in good shape for storage. If that happens, just tell the staff the next time you go and they'll make sure it doesn't happen again.

out exposing your blood to oxygen. And that refrigerator? Heat cooks things, so the lights have to go out! Any refrigerator that still has a light on is called an Easy Bake Oven.

Blood Part 2: **White blood cells** are the army. When a germ enters your **bloodstream**, white blood cells multiply and attack the germ. Actually, they eat it. There are six different kinds of white blood cells, but most of them are **neutrophils**, which are the germ eaters.

Why don't you see spots of white in your blood? White blood cells don't have a color until they are separated from the other cells. Then they are revealed as white. They are also too small to see with the naked eye.

Blood Part 3: **Platelets** build dams. They are sticky little cells, smaller than the other types, and when you have a cut, they come running. They group together to stop blood loss. They become connected by tiny threads and spread a thin veil over a cut. As it dries, it forms a scab. A scab is made of platelets.

Blood Part 4: **Plasma** is a clear, yellowish liquid that carries the cells through the system.

When you have your blood drawn as part of your yearly physical, the technicians will analyze your blood counts in the four groups. Your blood is separated into cells (parts 1, 2, and 3) and plasma (part 4) by spinning it in a contraption that creates centrifugal force, like a carnival ride.

Are You My Type?

There are four basic blood types. If you ever need a blood transfusion, there are only certain blood types that will work in your body. Before blood types were discovered, blood transfusions were often fatal. Blood types are not routinely tested in healthy people unless you need an operation or become pregnant (then one is done to find out whether your baby's type is compatible with yours). A good way to find out your blood type is to give blood. Then you can keep your donor card in your wallet with your type clearly shown.

This is how we identify the types: On your red blood cells, you have tiny bumps called **antigens**. Any substance that is foreign

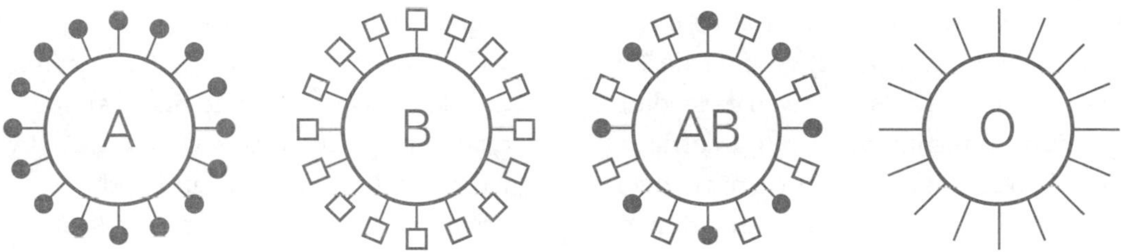

Red blood cells showing the antigens that help determine your blood type.

to your body and triggers your **antibodies** to attack is technically an antigen. The antigens on your red blood cells, however, are good antigens that determine what kind of antibodies you produce.

They are classified as antigens A, B, AB, and O, the four groups of human blood. (O means that your blood has neither A nor B antigens.) But there's a second step, which is to see whether you have an Rh factor. This is another antigen, discovered about thirty-five years after the first blood types. It was first found in a rhesus monkey and keeps the name Rh for that reason.

So let's say you are type A and you have the Rh factor. This makes you A positive, or A+ for short. Type B, with no Rh factor? Then you are B negative, or B– for short. Most people in the United States are Rh+.

Rh Factor and Pregnancy

We know which blood groups can be safely given to other blood groups. A person with Rh+ blood can receive blood from a person with Rh– blood without any problems, but a person with Rh– blood cannot receive blood from Rh+ people.

Your blood type and Rh status are tested early in pregnancy as part of routine blood work. When an Rh+ baby grows inside an Rh– mother, there is a chance that the mother may react to the presence of this foreign Rh marker by making antibodies against it. This happens during pregnancy if some of the baby's blood flows back into the mother's circulation, which is not very common. Usually, the mother's blood and baby's blood don't mix at all until birth; the placenta serves as a gateway that filters the mother's blood to deliver nutrients to the baby safely.

In a first pregnancy, there is very little danger of Rh disease because the baby is usually born before the mother develops antibodies. It's in the next pregnancy that the danger of Rh disease is greater. This is known as Rh sensitization. If blood tests early in pregnancy show that a woman is Rh–, she can receive an injection of Rh immune globulin to prevent sensitization in case the baby is Rh+. This is done at twenty-eight weeks of pregnancy and again within seventy-two hours after birth. This treatment is highly effective and safe. Rh immune globulin may also be given if bleeding happens during pregnancy; after a miscarriage, **ectopic** (tubal) pregnancy, or abortion; or when special tests such as **amniocentesis** are performed. Because of Rh immune globulin treatment, Rh sensitization is rarely seen today.

Not Your Type

You find yourself on a tour of Japan. You are introduced to a friend's Japanese cousin, who turns out to be interesting, funny, and good-looking. Everything is going really well. Then he blurts out, "What's your type?"

You stare at him in disbelief. "Well, honesty is important to me," you start to say, like you would fill in a form for a dating service. But then he says, kind of shyly, "I mean, what's your blood type?"

Don't run yet. He is not necessarily a vampire. Turns out that many people in Japan believe in blood type as a sign of personality. Asking, "What's your type?" is like asking "What's your sign?" Seriously. Everybody even knows the blood type of every celebrity. My favorite fact is that Japanese fictional characters have blood types, too. Check out manga characters and you'll see.

Go ahead, take a break from reading and Google a few websites to discover your blood type personality. If this were *Cosmo*, I would write a whole section about the personality types in an article like "What Blood Type Makes Your Man Go Wild." I know, it's fun, and there's nothing wrong with fun. But remember that there's no science behind this theory; please chalk it up to funny games.

Unfortunately, there's a long and very sad human history of using blood type as a weapon for and against people, and it all happened in the hundred years since the types were discovered. It was part of a field called eugenics, a bizarre chapter in semiscience in which dictators, fascists, Nazis, and even some scientists thought we should tamper with evolution by figuring out who was superior in "scientific" terms. Once people think they have a scientific way to prove themselves superior, they're usually one step away from wanting to keep all the "others" from spreading—or existing. It sounds like bad science fiction, but the history is real. Even a harmless dating game based on it makes me itch. I squirm when people talk about using blood type for anything but giving and getting blood.

REAL LIFE QUESTION: Does my cat have a blood type?

Yes! All mammals do. Dogs have twice as many blood groups as we do; cats have three types.

REAL LIFE FACT: Why You Should Donate Blood This Year

Donating blood is easy to do, and within twenty-four hours your body will replace the blood you gave. Think they don't need your common blood type? They do—it's in great demand, and you might be a universal donor. Every type is needed! They'll give you a little snack after giving blood, and drink plenty of liquids before and after you donate.

If there isn't a regular blood drive near you, call the Red Cross for locations at 1-800-GIVE-LIFE. It will take an hour from start to finish, but only ten minutes of that time will be the donation of blood. Imagine saving a life with one hour of your time.

What Can Go Wrong with Your Blood? Anemia

There are many types of anemia, but they all start with one problem: the blood doesn't have enough working **hemoglobin**. Hemoglobin is a protein, rich in iron, that carries oxygen from your lungs to the rest of your body. Your blood gets its bright red color when hemoglobin picks up oxygen in your lungs. As your blood travels through your body, the hemoglobin in red blood cells releases oxygen to your tissues, and the blood cells turn bluish.

Each of the many types of anemia has a different cause. We'll look at four types.

Iron-Deficiency Anemia

Iron deficiency is the most common cause of anemia, especially in young women. It happens when you don't have enough iron in your body to supply the hemoglobin in your red blood cells. Iron-deficiency anemia can leave you feeling tired and worn-out. Women are particularly vulnerable to iron-deficiency anemia because we lose blood during our period. It can also happen when you lose blood from **gastrointestinal** problems like **ulcers** (see page 159), colonic **polyps** (see page 177), or **hemorrhoids** (see page 174).

Pregnancy can also cause anemia because the amount of blood you have increases, and you need more iron to fuel that growth.

Add iron from foods such as beef, chicken, dark green leafy vegetables, lentils, and some beans and legumes, or by taking a supplement. To help your body absorb iron better, have foods and drinks that are rich in vitamin C when you take iron or eat iron-rich foods. Add some tomatoes to your burger or drink orange juice with your breakfast. This will help your body make the most of the iron you're feeding it.

Avoid foods and drinks that hurt your body's ability to take in iron, including caffeine and phytic acid. Phytic acid is found in seeds, grains, and beans. You can reduce it by soaking these foods and cooking them. You already know that caffeine is everywhere, from diet pills to soda. So limit your coffee, tea, caffeinated sodas, and (sorry) chocolate.

GOOD SOURCES OF IRON

- Apricots
- Beef
- Black beans
- Blackstrap molasses
- Broccoli
- Chicken
- Chickpeas
- Clams
- Collard greens
- Egg yolks
- Kale
- Kidney beans
- Lentils
- Navy beans
- Pinto beans
- Prunes
- Pumpkin seeds
- Shrimp
- Spinach
- Swiss chard
- Tofu
- Tuna
- Turkey

Megaloblastic (Vitamin-Deficiency) Anemia

Megaloblastic or vitamin-deficiency anemia is rare. It develops when your body doesn't get enough folic acid or vitamin B_{12}, two of the many vitamins in the B vitamin complex. Both help to maintain healthy blood and a healthy nervous system. With this type of anemia, your body makes red blood cells that can't deliver oxygen correctly.

Folic acid supplements can treat megaloblastic anemia. You can also get folate (the natural form of folic acid that is formed in foods) in your diet from leafy green vegetables, beans and legumes, citrus fruits and juices, whole grains, egg yolks, poultry, pork, and shellfish. B_{12} deficiency is more common in people with **autoimmune disorders**, like Crohn's disease (see page 171), or people who've had some of their intestine surgically removed or altered. Not getting enough B_{12} can cause numbness in your legs and feet, problems walking, memory loss, and vision problems. The treatment depends on the cause, and you may need to get B_{12} shots or take special B_{12} supplements.

GOOD SOURCES OF FOLATE

- Asparagus
- Beans
- Bread*
- Cereal*
- Citrus fruits and juices
- Collard greens
- Egg yolks
- Kale
- Legumes
- Pork
- Poultry
- Shellfish
- Spinach
- Sunflower seeds
- Swiss chard
- Tomatoes
- Turnip greens
- Whole grains*

*These items are typically enriched with folic acid.

GOOD SOURCES OF B_{12}*

- Cereal (fortified with B_{12})
- Eggs
- Fish
- Lean beef
- Pork
- Poultry
- Shellfish
- Yogurt

*Most B_{12} comes from animal sources, so vegetarians/vegans may need to take supplements.

REAL LIFE FACT: The Signs of Anemia

Most anemia develops very gradually. At first you may not have any signs, but symptoms, listed below, may increase over time:

- **Dizziness**
- **Fatigue**
- **Headache**
- **Rapid heartbeat**
- **Not doing well in work or school**
- **Pale skin**
- **Weakness**
- **Shortness of breath from even minor activity**

Sickle Cell Anemia

Sickle cell anemia is a genetic disease that causes many red blood cells to change shape. Instead of a round cell that can move through the system easily, these cells are shaped like sickles, a curved farm tool. Picture the shape of a shrimp, and you can see that these cells might get stuck. When they do, your blood's oxygen delivery system can't work as well.

This is a serious disease requiring lifetime management, preferably starting in infancy. Some of the other anemia measures will help, such as getting more folic acid in your diet. But several lifestyle decisions have to be made. Because sickle cell anemia can damage the lungs, smoking is even more dangerous. Because you're more vulnerable to illness, you must be sure to have the vaccinations your doctor recommends. Call your doctor immediately if your temperature rises above 101 degrees Fahrenheit. Avoid travel to places where oxygen may be lower than you are used to, such as high-altitude cities and mountains.

Sickle cell anemia affects people of African descent as well as some Mediterranean and Asian groups. It is inherited from both parents, but they may not be sick. If you receive the sickle cell anemia gene from only one parent, you may carry the anemia trait without your knowledge until you have children.

It's a good idea for babies to be tested for sickle cell anemia. The earlier the diagnosis, the better we can manage the disease.

Screening for Anemia

Few medical societies or organizations recommend screening for anemia (except for sickle cell anemia) as part of routine physical exams. The U.S. Centers for Disease Control and Prevention recommends anemia screening only for adult women at five- to ten-year intervals (more often for those at risk of iron deficiency because of heavy menstrual blood loss or poor iron intake), and for pregnant women at the first prenatal visit.

REAL LIFE FACT: Why People of African Descent Have a High Rate of Sickle Cell Anemia

Sickle cell anemia gives people a stronger than average resistance to malaria, a mosquito-borne disease that's a serious problem in sub-Saharan Africa. Over the centuries, each new wave of malaria caused fewer deaths in sickle cell sufferers than in people without anemia. Eventually, as a result, a higher percentage of the African population carried the sickle cell gene and unknowingly passed it onto their children.

Testing for anemia is important during pregnancy because anemia is associated with preterm delivery and low birth weight in newborns. But even if you are not pregnant, if you are having symptoms of anemia, have heavy periods, or have been anemic in the past, periodic testing is worthwhile.

How Do I Find Out If I Have Anemia?

To find out if you have anemia, you have a blood test called a complete blood count (CBC) to measure your hemoglobin and your hematocrit. Your **hematocrit** tells what percentage of your blood is made up of red blood cells, normally about 36 to 44 percent. Hemoglobin makes up about one-third of your red blood cells.

Other tests include measuring the iron stored in your body. Sometimes a **reticulocyte** count is helpful. We measure these young red blood cells to see if you are producing new red blood cells normally.

Other forms of anemia require a **hemoglobin electrophoreses**—a blood test to identify abnormal hemoglobins in the blood and to diagnose sickle cell anemia, **thalassemias**, and other inherited forms of anemia.

Treating Anemia

Treatment for anemia depends on its cause. You should never assume that symptoms you have are due to an iron deficiency. It's important to be checked by a doctor before you start taking an iron supplement.

If you do have iron-deficiency anemia, your doctor may prescribe an iron supplement and recommend that you add iron-rich foods to your diet. If your anemia is caused by heavy or irregular menstrual periods, birth control pills may help to regulate the bleeding. Folic acid and vitamin B_{12} supplements may be prescribed if the anemia is traced to a deficiency of these nutrients, although that's rare in our country.

REAL LIFE QUESTION: Am I at risk for anemia if I'm a vegetarian?

Vegetarians are sometimes at risk for iron deficiency anemia, and sometimes not. It depends on your diet. Because it's easier for your body to get iron from meat than from plants, some vegetarians may need to get a higher amount of iron each day than what is recommended for other people. But if you are careful about your iron intake and try to take vitamin C with iron-rich foods, enough iron can be found in a vegetarian diet. A more rare type of anemia caused by B_{12} deficiency can result from a vegan diet (one that contains no animal products). Vegans may need to add nutritional yeast or supplements to their diet to obtain adequate B_{12}.

What Else Can Go Wrong with Your Blood? Iron Overload

Healthy people use about 10 percent of the iron in the foods they eat. However, people with a disease called **hemochromatosis** can soak in up to 20 percent or more from their diet. The body has no natural way of getting rid of iron, except through your period or a very tiny amount everyone loses in dead skin. The extra iron is dumped into tissues and vital organs, especially the heart, **liver**, and **pancreas**, where it can accumulate and cause permanent damage.

Hemochromatosis is a genetic disorder that appears to increase iron absorption from the intestines. If the iron overload is discovered early, phlebotomies, or bloodletting, will prevent illness. Left untreated, the excess iron can turn the skin a grayish color and clog vital

REAL LIFE QUESTION: No chocolate and coffee, really?

It's easy for me to tell you to limit coffee, tea, and chocolate if you are anemic. But I don't say it lightly. I know that these are among life's pleasures and addictions and are hard to cut out. But please try to reduce them while you are working on your anemia problem. If you have iron-deficiency anemia, for instance, make a real effort to cut out coffee on a day when you want chocolate. You really will feel better.

REAL LIFE FACT: The Convenience of Donating Blood

Once upon a time, we didn't know how to store blood, so it always had to be fresh. In 1922, the telephone numbers of blood donors in London were kept in a registry created by librarian Percy Oliver. Donors would often be called to the hospital in the middle of the night to donate blood for emergencies. By comparison, donating blood today is a snap!

internal organs to such an extent that diseases such as **diabetes**, **cancer**, heart disease, and cirrhosis of the liver can develop. Bloodletting sounds like a primitive medical practice from ancient times, and it is. It was used by doctors from early civilizations until the discovery of germs and the other real causes of disease in the nineteenth century. It is very rarely used these days, but hemochromatosis is one disease for which it is effective.

In women, symptoms commonly develop after **menopause**, because the iron loss during our periods and pregnancy provides some protection. Screening by blood testing is recommended for those who have relatives with hemochromatosis, but not for the general population.

What If I Need Blood?

Lucky for you, we have a safe national blood supply and a safe way to give it to you. You may have images in your mind, from movies you've seen, of down-and-out sick people selling their blood to an unsuspecting public, but that's not how it works.

After you give blood, your unit is tested for blood-transmitted diseases such as hepatitis and **HIV**. They look at liver **enzymes**, antibodies, and antigens that would indicate infection. You will be notified if they find anything wrong. Otherwise, your blood donation is separated into its parts. Before any blood is

REAL LIFE QUESTION: Why does blood stain?

It's that pesky protein with a little iron that seems to grab onto your clothes and bond forever. You'll find plenty of products to remove bloodstains, but only one that is all-natural and recommended by Grandma.

According to Grandma, if this substance can digest food, it can digest blood. Yep, I'm talking about spit. (I have not tried this method.)

used, it is held for forty-eight hours, until the safety tests are complete. The parts are then distributed to hospitals. The Red Cross estimates that every donation has the potential to save three or four lives.

Plasma, for example, is used for patients who have trouble clotting. Platelets are used to clot blood from cuts and open wounds. The Red Cross says that cancer patients and transplant patients often need more than one transfusion of platelets.

What Does My Blood Say about Me?

So why does your doctor request so many blood tests on that lab form? Results of your blood tests will give your doctor a good snapshot of your health. Although blood tests can't catch everything that can go wrong—there's no blood test for breast cancer, for example—they can set off alarm bells.

The CBC test can show infection and anemia. Blood **glucose** testing will catch early warning signs of diabetes. Blood tests can also check your **thyroid** function, your **electrolytes** (such as sodium and potassium), your liver function, your **heart disease** risk, your **cholesterol** levels, your hormone levels, pregnancy, kidney problems, and a long list of other major and minor facts about you.

Your doctor will probably order basic blood tests as part of your physical and will add on other tests depending on your family history or any symptoms you have. The good news: Once you've got the needle prick over with, they can fill a bunch of tubes from that one prick.

To be an advocate for your own health, be familiar with your blood test results. If your glucose level is high or your cholesterol spikes, you want to know why. My advice is to pay attention, test by test—but don't make a full-time job out of knowing all of the tests and abbreviations and normal ranges. Just review your results when they come in. Many hospitals and doctors have patient sites where you can look up your test results.

If you were relatively young when you had your first physical and CBC test, the results were probably all normal. Unless you eat well, exercise, and take care of your body, the likelihood that your results will stay normal as you age gets smaller. But luckily, with this book's help, you are now starting to eat an even healthier diet, right? And the amount that you exercise is increasing, yes? You're making one small change at a time, and each will benefit you for life.

Healthy Blood for Life

The result of all this hard work? Your blood will stay healthy as you age. You'll never know what your numbers might have been like if you just coasted through the years on junk food and recliners. You just know that you feel great!

In the next chapter, we'll talk about your bones and joints. Your bones are where your blood is made (in the bone marrow); they provide a strong foundation for your body.

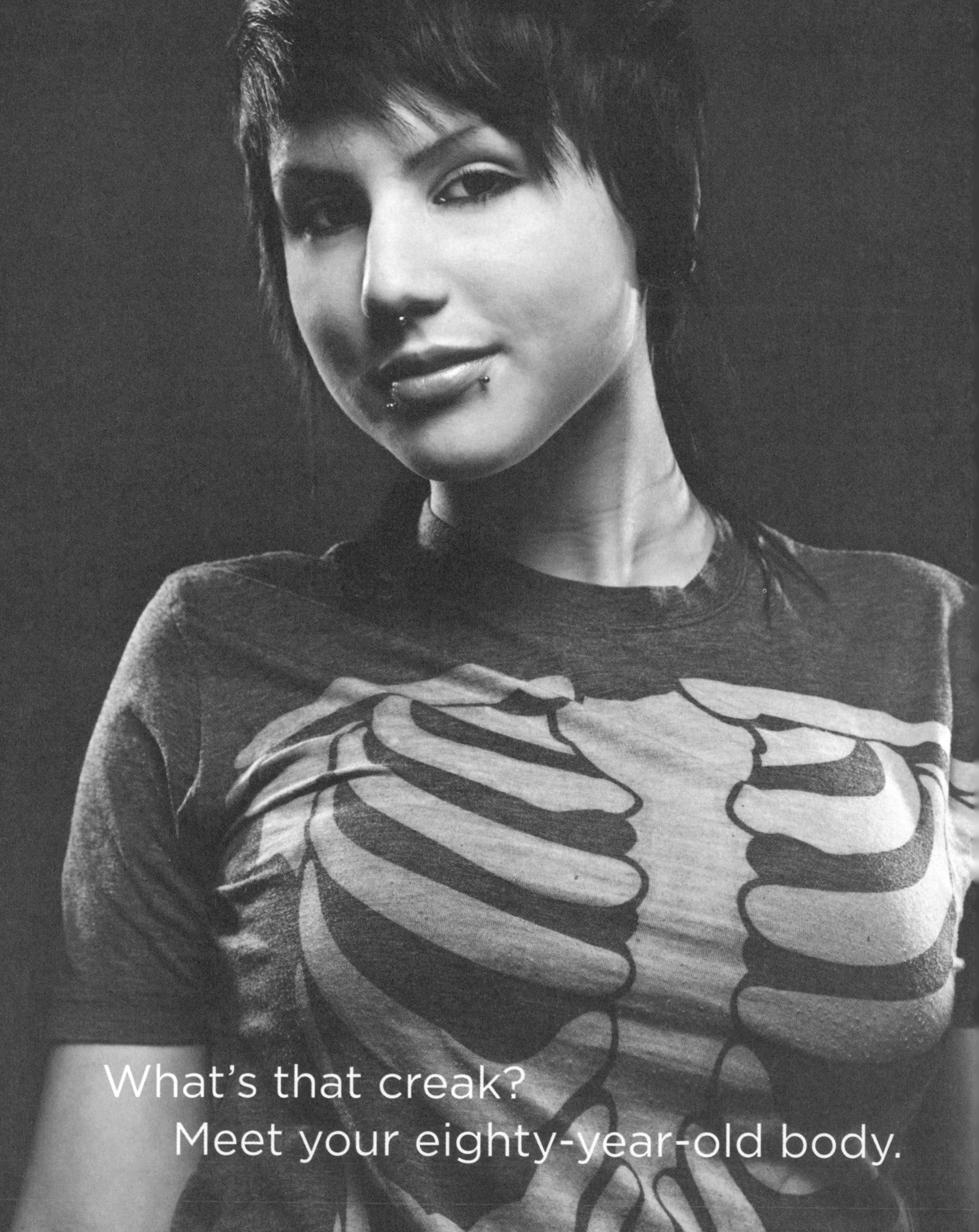
What's that creak?
Meet your eighty-year-old body.

your bones and joints

You probably don't give much thought to your bones and joints—

they're simply there inside your body to make sure you don't collapse into a heap, right? They get you where you want to go and let you do what you want to do. But if you visit a senior center, you are likely to notice that the elderly have two major body types: some walk with a straight back like they're fresh out of boot camp and others are bent over as if they carry the weight of the world on their shoulders.

The most important thing you can do to feel great at eighty is to pay attention to your heart and brain health. But if you want to feel good, be active, and *look* great too, think bone and **joint** health now. Why do you have to act now? Because your bone density stops increasing at age thirty.

I don't know why we're made this way. It probably has something to do with the fact that our ancestors didn't used to live as long as we do now. Because our life span has greatly increased, we are constantly searching for ways to make our later years healthy and happy ones. One major

NOTE TO SELF

Although you can always work to increase the strength of your bones, you can never build your bone density beyond what you have achieved by age thirty. So work to build bone density early in life to prevent problems later on.

tool: build up your bone density until age thirty. After that, be kind to your joints and continue to strengthen your bones for life.

Bones: More than Just a Skeleton

Your bones do so much more than simply keep you from falling down in a heap. You may not think about your bones as a storehouse, but that's exactly what they are: a storehouse for calcium, a mineral that's essential for your body. Ninety-nine percent of the calcium in your body is stored in your bones and teeth.

Do you know that you need calcium for many bodily functions, including blood clotting, transmitting nerve impulses, contracting muscles, and regulating your heart's rhythm? Calcium is important at every stage of life.

Your body gets the calcium it needs when you eat foods that contain calcium, but if you don't get enough calcium in your diet, your body will draw it from your bones. Your bones are kind of like an ATM that dispenses calcium. As long as you replace the calcium withdrawn from your bones by eating calcium-rich foods, getting enough vitamin D, and doing weight-bearing exercise, you're fine. But if you don't replace the calcium in your bones, eventually they stop working properly, just like an ATM that runs out of money. When your bones don't get enough calcium, they can become weak, thin, and easier to break. If you don't refill them regularly, you may even get **osteoporosis**: thin and weakened bones that break far more easily than healthy bones.

NOTE TO SELF

Ninety-nine percent of the calcium in your body is stored in your bones and teeth. If you don't get enough calcium in your diet, your body will draw it from your bones.

The Biology of Bones

Your bones are living tissues that are constantly being broken down and built up again in a process known as **remodeling**. Cells in your bones called **osteoblasts** build your bones; other bone cells called **osteoclasts** break down bone. The breaking-down process is called **resorption**.

Until you're about thirty years old, as long as you get enough calcium and physical activity the osteoblasts work harder than the osteoclasts, meaning that more bone is built than is resorbed, or your body saves more than it spends. At age thirty, your bones reach their peak maximum bone density. From age thirty to fifty, the osteoblasts and the osteoclasts both work at about the same pace, keeping your bone density steady. But at around age fifty, the osteoclasts (the resorbers) begin to outpace the osteoblasts (the builders). More bone is resorbed than is newly made. That's what causes bones to become thinner and increases fracture risk.

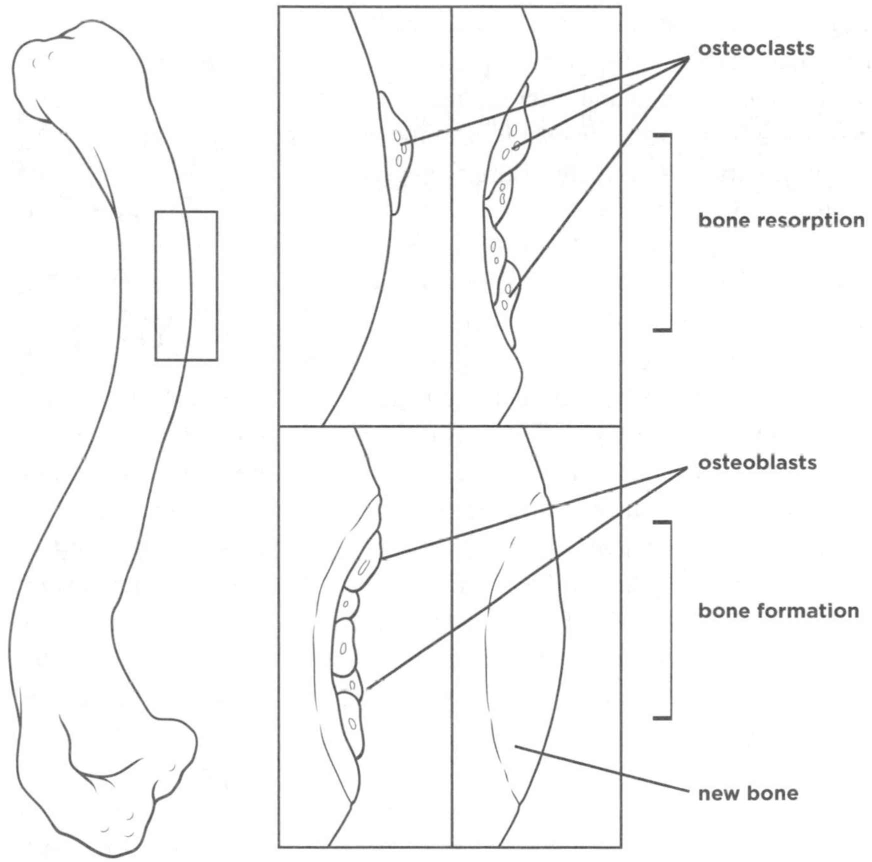

Bone remodeling: Osteoclasts break down bone (top two illustrations) and osteoblasts build new bone (bottom two illustrations).

REAL LIFE FACT: Your Bones Are Alive

They are living tissues that are built up and broken down (and built up again) over the course of your life.

Why the switch to more resorbing and less rebuilding? We don't understand it fully. One reason is the reduced **estrogen** that your body produces during and after **menopause**. Estrogen is important because it stimulates bone production, especially in the bones of your back, hips, and neck.

If your mom's bones have become thin, she can rebuild them through diet, exercise, and in some cases medications. But she can never build them higher than the peak bone density that she reached around age thirty. This is why it's important to start thinking about bone density early in life.

About 25 percent of your bone mass is added during your growth spurt at puberty. By age eighteen, 90 percent has been added; the final 10 percent is added between the ages of twenty-five and thirty. To fill your bone mass "bank account," you need to get enough calcium, vitamin D, and exercise to ensure strong bones. Building strong bones is important for both women and men, but women are more vulnerable to osteoporosis later in life because their bones usually are smaller and due to the drop in estrogen levels at menopause. Women also have a higher prevalence of eating disorders, which may cause a greater risk of bone loss.

No Bones About It: Osteoporosis Overview for Young Women

I know it's hard to imagine having a weak and vulnerable body. After all, you've had sports injuries and you've probably slipped on the ice or tripped off the curb, right? Chances are good that you've tripped, slipped, and fallen without breaking any bones.

But what if you were extra prone to breaking your bones? What if that trip on the curb or the slip on the ice put you in a cast every single time it happened? And what if your other limbs weren't strong enough to help out? Right now, you can break your foot and hop around on the other one. With osteoporosis, forget the hopping. You'd probably trip and end up with two casts—and in a wheelchair.

YOUR BONE BANK ACCOUNT

These are the "deposits" you make by different ages.

AGE	BONE MASS
Puberty	25 percent
Eighteen	90 percent
Nineteen to thirty	100 percent

REAL LIFE QUESTION: Can caffeine increase my risk of bone fracture?

Here's a good reason to limit your caffeine: When you increase caffeine in your diet, more calcium shows up in your pee. This may mean that caffeine is pulling calcium from your bones.

Am I trying to scare you? Absolutely. Look around you and you'll see the number of bent-over elderly people, inching along, head down, because they must look out for anything that might make them fall, or because they truly cannot straighten up. That's not where you want to be at eighty, is it? Or at seventy?

Premature Osteoporosis: Who Is at Risk?

Studies suggest that women who have no periods for a long time (**amenorrhea**) are at risk for osteoporosis. It's all about the hormone estrogen. Women who stop getting their periods are often low in estrogen, which is produced during **ovulation**. When ovulation stops, even if you get a normal amount of calcium and vitamin D in your diet, your bones can become thin and weak.

Women who do strenuous exercise, and women with very low body weight due to eating disorders, may stop getting their periods and therefore have low estrogen levels. (Please see chapter 2, Your Head, for more info about eating disorders.) Scientists have found that bone density in amenorrheic women is significantly lower than in women who have regular periods. And their bone density does not always return to normal after their periods return; some women are left with osteoporosis.

Premature osteoporosis has both short- and long-term consequences. In the short term, you're more vulnerable to injuries, particularly stress fractures. In the long term, women with premature osteoporosis are at increased risk for osteoporotic fractures.

Osteoporosis in Female Athletes

Before Title 9 was passed in 1972, there were only a few women's sports played in college. There were *some* options. Basketball was one, played in short dresses over short shorts. Field hockey was another, also played in short dresses over short shorts. (I think it still is!)

Well, Title 9 equalized sports funding for women and they flocked to the fields. However, along with this success have come some problems, one of which is called the female athlete triad. The triad consists of disordered eating, amenorrhea, and osteoporosis.

Disordered eating refers to eating behaviors that result in not getting enough calories and **nutrients** for good health. An athlete who eats this way may stop having her period, which leads to lower levels of estrogen and premature loss of bone density. In sports in which low body weight may be a competitive advantage—such as distance running, dancing, swimming, diving, gymnastics, and figure skating—there are more athletes with disordered eating and true eating disorders than in other sports. Though these athletes are physically active (which increases bone density) and may get adequate calcium and vitamin D, the low estrogen levels still put them at risk for osteoporosis.

Estrogen replacement using birth control pills can improve bone density in athletes who have stopped having periods. Significant bone loss can happen as soon as six months after losing your period, so it is important to seek treatment right away to prevent this.

Bone Density and Depa-Provera

Studies show a relationship between low bone density and use of the injectable, long-term **progestin**-based contraceptive Depo-Provera (generic name: medroxyprogesterone acetate), also known as "the shot." Luckily, the bone loss associated with Depo-Provera use appears to be reversible once the shots are stopped.

If you are considering using a contraceptive and you have risk factors for osteoporosis (smoking, a thin or small frame, prior broken bones, Caucasian or Asian ancestry, family history of osteoporosis, or a diet low in calcium), you should discuss the risk of bone loss with your doctor. Researchers estimate that women who use Depo-Provera continuously for four years experience bone loss comparable to what happens in menopause. Young women aged eighteen to twenty-one appear to be especially at risk. Having adequate calcium and vitamin D, either in your food or in supplement form, while you use Depo-Provera helps slow the bone loss.

Women who discontinue Depo-Provera show increases in bone density, although bone

REAL LIFE QUESTION: Do men get osteoporosis too?

They do, but science only discovered that in the last twenty years. Men can also develop weak bones, but at least a decade later than women do because men don't have the major hormone change of menopause. Osteoporosis in men doesn't appear to be hormone related, but we have much more to learn about it. Men are more likely to die within a year of having a hip fracture, for example, but that may be because men tend to be older by that point.

density returns at the hips more slowly than at the spine, and it takes about two and a half years after stopping Depo-Provera to regain your former bone density. Despite this problem, Depo-Provera can still be a good birth control option, especially for women who just can't remember to take a pill every day. (Please see chapter 15, Your Reproductive System, for more about contraception.)

Building Strong Bones

Here's the recipe you need to help you build strong bones for life:

Calcium + Vitamin D + Weight-bearing exercise = Maximum bone density

The recommended daily allowance of calcium for young women is 1,300 mg until the age of eighteen, then 1,000 mg until you reach menopause. If your mom is through with menopause, her recommended dose is 1,200 to 1,500 mg. (By the way, her iron supplement should usually decrease. Be sure Mom talks to her doctor about her supplements.)

The recommended daily allowance for vitamin D is 200 IU when you are under fifty. Three-quarters of young women today do not get adequate amounts of calcium or vitamin D. Maybe we are drinking more water, soda, and juice and much less milk (which has been fortified with vitamin D since the early 1930s) compared to twenty years ago.

Many doctors and scientists are recommending much higher levels of vitamin D—400 IU daily for young women—as evidence is mounting for many health benefits beyond bone health. If you and your doctor decide to increase your vitamin D, remember that the U.S. Institute of Medicine of the National Academy of Sciences sets the safety limit at 2,000 IU daily.

REAL LIFE FACT: Comparing Whole, Low-Fat, and Nonfat Milk

1 CUP	FAT (grams)	CALCIUM (mg)	CALORIES (kcal)
Whole milk	9	290	150
Reduced-fat milk (2 percent)	5	298	140
Low-fat milk (1 percent)	2	300	120
Nonfat milk	0	301	90

Source: Adapted from U.S. Department of Agriculture

NOTE TO SELF

Three-quarters of young women today don't have enough calcium in their diet.

Calcium: Think Outside the Milk Bottle

Most of us immediately think of milk when we think of calcium. By comparison, soy milk is fairly low in calcium—about 80 mg in an average glass compared to 300 mg in cow's milk. Although milk and other dairy products (that are fortified with vitamin D) are good sources of easily absorbed calcium, they are not the only sources. Nondairy sources of calcium include dark green leafy vegetables and tofu processed with calcium.

There is as much calcium in skim and low-fat dairy as in whole-milk dairy products. The calcium isn't in the fat part of the milk, so removing the fat does not remove any of the calcium. This, sadly, means that calcium cannot be used as an excuse to down a pint of ice cream.

Because the fat in dairy is **saturated fat** (an unhealthy fat), try to include more nonfat or low-fat dairy products in your diet. Choose nonfat milk and yogurt and low-fat cheese for most of your dairy products.

Keep this in mind: calcium from your diet must be dissolved in your stomach and then passed into your **small intestine**. The problem? To be absorbed in the intestine, calcium competes with magnesium, copper, and iron. If there's a lot of one nutrient, it's harder for the others to be absorbed. Other substances can interfere with absorption in different ways. For example, chocolate, Swiss chard, grains, and tea contain substances (oxalic acid in chocolate, Swiss chard, and spinach; phytic acid in grains and tea) that bind to calcium and keep it from being absorbed. Broccoli and romaine lettuce, on the other hand, give you a calcium boost. So a nice salad made with romaine lettuce and some shavings of Parmesan is a good thing.

Right about now you're probably thinking to yourself, "So why can't I just take calcium supplements? Remembering all of this info about absorption and levels of calcium is

REAL LIFE FACT: Too Much Protein in Your Diet Can Leach Calcium From Your Bones!

High-protein diets like the Atkins diet are bad for your bones. As your body digests protein, it releases acids into the bloodstream, which the body neutralizes by drawing calcium from your bones. Animal protein seems to cause more of this calcium leaching than vegetable protein does. Just how big a risk factor protein is for osteoporosis is still being researched.

COMPARING THE CALCIUM CONTENT OF FOODS					
Food	**Quantity**	**Calcium (mg)**	**Food**	**Quantity**	**Calcium (mg)**
Dairy products			**Vegetables and fruits**		
Blue cheese	1 ounce	150	Bok choy	1 cup	116
Cheddar cheese	1 ounce	204	Broccoli, cooked	1 cup	180
Cottage cheese	½ cup	68	Collard greens, cooked	½ cup	174
Cream cheese	2 ounces	46	Kale, cooked	½ cup	100
Ice cream, soft vanilla	1 cup	236	Orange	1 medium	52
Milk, whole	1 cup	291	Orange juice, calcium-fortified	1 cup	300
Milk, skim	1 cup	302	Romaine lettuce	1 cup	37
Mozzarella, part-skim	1 ounce	207	Spinach, cooked	1 cup	291
Parmesan	1 ounce	60	Swiss chard	1 cup	128
Ricotta, part skim	¼ cup	169	Turnip greens, cooked	½ cup	125
Romano	1 ounce	330	**Nuts and seeds**		
Swiss cheese	1 ounce	272	Almonds	1 ounce	70
Yogurt, frozen	½ cup	147	Pine nuts	1 ounce	38
Yogurt, nonfat	1 cup	415	Sesame seeds, unhulled	1 ounce	381
Beans and legumes			Sunflower seeds	1 ounce	33
Black beans, cooked	½ cup	30	Walnuts	1 ounce	27
Chickpeas, cooked	½ cup	45	**Other**		
Soybeans, cooked	½ cup	131	Canned salmon (with bones)	3 ounces	200
Soybeans, dry-roasted	½ cup	232	Sardines (with bones)	3 ounces	370
Soy milk	1 cup	46	*Source:* Adapted from U.S. Department of Agriculture		
Tempeh	2 ounces	47			
Tofu, firm	4 ounces	201			
Tofu, soft	8 ounces	111			

complicated." The truth is, you can. Your body doesn't seem to mind if you get calcium from supplements rather than from food. But getting your vitamins from healthy food is usually a better choice, because food can provide other nutrients too, such as fiber. Sometimes, however, the need is great and supplements are simple.

There are a few tricks to maximizing calcium absorption. For enough calcium to be absorbed, make sure you're getting at least 400 IU of vitamin D daily (from either your diet or a supplement). Some calcium supplements are already combined with vitamin D, which is ideal.

In supplement form, there are different types of calcium to choose from. Calcium citrate is a bit more easily absorbed than calcium carbonate (found in antacids) because you don't need a full stomach for calcium citrate to be absorbed. Calcium citrate seems to cause less gas than calcium carbonate. Calcium isn't easily absorbed in large amounts, so break up your supplement into two doses, and take it with meals. If you can't remember to take your supplement in divided doses, just take it all at once. It's better than not taking any at all or missing a dose.

Vitamin D Is Vital

Vitamin D also plays a big role in maintaining healthy bones. The relationship between calcium absorption and vitamin D is like a locked door and a key—vitamin D is the key that unlocks the door and allows calcium to be absorbed into your body.

Here's how it works: When your blood levels of calcium begin to drop, your body responds by converting vitamin D into its active form, which then travels to your **intestines** to encourage greater calcium absorption from food. Next, it travels to your **kidneys**, where it helps to soak up extra calcium that otherwise would be "thrown out with the trash" in your urine.

Vitamin D is produced in your skin when it's exposed to sunlight. But not all sunlight is created equal. In many parts of the world, especially in winter, there is not enough direct sunlight for your body to make all of the vitamin D it needs. For example, in the United States above 40 degrees latitude (north of San Francisco, Denver, Indianapolis, and Philadelphia), the winter sunlight isn't strong enough for vitamin D production. Also, darker skin color, sunscreen, window glass, clothing, and air pollution all decrease vitamin D production.

The major food sources of vitamin D are egg yolks, vitamin D–fortified dairy products, fish, and liver. Some calcium supplements and most multivitamins contain vitamin D; check the labels to learn how much each contains. Remember that many doctors are recommending much higher doses of vitamin D for health reasons besides bone health. To explore the issue of taking higher levels of vitamin D, visit www.vitamindhealth.org.

NOTE TO SELF

You need vitamin D in your diet to absorb calcium.

GOOD SOURCES OF VITAMIN D

- Fortified dairy products
- Egg yolks
- Fish
- Liver
- Sunlight
- Vitamin supplements

Exercise and Your Bones

The good news is that you can do a lot to improve your bone density, starting now. Weight-bearing exercises help to increase bone mass when you are young and maintain bone mass later in life. A weight-bearing exercise is anything in which your body works against gravity or your muscles lift weights. The higher the impact of the activity, the more it does for your bones. Running, fast walking, stair climbing, dancing, skiing, tennis, and aerobics are all excellent. The very best bone-building exercises for bone strength are resistance training—free weights, resistance machines, Pilates, and yoga.

Swimming is a great exercise to build the heart and **cardiovascular system**, but because water supports the bones rather than putting stress on them, it's not considered a good weight-bearing exercise for bone strengthening. Patients tell me, however, that you can do weight training in the water using foam-padded weights, and that it's actually very challenging. Regular swimming exercise won't do that for you, so if you are a frequent swimmer, you might consider adding on a weight-training class in the pool or on land.

Bone density that you build when you are young does not last a lifetime. To maintain the bone-strengthening benefits of weight-bearing exercise, you need to keep up the exercise regularly. If you stop exercising, the benefits wear off. Try to perform thirty minutes of weight-bearing exercise every day to build and maintain bones. Just as muscles grow stronger the more you use them, bones become denser the more demands you place on them.

Keep in mind that you need to do a variety of physical activities to strengthen all of the bones in your body. Change up your exercise routine often to keep your whole body healthy and to prevent boredom so you can stick with the program.

NOTE TO SELF

Swimming is good for your heart, but does not improve bone strength unless you also do aquatic weight training.

Your Joints: It's All About Connections

Your body has a few hundred joints that help you move. A joint is simply where two bones meet, but there's a lot more between them that gives your bones the ability to move in so many ways.

First, at each joint the two bones are shaped to work together, like puzzle pieces. The two bones are connected to each other with tendons and ligaments. They also have to be protected from rubbing against each other, so you'll find cartilage and lubricating fluid (synovia) between the bones, like cushions.

What Can Go Wrong with Your Joints?

You have four types of joints in your body, and each allows you to make a different kind of motion. Ball-and-socket joints, found in your shoulder and hip, allow lots of all-around movement. Gliding joints, found in your wrist and foot, allow somewhat less. Hinge joints, found in your elbows and knees, only move in one direction. And suture joints, found in the skull, allow very little movement at all.

What can go wrong? Injuries, disease, and erosion. All three can happen to your joints at any age. Let's look at these problems in detail to give you your best chance at having strong, flexible, and pain-free joints for a lifetime.

Arthritis Is for Old People, Right?

Inflammation and damage in the joints is known as **arthritis**. It's true that most arthritis happens to older people, but are you doing everything you can to protect your joints now? There are many different sources of arthritis, which is the leading cause of disability for people over the age of sixty-five. Some types of arthritis come from wear and tear on the joints over time and can be prevented in part. Other types of arthritis are caused by **autoimmune disorders** or infection and are not preventable. It helps to understand the causes, because a bit of attention to your joints when you are young can help you to keep them healthy as you age:

- **Juvenile rheumatoid arthritis:** This is the most common form of childhood arthritis, causing pain, stiffness, swelling, and loss of function of the joints. It usually appears before the age of sixteen and may come with rashes and fevers.
- **Rheumatoid arthritis:** If you have rheumatoid arthritis in your family history, please let your doctor know. This is an autoimmune inflammatory disease of the synovium—the lining of the joint. It causes joint pain, stiffness, swelling, movement restriction, and damage to the joints. It most often affects joints of the hands and feet, usually on both sides of the body equally. Rheumatoid arthritis occurs two to three times more often in women than in men. The difference might be due to some interaction of hormones and the immune system. The average age for the development of joint problems from rheumatoid arthritis is forty-five, but it can happen at any adult age.
- **Osteoarthritis:** Osteoarthritis is known as wear-and-tear arthritis, because the cartilage begins to fray and wear away from use. This is the most common type of arthritis, and it affects cartilage, the tissue that cushions the joint between the bones. Joint damage from osteoar-

thritis can cause pain and stiffness. This is probably the form that your parents and grandparents are getting.

Fibromyalgia and Why You Should Know the History of It

Imagine that it's 1980. You can't sleep even though you're exhausted. Pain in every joint and muscle follows you everywhere. You start to have trouble remembering things. You also start to feel depressed. You know that your pain isn't arthritis because your doctor has already looked for deteriorating joints and not found any. So s/he starts doing blood tests, radiology scans that are primitive by our standards today, and then more blood tests—but doesn't find anything specific. S/he gives you some painkillers. They don't work, so you ask for a higher dose. Now your doctor is worried that on top of having a problem that s/he can't figure out, you are now getting addicted to painkillers. The truth? Painkillers don't really work on fibromyalgia so the pills don't help. Nobody knew that back then though.

Having ruled everything else out, the doctor announces that you have fibromyalgia. Fibromyalgia is a chronic pain disorder in the bones, joints, and muscles. Pain, stiffness, and localized tender points occur especially in the neck, spine, shoulders, and hips. Although there is pain in the joints, there is no arthritis. Many people who have fibromyalgia also have fatigue and sleep disturbances. Nine out of ten of those who have it are women. We don't yet know why.

Fibromyalgia means "pain." *Fibro* means "fibrous tissue," like in your ligaments and tendons; *my* means "muscle;" and *algia* means "pain." But back in the 1980s, a diagnosis of fibromyalgia meant "you are crazy and this is all in your head." The government thought so too, which you found out when you applied for disability payments and were turned down. Even today, some women report that applying for disability payments is a longer battle than it is for "normal" disabilities.

It wasn't until 1990 that scientists developed specific diagnostic standards for fibromyalgia, and even then many people continued to believe that it wasn't real. Some still do. Why? Fibromyalgia doesn't show up on X-rays or in blood tests, so the diagnosis is based on the symptoms you report to the doctor, as well as tenderness the doctor elicits when examining your body's tender point sites. Probably, too, because it's mostly women who get fibromyalgia—we more often get the "crazy" label before a disease is identified.

Why is this history important? Because it shows how important it is for you to demand good health care and fight for a diagnosis. Don't let your problems go undiagnosed just because your doctor is biased, uneducated, out of date, or even lazy. And remember that female doctors can be biased, too. It wasn't only the male doctors and scientists who treated fibromyalgia sufferers so poorly. (And to be fair, it's not only women who are treated with suspicion when there's a newly identified illness. Think about how our veteran soldiers have been treated after the past few wars. Many have come home with unidentified physical ailments, initially labeled as reactions to stress, that were later found to be real diseases caused by exposure to war-related toxins.)

Doctors now have specific criteria from the American College of Rheumatology to diagnose fibromyalgia, and there is medicine to treat it that has been approved by the U.S. Food and Drug Administration. We still don't know what causes fibromyalgia, but new work is finding some common threads in infection, previous injury, and genetics. And we're doing a better job managing the symptoms.

Systemic Lupus Erythematosus

Lupus is a challenging autoimmune disease in which the immune system damages the body's own cells and tissues, harming the joints, skin, kidneys, heart, lungs, blood vessels, and brain. Nine out of ten people who have lupus are women. Lupus is three times more common in African American women than in Caucasian women. The gender difference may be caused by hormones. The racial difference may be due to a genetic component. Nobody knows how lupus starts or why. We only know that it is not contagious.

People who have lupus experience what are called flares of the illness, followed by remission. These flares can be very difficult and even life threatening.

It's possible to live a long and vibrant life with the right medical care for lupus, but even working with the very best doctors is not a guarantee. If you have lupus, be sure that you are seeing a doctor who stays up to date on the latest developments. The Lupus Foundation of America (LFA) estimates that some 1.5 million Americans and about 5 million people worldwide have lupus. It affects primarily women of child-bearing age, which the LFA defines as fifteen to forty-four years old, but anyone can get lupus—men, children, teenagers, and all races and ethnic groups.

What Can You Do to Protect Your Joints?

Picture yourself as an older woman. Imagine yourself climbing stairs easily, moving your shoulders and arms without pain, and going for long walks without your knees complaining. How can you get from here to there?

Watch Your Weight

You can protect your joints by keeping your weight in a healthy range. Every pound of your weight puts four pounds of pressure on your knees and hips! The good news is that even a small weight loss can lead to a big reduction in risk. One study showed that women who lost an average of eleven pounds over ten years cut their risk of osteoarthritis in the knee by half.

Avoid Injuries

Take good care of those joints. Although exercise is really important, injuring your joints, ligaments, or cartilage or breaking bones can lead to arthritis later in life. Young people with knee injuries are nearly three times more likely to have arthritis by the time they reach age sixty-five. Football, basketball, soccer, and gymnastics are especially likely to cause joint injuries. But just about any type of exercise can be dangerous if you aren't careful.

To avoid injuries, be cautious when you start anything new. The American Academy of Orthopedic Surgeons recommends following the 10 percent rule when you start a new exercise routine: increase your physical activity by no more than 10 percent at a time. For example, if you normally run 1 mile a day and you want to increase it, try running 1.1 miles the next week. This gradual increase will allow you to get fit and avoid injuries.

Variety in exercise helps with the boredom factor and also reduces repetitive-stress injuries by varying the way the body moves. A fitness routine that combines several different kinds of exercise—including aerobic activity and strength training—will help keep your joints strong and flexible while reducing the risk of injury, especially from overuse.

NOTE TO SELF

Follow the 10 percent rule: increase your involvement in any activity no more than 10 percent at a time. If you are comfortable jogging for 10 minutes, add 1 minute when you want to improve—not another 10 minutes!

Your Bones and Joints: A Solid Investment

Don't take your bones and joints for granted because they feel strong and healthy today. Invest in them like you would a savings account when you're young, and they'll pay you back with a strong, solid, and flexible skeleton for life.

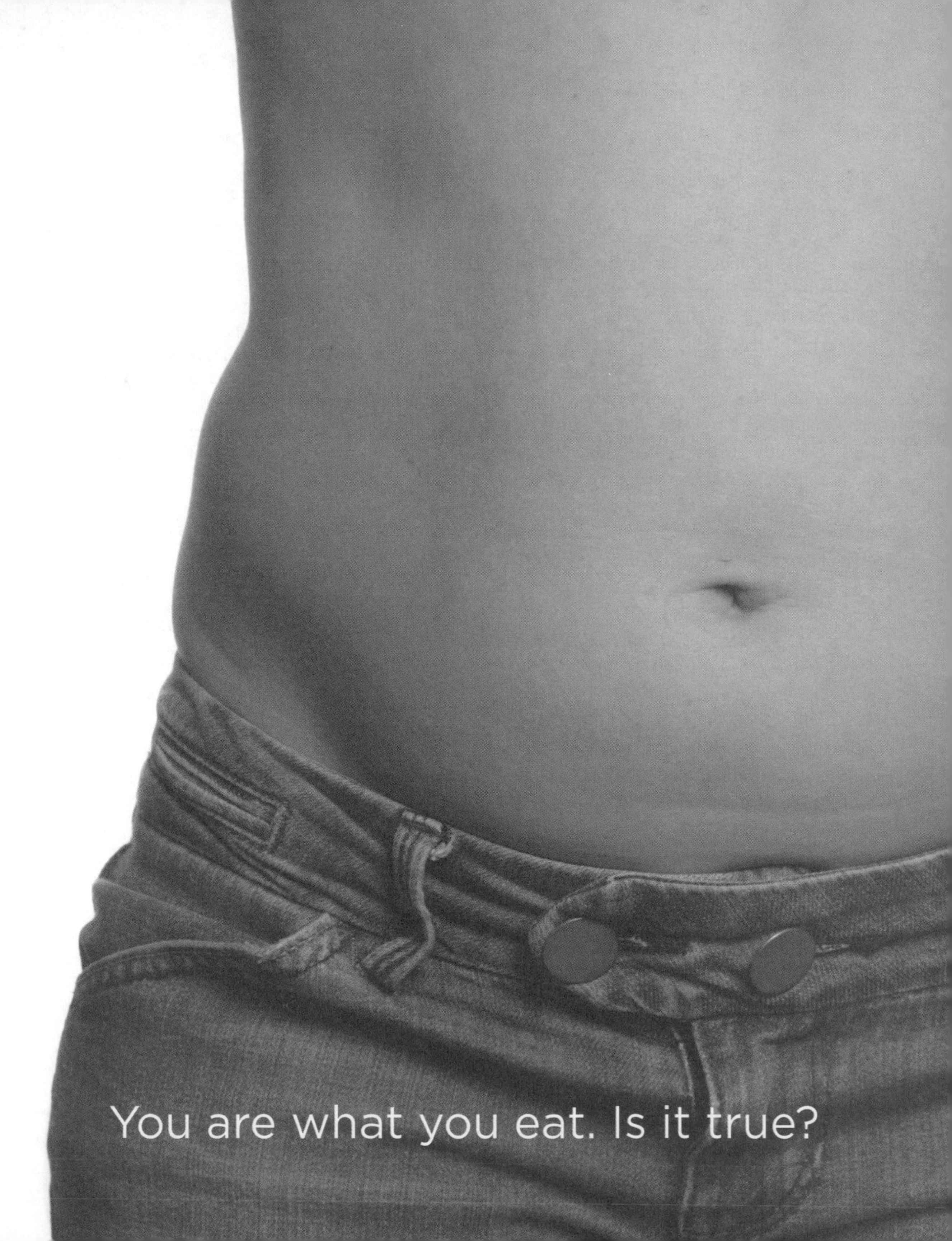
You are what you eat. Is it true?

your stomach and intestines

To find out whether you really are what you eat, don't ask your friends.

Just sit down with Grandma. You'll find out that modern life gives your innards a beating—and if you don't eat well, you'll pay for it in about fifty years. How? Listen to Grandma and count how many times you hear her say something like "I'd give my life for a bowel movement." If drinking games weren't such a bad idea, this would be a good one.

Your digestive system is the route your food takes from your mouth to the toilet. This system hasn't changed since humans first arrived on the scene. It was made for people who had short lives, no lattes, and no doughnuts. It wasn't built to last for people who eat the way we eat. The good news: You can take care of your innards now and have a healthy body later.

Let's start by understanding what happens to your food after you eat it. This is a short summary of everything your high school biology teacher tried to teach you about digestion.

The Long, Strange Trip of a Chicken Caesar Wrap

You unwrap your wrap and dig in. You just flicked on your digestion switch by taking a bite. First, your **saliva glands** turn on the shower, wetting the food and breaking it down with **enzymes**. The **carbohydrates** are already turning into sugar.

Now your tongue pushes the clump of food to the back of your throat, where a trapdoor called the epiglottis covers your windpipe, or **trachea**. The food goes down the hatch, which is your **esophagus**. Your esophagus does its work now, moving the food along with a muscle action called **peristalsis**. It's kind of like when you squeeze a tube of toothpaste.

At the bottom of the esophagus, another trapdoor (the lower esophageal sphincter) opens and the food lands in the stomach—all in less than a minute from the time you took your first bite. Wow!

Your stomach is a wrinkly, muscular bag. It tosses the food around like a washing machine, adding digestive chemicals including **stomach acid**. Your stomach's inner surface is covered with **mucus** to protect it from the acids, because otherwise it would, honestly, eat itself.

Later we'll talk about how important it is to keep stomach acid in the stomach and nowhere else. It is powerful stuff, and you want to have as little contact with it as possible over a lifetime. You already know this from what you see when you throw up. When stomach acid travels back up the esophagus, we call it **heartburn** or **acid reflux**. Controlling these now can help you to avoid very serious problems later.

Along the digestive path, the gallbladder, liver, and pancreas all have jobs to do. The **liver** is your body's filter for everything bad you expose it to—alcohol, drugs, **bacteria**. It is your largest organ, and you can't live without it, so you should limit the filter work it has to do. When your liver works too hard—to the point of damage from excessive alcohol, for example—you can develop an extremely serious problem (cirrhosis) that may be fatal. Your liver also makes **bile**, which your body needs to break down fats.

Your **gallbladder** stores the bile, a couple of ounces at a time. At some point in the life of many women, the gallbladder will make **stones**. These can be a minor or major problem. If you find yourself with pain, nausea, vomiting, fever or chills, and jaundice—a yellow color in your skin or eyes—call your doctor right away. Women are more likely to develop gallstones than men. Other risk factors for gallstones include being overweight, being pregnant or on the Pill, taking **estrogen**, having a family history of gallstones, having **diabetes**, taking drugs to lower **cholesterol**, or being of Native American or Mexican American heritage.

Your **pancreas** produces some of your digestive enzymes and **insulin**. (Diabetes is caused when the pancreas can't produce insulin.)

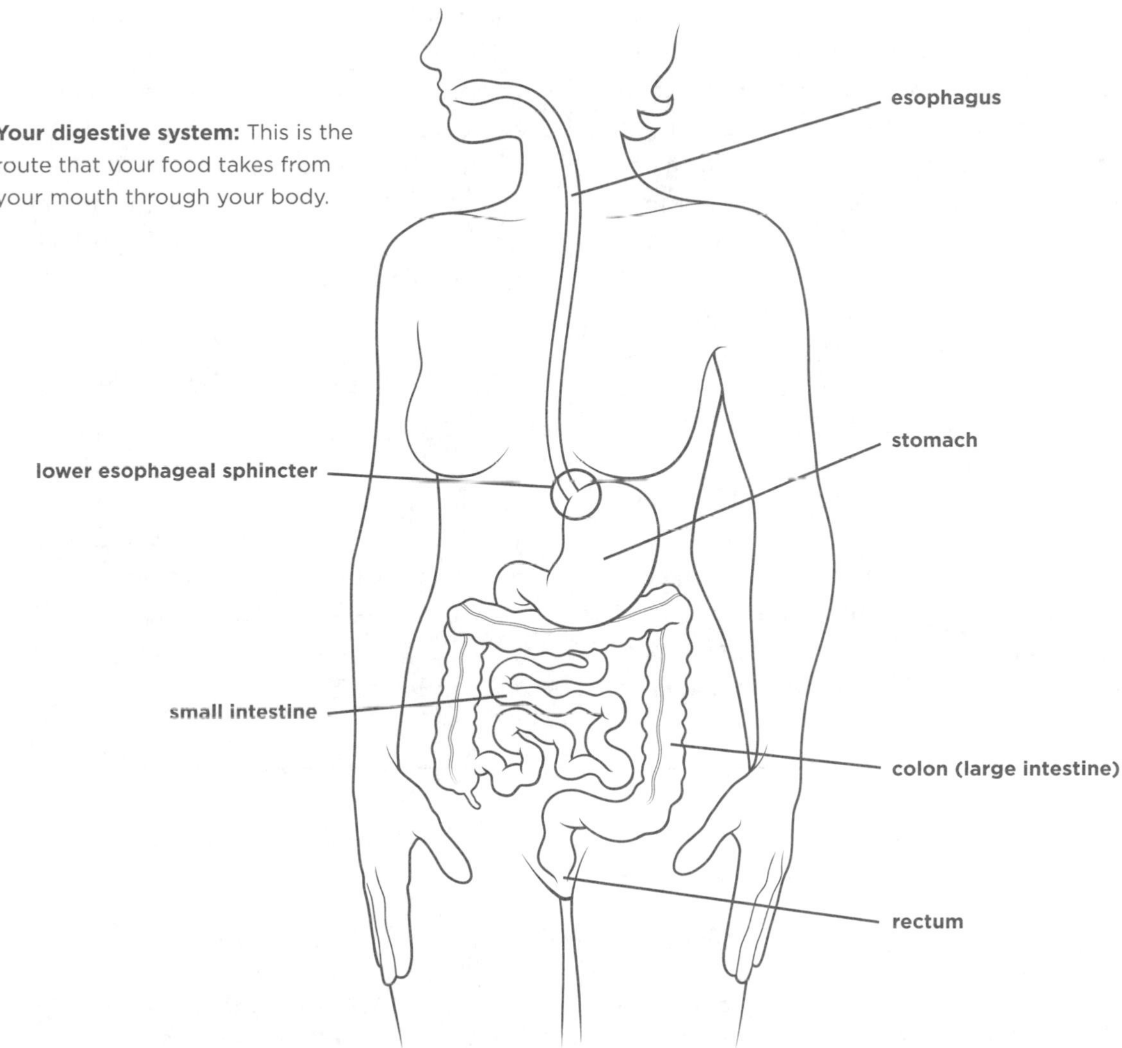

Your digestive system: This is the route that your food takes from your mouth through your body.

Back to the chicken Caesar wrap, which has now been doused with digestive acids in your stomach. Another trapdoor will open and your food will move into your **bowels**. These trapdoors are usually called **sphincters** (pronounced SVINK-ters)—this one is the duodenal sphincter. You have probably also heard the word *sphincter* used by boys to mean "stupid person," as in "Ask her out, Sphincter!" or "A sphincter says what?"

The first stop for your wrap is the **small intestine**; just below the stomach. The small intestine is a long, twisty tube. Why is it so big and curled up? It takes a lot of surface area to do its job. This is where food really starts to feed your body. If you had just a short straight tube to the toilet from here, you would be unable to absorb vitamins, for example. This process takes time, and a slow, winding road is better for the job.

In the small intestine, more chemicals and liquids mix up the food. The walls of the intestine are covered with **villi** (rhymes with "Will I"), which are like the hundreds of bristles on a soft brush. These villi absorb the good stuff, the **nutrients**, from your food and pass them into your **bloodstream**.

Your Caesar wrap has now traveled twenty feet in about three hours. Your body has used everything it can from the wrap and sends its leftovers into the **large intestine** or **colon**. It's wider and shorter than the small intestine, and drier inside. It's where poop is made. It will take between eighteen hours and two days for what's left of the wrap to travel five feet, getting drier, smaller, and harder as it goes. Now it will wait at the **rectum** until you go to the bathroom, when it will be pushed out through your **anus**.

Keep Your Digestive System Flowing

The tale of the chicken Caesar wrap shows you how the system is *supposed* to work. You already know that it doesn't always happen so smoothly, so let's take a look at how to care for your digestive system and what to do when it has problems.

REAL LIFE FACT: Put Out the Fires of Heartburn and Acid Reflux

- **Rev down by revving up your stress-reducing techniques.**
- **Limit alcohol or avoid it completely.**
- **Do not eat lying down or lie down after you eat.**
- **Eat small meals and eat them slowly.**
- **Cut your use of coffee, tea, and soda.**
- **Cut down on deep-fried food, red meat, high-fat food, sugar, peppers, onions, and hot spices.**
- **Limit chocolate and dairy products.**
- **Replace high-acid foods (citrus fruit and tomatoes).**
- **Wait a couple of hours after a meal before you exercise.**
- **Quit smoking; it causes heartburn.**
- **Take an over-the-counter antacid, but if you need one more than once or twice a week, call your doctor.**
- **Sleep with your torso elevated.**
- **Obesity worsens heartburn, but even a small weight loss will improve it.**

Heartburn and Acid Reflux

Let's start with your stomach. Your stomach is designed to make a powerful acid to break down food, but the modern diet piles on even more acid. If your typical day includes juice, a hot dog, cheese, fish and chips, fried onion rings, and a soda, your stomach is turbocharged.

Sometimes that acid goes up your esophagus, which may be a sign of **acid reflux** disease. Because you know acid could digest your stomach if it wanted to, you know it's not good to let it eat away at your throat. That can cause difficulty swallowing, hoarseness, and even **asthma**. You want to keep your stomach acid controlled, which means you want to reduce episodes of **heartburn**. Heartburn is the burning feeling that means you just threw up into your mouth a little bit.

How do you control stomach acid? Eat smaller meals and eat slowly. Chew each mouthful well (and really savor your food). Fat and sugar get heartburn raging—minimize the amounts you eat. Do not lie down when eating or after eating. Avoid alcohol. Avoid high-acid foods. Control acid with antacids if necessary. If your heartburn doesn't get better, call your doctor. Heartburn really can cause damage if you don't take care of it.

Many women who have never had heartburn develop it during pregnancy. Be sure to discuss yours with your doctor and see what approach you should take. For my patients, I recommend a combination of smaller, more frequent meals, stress reduction, sleeping with the torso elevated, and taking antacids and other medications to lower stomach acid. My pregnant patients remind me that they don't sleep anyway, but I still want them to try.

Ulcers

An **ulcer** is any sore in the stomach, lower esophagus, or intestine. When you have an ulcer, you may experience nausea, heartburn, weight loss, stomach pain, stomach pain during the night, stomach pain that goes away when you eat or chew antacids, or a burning sensation at the back of your throat.

We used to think that ulcers were caused by stress or a poor diet, either one increasing

REAL LIFE QUESTION: When should I call the doctor about digestive problems?

- **When your problem is getting worse.**
- **If you have nausea and vomiting.**
- **If you have new symptoms.**
- **When you have chest pain. Heart problems and even heart attacks in women can be disguised by heartburn—although rarely at your age.**

your stomach acid. People still say, "That's giving me an ulcer." Now we know that a certain bacteria can live in the lining of your digestive system and irritates the lining, making it much more likely to be damaged by stomach acids. The good news: **Antibiotics** and medicine to reduce your gastric juices can treat most ulcers.

Lactose Intolerance: Can You Banish the Bloat?

Many people have some degree of lactose intolerance. Lactose is a sugar found in milk that is too big a molecule to pass through the wall of your small intestine and enter the bloodstream. To digest milk, your small intestine produces an enzyme called lactase, which breaks lactose down into smaller pieces so your body can absorb it. If you don't have enough of this enzyme, you have lactose intolerance. Some people have a little lactase, some have almost none. Lactose intolerance is not an all-or-nothing issue. Some of us produce just enough lactase to have a glass of milk without suffering, while others can't even have milk in their coffee.

Why? The lactose is left behind in your intestines, unabsorbed. The normal bacteria in the intestine go to work on it. This is a bit like adding sugar and yeast to wine to make champagne bubbly. The bacteria ferment the lactose, making bubbles of gas in your bowels. Welcome to the stomach bloating, gas, cramps, and diarrhea you get after eating dairy products. These symptoms may be mild or severe, depending on the degree of lactase deficiency and the amount of lactose you eat.

The amount of lactase you make can change as you age; many people produce less of it as they get older. Lactase deficiency may also be inherited. It seems to be more common after adolescence and in certain ethnic groups, including people of African, Asian, Mexican, Mediterranean, or Jewish descent. Some digestive diseases or injuries to the small intestine can also cause your body to produce less lactase.

Lactose intolerance is not the same as milk allergy, in which your body responds with hives and other symptoms of an allergic reaction. If you suspect that you're allergic to milk products, tell your doctor so that you can find out how severe your allergy is.

REAL LIFE FACT: Symptoms of Lactose Intolerance or Lactase Deficiency

These happen after you eat milk products:

- **Abdominal cramps**
- **Bloating**
- **Diarrhea**
- **Gas**
- **Nausea**

REAL LIFE QUESTION: Should I be tested for lactose intolerance?

If you think it's necessary, sure. Or just go dairy free for a few days and then eat some milk products. Keep a food journal of how you feel. Most people get a clear diagnosis one way or the other.

How do you know that you have lactose intolerance? Let's say that about an hour after chowing down on pizza and ice cream with a group of friends, your stomach rumbles and you begin passing gas. To find out if lactose intolerance is the culprit, your doctor may recommend a few tests:

- **Breath hydrogen test:** When the bacteria in your colon ferment lactose, hydrogen gas is released, which then passes out through your lungs. During a breath hydrogen test, you drink a lactose solution. A few hours later you blow into a special mouthpiece and your breath is collected for analysis.
- **Lactose tolerance test:** Your doctor will measure your lactose absorption by taking multiple blood samples before and after you drink a solution of lactose.
- **Simple home test:** Avoid milk products for several days. Then, when you have a morning off, skip breakfast and drink two large glasses of milk. If you have symptoms in the next four hours, lactose intolerance is likely.

What can be done? First, you'll adjust your diet to figure out how much lactose you can tolerate. The strictness of your low-lactose diet depends on how much the symptoms bother you. This is a good time to keep a Digestion Journal (see the appendix, Tools to Use).

A low-lactose diet restricts milk and milk products. Many common foods contain hidden sources of lactose, so check labels to see whether foods contain milk derivatives such as casein, whey, skimmed milk, nonfat milk solids, and hydrolyzed whey. By the way, nonfat milk and low-fat milk trigger lactose intolerance symptoms just as whole milk does. The amount of lactose is the same in low-fat milk.

Fortunately, most people with lactose deficiency can tolerate small amounts of lactose, such as half a cup of milk, and don't need to follow a diet that is completely lactose-free. Following are some tips for dealing with lactose intolerance.

- Small amounts of lactose-containing foods eaten several times a day may be better tolerated than a large amount taken all at once.

- Foods and drinks containing lactose are better tolerated if they are taken with other foods.
- Heated milk products such as cream soups, cocoa, custard, or cooked puddings are tolerated better than unheated foods.
- Yogurt that is labeled "contains active culture," aged cheeses such as Cheddar or Swiss, and processed American cheese have reduced amounts of lactose. So do certain brands of milk, such as Lactaid, which you'll find in the supermarket.
- Goat's milk is lower in lactose, so it can be a good alternative to cow's milk. You either like the taste or not.
- Nondairy milks, such as soy milk and rice milk, generally don't contain any lactose.
- Butter and margarine (which may contain whey or other dairy components) in moderation are usually not a problem.

For occasional use, an over-the-counter lactase medicine can be helpful, especially for travel and special occasions. It can keep a family wedding trip from becoming a nightmare.

Chanel No. 2: Mommy, I Burped in My Pants

Every human on earth, and most of the animals, produce gas. The word *fart* has ancient roots in every language and culture and can be found in Chaucer and plenty of other writers you had to read in school. I don't know why we all need to pretend that it never, ever happens to us. There must be a reason, something from our hunter-gatherer past, but who knows? The cultural pressure is so strong that when your mother is alone and she farts, she says, "Oh, excuse me," out loud.

Some farts, gas, tooters, trouser coughs, and butt trumpets start as air. You swallow air all day, especially when you chew gum, drink through a straw, or drink a soda. Air is odorless. If the air makes it all the way to the rectum without passing much food along the way, the gas you pass may be odor free, too. If gas could be measured, we would find that even the Queen of England produces at least two cups of it a day and passes it at least a

REAL LIFE QUESTION: Are eggs dairy products?

You may think this is a trick question, but it's not. So many stores put eggs where the milk is—because that's where the refrigeration is—that many people think eggs are a dairy product in some way. They're not; they just need to stay cold.

REAL LIFE FACT: The Shy Pooper

Could this be you? In your innocent days, you thought everybody else's leave-behinds in the bathroom smelled like a sewer except yours. Then one day you left your wallet in the bathroom and went back. It took you a while, but because you knew you were the only one who had been in there, you realized the truth: Yes, you made that smell. Your nose, like everyone else's, couldn't smell your own smell because of sensory adaptation. That was the last time you pooped anywhere but your own house when nobody was home.

Some of us couldn't care less. We know that every human in history has pooped, so who cares? Or we think the whole process is kind of funny and we make jokes about it. But if you are a shy pooper, you will go to great lengths to pretend that no such thing ever comes out of you. Staying with the boyfriend's family? You'd rather creep out to the woods than use the toilet. Nobody knows why some of us are this way, but you feel nobody can help you. To you, spraying the air or lighting a match merely advertises your sins.

Today, there are toilet drop products that you can add to the toilet before you go. These can help to eliminate odor. Plenty of women are going to use these, and it will no doubt make many of us feel more comfortable sharing bathrooms with the world. But if you find yourself at the boyfriend's house and you didn't know there was that much milk in Mom's cooking, you're going to have to relax. Roll your eyes, say excuse me, and ask if they have a dog you can blame—and smile. Seriously, who wouldn't love you?

dozen times. This may be the reason she has so many dogs—to blame it on.

The normal bacteria in your colon, however, release gas that contains sulfur. Bacteria in your colon is a good thing that helps to keep it healthy, but sulfur is a nonmetal element that's common throughout nature and smells just awful. Certain foods, usually carbohydrates, help gas-producing bacteria to thrive in your colon. That's when you'll clear the room.

Beans (all types), milk, and milk products may be the worst offenders. Onions, celery, carrots, raisins, apricots, prune juice, wheat products, and brussels sprouts take second place. You can reduce gas by avoiding them, but you may not have to cut out these foods completely. Sometimes you can tolerate them in smaller amounts. Three glasses of milk a day may give you trouble, but one glass may not. Sometimes adding foods to your diet slowly can build tolerance. Many people complain that adding fiber to the diet causes gas, for example. But adding fiber gradually over

NOTE TO SELF

If you are nervous about gas as you adjust to a high-fiber diet, occasional use of over-the-counter antigas products (such as Beano) may help.

a period of several weeks can usually reduce the problem.

Burp Basics

Burping is your body's way of releasing the air you swallow each time you eat or drink something. Your stomach does not make air or gas on its own. If burping is a problem for you, you can try to reduce the number of times you swallow air when eating or drinking. Avoid chewing gum and hard candy (lots of swallowing, lots of air). Avoid sipping through straws and drinking from bottles. Avoid food or drinks that contain air, such as sodas or whipped cream, and fizzy medicines that you plop into water. Eat slowly. Gulping brings a lot of air into the stomach, as any teenager who can burp the alphabet will demonstrate.

Bloated Belly

You feel like a small balloon that has been blown up too much. You feel swollen, filled with air. The first time you feel this way you will think you have a serious disease because you feel so uncomfortable.

The good news: Bloating by itself is not serious, and it can be treated with medications that stimulate contractions in the stomach and upper intestine, moving the food and fluid along and reducing abdominal bloating.

Bloating usually happens when the normal contractions of your stomach and upper intestine aren't working well, and it happens more often in women than in men. Certain foods, eating too quickly, anxiety, even your menstrual cycle can cause bloating. Irritable bowel syndrome and inflammatory bowel disease (coming soon, later in this chapter) can also cause bloating, so it's important to discuss it with your doctor and to see if dietary changes can help.

Bloating may also be caused by delayed emptying of the stomach, called **gastroparesis**. Your doctor may order certain tests such as **X-rays** and **endoscopy** to see what's going on. Endoscopy is a visual scope examination of the stomach using a flexible, lighted tube. There are other medical conditions, such as malabsorption and certain types of bowel surgery, in which excessive gas may be produced. These conditions need to be treated by your doctor.

REAL LIFE FACT: The Gassiest Place on Earth?

I don't know why this is true, but try walking into a yoga class full of middle-aged women. After an hour of twisting and holding poses, the women will stand up for the first time and it's like fireworks in there.

NOTE TO SELF

It's true: a rapid change to a high-fiber diet is going to give you more gas. Add fiber slowly and your body will adapt. Start your high-fiber diet when you have a few days to see how much gas it will give you. A patient once reported, "My high-fiber diet provided the entertainment during a conference call at work this morning."

Addicted to white rice? Start by mixing a half portion of brown in with your white. Eventually you'll like the nutty flavor of brown rice. Maybe you can limit the bowl of white rice to nights out for Asian food. And no, fried rice is not whole-grain rice just because it's brown.

The Challenges of a Low-Fiber Diet

Your large intestine is designed to be filled with waste from the fiber you eat. All of those indigestible bits of whole grains hold water in the large intestine, where it passes through the body. Now imagine a typical American low-fiber diet: scrambled eggs with white toast, a beef burger with a white bun, chicken and mashed potatoes.

Your large intestine becomes as parched as a desert. It will keep trying to find water to soak up for your body, but it can't find any. Your poop will become harder and harder, which will make you **constipated**, which will foster **hemorrhoids**. About 80 percent of us will have constipation someday, and of course an occasional problem is normal. But throw in a few bubbly sodas and it's amazing we don't explode.

What to do? Fiber, water, and more fiber. Eat whole-grain breads, brown rice, beans, fruits, and vegetables, with plenty of water. A high-fiber diet adds bulk to your poop, which keeps more water in there and stimulates your colon to move things along.

It also helps to have a routine, with a particular time that you relax and go to the bathroom. Yes, people bring newspapers and magazines in. There are plenty of us who wouldn't know a thing about the world if it weren't for the daily bathroom time. You don't want to overdo sitting on the toilet, because that can cause hemorrhoids. But the simple step of making an appointment with your toilet can help with constipation.

Can't I Just Take Fiber Pills and Powders?

If you want your digestive system to work for a lifetime, you can't fill it with processed junk food every day and expect a fiber pill to push it all along. Taking fiber supplements occasionally is fine, but you are better off changing your diet first. You'll be getting more of the nutrients you need instead of living a low-fiber life and then letting the supplements repair the damage.

What about laxatives? Never depend on them. They are for urgent problems. Laxatives stimulate your bowels to move, yes. Unfortunately, your bowels are lazy, and laxatives are like having a personal assistant. Your body will get used to laxatives quickly, and then you'll have a hard time without them. Laxatives should be reserved for very occasional use when even a high-fiber diet isn't working. It's a lot like using water to put out a fire. It works, but it's much better to keep the fire from starting in the first place.

Do yourself a very big favor and start adding fiber to your diet now. Sure, your young system can tolerate the abuse of a modern junk-food diet. But get ahead of aging by having a healthy diet now, and your body will thank you for it.

NOTE TO SELF

Start on the high-fiber path today. Add just one piece of fruit to what you normally eat every day. Pick a portable fruit—apple, orange, clementine, pear, peach, plum, banana—so it will be easy to eat when you're on the go. And no, coconut milk in a frozen drink is not a fruit serving.

Will Yogurt Keep Me Regular?

Here's another one of those science versus experience versus advertising problems. There was a zillion-dollar ad campaign promoting yogurt as a way to keep you regular. It was targeted at women. The campaign used an actress we all love.

Well, the company was sued for promoting a medical use of food without any scientific evidence. It turns out that the claims they made couldn't be proven. They settled for $35 million to reimburse women up to $100 per person. That's probably worth it for the company, because their business made giant gains. And most women never saw the news that the claims can't be proven.

Worst of all, the company that advertised its yogurt said that it did scientific studies. According to court reports, they did do studies, but the studies didn't actually prove their own claims!

But if it's working for you, then keep eating it. Yogurt is healthy food, it's good for you, and if it keeps your bowels humming, go ahead.

What about eating yogurt to prevent diarrhea? When you're taking antibiotics, everyone, including some doctors, will recommend that you eat yogurt or take pills containing certain of yogurt's ingredients. This is supposed to balance your normal intestinal bacteria that have been killed off by the medicine. The problem is that there isn't any scientific evidence to prove that this works. Does it work for you? Again, yogurt is good for you, so go ahead.

So why is scientific study so important? When I recommend a treatment to my patients, I want to know that it's been proven to work, that it's safe, and that the manufacturer is making the same dose every single time. Many "natural" medicines are not quality controlled, and you have no way of knowing what dose you're getting, no matter what the label says. Yogurt is at least controlled by the food part of the Food and Drug Administration. So eat yogurt frequently if you like it, but when a company starts making big claims, be skeptical.

REAL LIFE QUESTION: What is a normal bowel movement anyway?

You've seen them all. You produce a wide range of sizes, colors, textures, frequency, odor, and floatability. Yes, these are all catalogued on the Internet. I have my own favorite category, "poops at other people's houses." You produce something so big that it cannot be flushed, and you stand there panicking as the water level rises. By now, another guest is knocking at the door. "Will you be out soon?" says a desperate sounding fellow guest.

These variations are not a medical problem. But if you have black or very dark poop, tell your doctor as soon as possible. S/he will want to look for any fecal occult blood (more about that later). Other than that, tell your doctor if you have frequent diarrhea or constipation. Tell your doctor if you have changes in your bowel habits or poop that don't go away. Green poop that lasts for a day does not need to be called in, but a change like this that lasts for a week should be.

(Need a solution to the wide poop problem? You can let it sit until it softens, then flush it. In a pinch, honestly, you can cut it up, preferably with a disposable knife, then flush it down—and throw that knife away wrapped in toilet paper.)

Diverticula: -Osis and -Itis

In medical terminology, *-osis* indicates a condition, and *-itis* indicates an infection. You can blame a low-fiber diet for the first problem: **diverticulosis**. This starts when the small, hard poops of a low-fiber diet arrive in the large intestine. When the inner layer of the large intestine makes a bulge through the outer layer, it is called diverticulosis. The large intestine has to work harder, tightening in on the poop and weakening the muscles of the outer wall.

You probably won't know that you have any diverticulosis until a hard poop or some food waste or germs get stuck. It will become infected and will cause pain and fever. Now you have **diverticulitis**. If you have intestinal pain and fever, always, always call the doctor. Diverticulitis can be treated before it gets any worse. You'll give your colon a break from food, take medication to stop the infection, and then start a high-fiber diet. A case of diverticulitis can be a powerful motivator for you to increase your fiber.

Ever traveled with friends? You'll notice quickly how different we all are from each other. One friend stuffs her colon with a low-fiber, high-acid, all-meat diet all day, topped off with high-sugar alcohol drinks at night, yet spends just a minute in the bathroom once a day. Friend number two? Her troubles start at the airport. "Flying wrecks me. I'll be constipated all day and then have diarrhea for the rest of the week." She is true to her word. Her bowels are a big part of her life, and now you know why everyone else lets her have the one single room.

The rest of your group is different every day. Spicy food might trigger some trouble. You might be eating at restaurants for every meal, which means you're getting a lot more butter in your diet than normal, whether you can see the butter or not. At least one of your friends will be lactose intolerant yet want to try every new cheese she sees. Twenty minutes after leaving a restaurant, at least two of you will be racing for any bathroom you can find, with a case of explosive diarrhea that just can't wait.

These problems—short-term issues with a cause you can figure out—happen to everyone. Never been constipated, you say? Wait until you are breastfeeding and forget to drink your water that day. No trouble with diarrhea? Maybe you haven't traveled much. Other issues are longer term. And that's our next subject: colon problems that don't go away.

Irritable Bowel Syndrome

If you hve irritable bowel syndrome (IBS), your bowels just don't work right, and it can be pretty bad. You'll be constipated one day and racing to the toilet with diarrhea the next, or both on the same day. Then you'll have a crampy urge to go but be unable to.

IBS means that your bowels are extra sensitive to change and cause you discomfort. It is **chronic**, and you may have good days and bad.

No one has proven the cause of IBS. It may be that the nerves and muscles of the large intestine are just not working as they should. For some people, it means a minor inconvenience. For others, it keeps them housebound, unable to travel even short distances for fear of an emergency bowel movement.

IBS often runs in families and often begins before age thirty-five. It's much more common among women, who make up 75 percent of IBS cases. Many of these women notice either a flare-up or some relief from IBS just before their periods.

REAL LIFE QUESTION: Why do some people need a colostomy (a bag to collect their poop)?

If your bowels won't function, you may eventually have to have part of them removed. You may have older relatives who have had a colostomy. If this happens to you, part of your bowel will be removed and your poop will come out into a little plastic bag that you carry at your waist and have to empty yourself. So keep your bowels healthy. Keep them moving.

REAL LIFE QUESTION: What is constipation?

Constipation is having fewer than three bowel movements a week, or having difficult bowel movements frequently. Call your doctor if this doesn't go away or if you also have bleeding, cramps, nausea, vomiting, or unexpected weight loss.

Testing for IBS

There is no medical test that confirms IBS, but your doctor still may want to run a few tests to make sure that you don't have something else. You may have **polyps** in your colon, you may have trouble tolerating **gluten**, or you may have an **inflammation** brewing.

These tests may include a few ways of looking into your colon. In a lower GI (gastrointestinal) series you'll be given a barium enema, which means you'll have a thick liquid put into your bowels through, yes, your **anus**. The liquid helps an X-ray to see problems. If you are the first of your friends to have a **barium enema**, you'll be telling them about it later and probably laughing quite a bit. Your job on the exam table is to keep that barium in, which is not easy, so you'll notice that the X-ray technicians move pretty quickly to finish up before you can't hold it anymore. Want to make them run faster? Just say, "Oops."

If your doctor recommends an endoscopy, a thin tube that has a tiny camera on it will be threaded up into your bowel, viewing along the way. At your age, it is less likely that you would have a **colonoscopy**, in which the whole colon is reviewed by the tiny camera, but it's possible.

These tests all require preparation. You may have to fast after midnight, or spend a day on a liquid diet, or drink medicine that clears your bowels. You may have to take a day off. Please be sure to follow the instructions carefully, even if you have to spend a day on the toilet. If you don't and your bowels are not completely empty, you will just have to go back again.

If you have to have a colonoscopy, you cannot do the prep and leave the house, because you don't want to be more than ten feet from a toilet. Anybody who tells you otherwise has a very twisted sense of humor. I recommend trying to get an early Monday morning appointment for bowel testing, so you can do your prep work on the weekend and not have to fast too long on the day of the test.

There is no cure for IBS, but there is plenty of diet-based treatment. Everyone's IBS is triggered by different foods, so the best way to develop your food plan is to keep a notebook. You might start by eliminating the usual suspects, which are milk products (cheese, ice

REAL LIFE QUESTION: What is diarrhea?

Diarrhea is a noticeable increase in the frequency of your bowel movements and a liquid consistency. For most people this means four or more movements a day, but for you it may be fewer if you normally go only a few times a week. Call your doctor if it doesn't go away, you have pain or fever, you are vomiting, you are becoming dehydrated (dry mouth, dizziness, darker urine), you are pregnant, or you have recently traveled overseas.

cream, yogurt, milk), chocolate, alcohol, caffeine, soda, beans, broccoli, and cabbage. You can try adding foods back in one at a time and keep track of any symptoms. You might also start by taking notes before making any changes. By writing down when, what, and how much you eat, what symptoms you have, and when you have them, you and your doctor may identify which foods bother you most.

Some foods make IBS better. If you have constipation, add fiber: bran, whole wheat bread, cereal, fruits, and vegetables. Add these to your diet a little at a time to let your body get used to them. Too much fiber all at once may cause gas, which can trigger symptoms. Large meals can cause cramping and diarrhea in people with IBS, so try eating four or five small meals a day.

If necessary, your doctor may give you medicine to help with symptoms, such as laxatives to treat constipation or antispasmodics, which slow contractions in the bowel and may help with diarrhea and pain. Although you don't want your lazy bowels to become

REAL LIFE FACT: Some Symptoms of Irritable Bowel Syndrome

Contact your doctor if these IBS symptoms sound like yours:

- **Crampy pain in the stomach area**
- **Hard, dry, infrequent stools (poops)**
- **Frequent loose poops**
- **Mucus in the poop**
- **Swollen or bloated stomach area**
- **Feeling like you haven't finished a bowel movement**
- **Gas**
- **Heartburn**
- **Feeling uncomfortably full or nauseated after eating a normal-size meal**

dependent on medicine, having treatments available can give you peace of mind on special occasions or when traveling.

Stress and IBS

Although stress may not cause irritable bowel syndrome as far as we know, it can worsen symptoms. Meditation, acupuncture, yoga, massage, exercise, hypnotherapy, counseling—any and all of the stress-reduction methods described in chapter 3, Stress and Your Body, may help.

You'll need to try different activities to see what works best for you. Staying well-hydrated by drinking six to eight glasses of water each day can help, and exercise is the magic pill for both stress reduction and energy improvement. A holistic approach that takes the whole body into consideration is the best way to deal with this chronic problem.

Inflammatory Bowel Disease

Although IBS is hard to live with at times, inflammatory bowel disease (IBD) is a more chronic and lifelong problem. It is an **inflammation** of the lining of your bowels. Think about when you have a cut on your finger. The skin around the cut becomes a little red and puffy as it heals. That's inflammation, caused by an increase in blood and **white blood cells** that are rushing in to stop infection. Now, imagine if an inflammation started up on its own, but not because you had a cut. Blood flow increases and **white blood cells** fly in, but there are no invaders to fight and they don't stop. That's IBD. There are also two related intestinal disorders, ulcerative colitis and Crohn's disease, that are together known as inflammatory bowel diseases.

IBD starts with diarrhea, crampy abdominal pain, bloating, gas, and bloody poops. These symptoms often happen daily, and because these are symptoms that can apply to many conditions, including IBS, people often suffer for years without being diagnosed. Usually, looking inside the bowel with a colonoscope and taking a few biopsies of the lining confirms the diagnosis. Most people are diagnosed in their twenties or thirties. Although anyone can get IBD, people of eastern European Jewish (Ashkenazi) descent are more prone to it.

Ulcerative colitis is confined to the lining of the colon and can often be cured by surgery. Crohn's disease can be a disease of either the small or large intestine or both. It inflames the full thickness of the bowel. Fistulas, the name for any openings in the bowel to the skin or other organs, can develop. The inflammation can block the bowel. With Crohn's there can even be disease outside the bowel, such as in the eyes, **joints**, and skin. Surgery can treat but not cure this problem.

IBD is like other chronic diseases, such as diabetes and asthma. With proper care, most people lead normal and active lives. It's another reason to call your doctor if you are having trouble with bowel movements—crampy abdominal pain, bloating, gas, diarrhea and/or constipation, or bleeding. (Blood in your poop—not just on your toilet paper—should always be checked. More on this later in the chapter.)

I encourage any patient with IBD to stay informed about developments in the field. There are very active advocacy groups, support groups, and ongoing research efforts to understand and treat IBD. The Crohn's and Colitis Foundation of America (www.ccfa.org) is a good place to start.

Celiac Disease

Celiac disease, also known as gluten sensitivity, is one of the most underdiagnosed bowel disorders, yet one of the most common. It is a chronic, inherited disease and, if left untreated, can ultimately lead to malnutrition.

Gluten intolerance is the result of an abnormal immune response to the ingestion of gluten—found in wheat, rye, and barley—that damages your small intestine. Instead of being absorbed by your body, nutrients pass through the small intestine, resulting in pain, bloating, cramps, and, ultimately, malnutrition. Common triggers include stress, surgery, pregnancy, and viral infections.

Celiac disease can start in childhood or in adulthood. Anyone can get celiac disease, but a northern European or Celtic heritage can be a factor.

Symptoms

Celiac disease is a multiple-symptom, multisystem disease. It's difficult to diagnose, because it presents symptoms that can mimic other problems. The classic symptoms of celiac disease are diarrhea, bloating, weight loss, anemia, chronic fatigue, weakness, bone pain, and muscle cramps. Other symptoms can include constipation, constipation alternating with diarrhea, and premature **osteoporosis**. Overweight people may also have undiagnosed celiac disease.

Children may show behavioral, learning, or concentration problems; irritability; diarrhea; a bloated abdomen; growth failure; dental enamel defects; or projectile vomiting. Others will have symptoms such as weakness, **migraine** headaches, nerve problems such as tingling of hands or difficulty walking, or other conditions that are unexplained or do not respond to usual treatment. Patients are frequently misdiagnosed as having IBS, spastic colon or bowel, or Crohn's disease.

Diagnosis and Treatment

Initial testing for celiac disease is a blood test. (In case you are wondering, they are looking for antiendomysial **antibody**, antigliadin antibody, and tissue transglutaminase.) If these tests suggest that you have celiac disease, a digestive system specialist (a **gastroenterologist**) will then take small intestine tissue biopsies during a colonoscopy to confirm the diagnosis. S/he is looking for damaged **villi**.

If your doctor believes that you are likely to have celiac disease because you have the symptoms and a family history, you might start with a gluten-free diet before testing begins. If this stops your symptoms, the diagnosis is likely.

Having a gluten-free diet means cutting out wheat, rye, barley, and all forms of these grains. Medication is not normally required, unless there is an accompanying condition, such as osteoporosis. You'll notice improvement within days of starting the diet.

The small intestine is usually completely healed in three to six months in children and younger adults and within two years for older adults. When I say "healed," this means the person now has villi that can absorb nutrients from food into the bloodstream. To stay well, people with celiac disease must avoid gluten for the rest of their lives. Eating any gluten, no matter how small an amount, can damage the small intestine. The damage will occur in anyone with the disease, including people without noticeable symptoms. Depending on a person's age at diagnosis, some problems, such as delayed growth and tooth discoloration, will not improve.

What Is a Gluten-Free Diet?

A gluten-free diet means not eating foods that contain wheat, rye, and barley or anything made from them—that means most bread, pasta, cereal, and many processed foods.

The good news: Gluten-free products are increasingly available from regular stores, and people with celiac disease can eat a well-balanced diet. They can use potato, rice, soy, amaranth, quinoa, buckwheat, or bean flour instead of wheat flour. They can buy gluten-free bread and pasta, and can order a wide variety of products from specialty food companies.

I'll be honest. Some of the foods taste awful, and many people just end up switching to rice and potatoes instead of having gluten-free bread. But I suggest you try them, because these foods are improving all the time. By the time you are reading this, there may be some delicious options.

Checking labels for "gluten free" is important, as many corn and rice products are produced in factories that also manufacture wheat products. Hidden sources of gluten include additives such as modified food starch and stabilizers. Wheat and wheat products are often used as thickeners, stabilizers, and texture enhancers in foods. Gluten is also used in some medications. Meat, poultry, eggs, fish, rice, fruits, vegetables, dairy products, nuts, seeds, beans, and legumes do not contain gluten, so people with celiac disease can enjoy them.

NOTE TO SELF

Recommending that people with celiac disease avoid oats is controversial because some people have been able to eat oats without triggering symptoms.

Prevention

There is a clear genetic link to celiac disease, so it can't be completely prevented. Three factors seem to play a role in when and how celiac disease turns up: the length of time you were breastfed, the age at which you started eating gluten-containing foods, and the amount of gluten you eat. Some studies have shown, for example, that the longer a person was breastfed, the later the symptoms of celiac disease will appear and some symptoms may not develop. So if celiac disease runs in your family, consider this one more reason to breastfeed your children.

A Pain in the Sit-Upon: Hemorrhoids

Hemorrhoids (pronounced *HEM-er-oids*) are common and usually not serious. They are also annoying and painful. Hemorrhoids are **veins** in your anus and rectum that are swollen and inflamed. About half of U.S. adults have hemorrhoids by age fifty.

The modern diet is a big culprit. Low-fiber diets cause harder poops, which result in straining to have bowel movements. This increased pressure causes engorgement of the hemorrhoids. Pregnancy is another suspect, causing increased pressure on the veins.

The most common symptoms of hemorrhoids include itching, bleeding, and pain, as you know from the many TV ads (which make you squirm when you actually have hemorrhoids). Fortunately, effective treatments are available for hemorrhoids. In many cases self-care and lifestyle changes will do it. More serious cases might require surgery. Hemorrhoids need to be treated only when they bother you. If you notice external hemorrhoids but they don't bother you, you can leave them alone.

NOTE TO SELF

While hemorrhoids are no fun, they are both common and treatable.

Types of Hemorrhoids

Internal hemorrhoids can't be seen or felt because they are inside your rectum. You don't have pain-sensitive nerve fibers in your rectum, so these don't usually cause pain.

Straining or irritation from your poop can injure a hemorrhoid's fragile surface and cause it to bleed. The most common sign of internal hemorrhoids is a small amount of bright red blood on your toilet tissue or in the toilet bowl after you poop. One patient "popped" an internal hemorrhoid and saw so much blood in the toilet that she paged her doctor in the middle of the night. This is one of those body events that is scary-looking but normal.

Occasionally, straining can push an internal hemorrhoid through the anus. If a hemorrhoid sticks out like this, it can cause pain and irritation, and you may feel as if your rectum is still full when it's empty.

External hemorrhoids can be felt as a little grapelike projection right around your anus. These hemorrhoids tend to be painful. Sometimes blood may pool in an external hemorrhoid and form a clot (thrombus), caus-

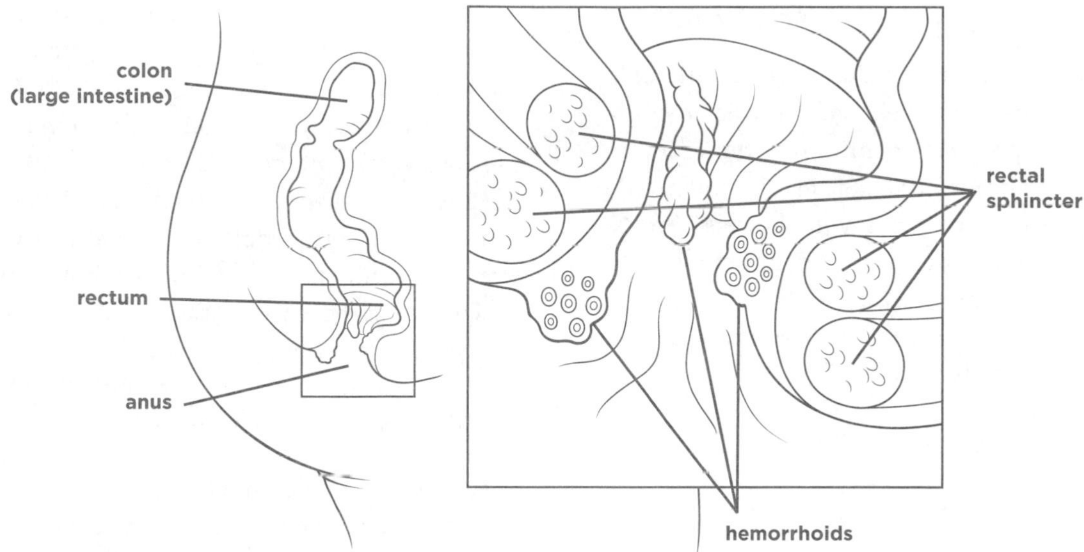

Hemorrhoids are swollen and inflamed veins in your rectum and anus. They can bleed or cause pain with bowel movements.

ing severe pain, swelling, and inflammation. When irritated, external hemorrhoids can itch or bleed.

Hinder Your Hemorrhoids

To reduce the chance of hemorrhoids:

- **Eat high-fiber foods:** fruits, vegetables, and unrefined grains. This softens the poop and increases its bulk, which will help lessen the straining that can cause hemorrhoids.
- **Drink plenty of liquids:** This keeps poops soft.
- **Use fiber supplements if necessary:** Over-the-counter fiber supplements can help, but you should not use them in place of fiber in your diet. Be sure to drink plenty of water when you take a fiber supplement, or it might make things worse!
- **Exercise:** It stimulates your bowels and keeps things moving. The longer that poop sits in your intestine, the harder the poop will be.
- **Go as soon as you feel the urge:** If you wait to pass a bowel movement and the urge goes away, your poop can become dry and be harder to pass.
- **Ask your doctor about stool softeners:** Under some conditions (after surgery or when taking certain pain medications) stool softeners are very important.

Making Hemorrhoids Worse

Hemorrhoids can develop from any increase in pressure in the veins in the lower rectum. It's also possible to inherit a tendency to develop hemorrhoids. Sit on the toilet only long enough to move your bowels. Persistent straining or prolonged sitting can lead to engorged hemorrhoids.

Common sources of pressure that can cause hemorrhoids include:

- Constipation and extra straining
- Diarrhea
- Sitting or standing for a long time
- Obesity
- Heavy lifting
- Pregnancy and childbirth

When Rectal Bleeding Isn't Hemorrhoids

Not all rectal bleeding is from hemorrhoids. It can also be caused by other, more serious conditions such as colorectal **cancer** or bleeding from other parts of the **gastrointestinal** system. If rectal bleeding occurs along with a marked change in bowel habits or if you're passing black or maroon poops, call your doctor right away. Get emergency care if you notice large amounts of rectal bleeding, lightheadedness, dizziness, or faintness.

Treating Your Hemorrhoids

If you have mild discomfort, you can try over-the-counter creams, ointments, or pads containing witch hazel, or a topical anti-inflammatory agent containing hydrocortisone. Soaking in a warm bath can help. The warm water relaxes the anal sphincter muscle spasm, which can reduce pain.

Ice can relieve the pain of a blood clot in an external hemorrhoid. If a blood clot has formed within an external hemorrhoid, your doctor can remove the clot with a simple incision, which may give you relief.

For persistent bleeding or painful hemorrhoids, treatment options include:

- **Banding hemorrhoids:** Your doctor places one or two tiny rubber bands around the base of an internal hemorrhoid to cut off its circulation; the hemorrhoid "dies" and falls off. This simple procedure—called rubber band ligation—is done in the doctor's office and is effective for many people.
- **Sclerotherapy:** A chemical solution is injected around the blood vessel to shrink the hemorrhoid.
- **Infrared light:** A one- or two-second burst of infrared light can cut off circulation to small, bleeding internal hemorrhoids.
- **Surgery:** If other procedures haven't been successful or if you have large hemorrhoids, your doctor can remove tissue in a procedure called hemorrhoidectomy. The surgery is done with either local anesthetic combined with sedation, a spinal anesthetic, or general anesthetic. It's usually done as an

outpatient procedure but could require an overnight hospital stay. You may hear that this is a very painful procedure to recover from, but some newer surgical techniques may decrease the amount of pain that some people experience.

Colon Cancer

Why does Katie Couric keep telling everyone to get a colonoscopy? Because she lost her husband to colon cancer. Early detection of colon cancer catches it when it's most curable.

Most women do not need to be screened for colon cancer until they are fifty or older, because colon cancer doesn't usually happen until later in life. Your doctor may recommend screening for colorectal cancer at your age if you have any of the following factors:

- Parents or siblings who had colon cancer before the age of fifty-five.
- A personal history of colon polyps or having a close relative with multiple colon polyps (familial polyposis). Polyps are **benign** growths. They are removed because there is a chance that cancer may be in them.
- A history of inflammatory bowel disease, such as ulcerative colitis or Crohn's disease.

If your doctor recommends that you have a colonoscopy at your age, you should do it. Many deaths from colorectal cancer can be avoided if screening tests are done. When colorectal cancer is found at an early, localized stage, the five-year survival rate is about 91 percent. The trouble is, only about 40 percent of people are getting properly screened.

How do we screen for colon cancer? In the years before you have a colonoscopy, we have a couple of screening methods for young women. These don't tell us if you have colon cancer, but they tell us when it's a good idea to do more tests.

Digital Rectal Exam

You may or may not have a rectal exam as part of your physical, depending on your family history and risk factors. This exam is useful in detecting some polyps and cancers, but it's limited only to the rectal area. Unfortunately, the word *digital* here does not mean "electronic." It means "with a finger." Your doctor inserts a gloved, lubricated finger into your rectum to look for any abnormalities.

Fecal Occult Blood Test

The name fecal occult blood test sounds like a Wiccan ritual, but it just means to look for blood hidden in your poop. Your doctor will ask you to do this if your family history, risk factors, or any symptoms make it necessary. You take home a test kit and collect tiny samples from three bowel movements in a row, then mail the kit to a lab for analysis. Traces of blood in your poop are a possible sign of cancer or benign polyps, which may be very early warnings of cancer. If the test shows blood, you should then get a colonoscopy.

Colonoscopy

The colonoscopy is another test not usually needed before age fifty, unless your family history or risk factors call for it. I'm including this information here because if you do need one at your age, I want you to have the information you need.

Let's start with the preparation. Your doctor will give you complete instructions. Everything you have heard about this test is true. You don't eat, you drink special liquids, you take some medication, and you make a zillion trips to the toilet with diarrhea (and finally, pure liquid). Do not plan to go to work or anywhere else. There's really nothing you can do about this, except keep reminding yourself that this is important and if all goes well, you won't need another one for a long time.

Try to get the earliest appointment of the day for your colonoscopy if that's convenient for you. It's harder to avoid hunger pangs when you're awake, so I usually recommend that you always try for the earliest appointments for any procedure that requires fasting.

You'll be sedated before the procedure. This is not general anesthesia at all. It is a gentle sedative that puts most people into a twilight sleep. If you are feeling pain, tell the doctor!

The colonoscope is a long, flexible, lighted tube that is inserted through the rectum to examine the entire colon. If a polyp is found, it can be removed and examined. The doctor may also find an adenoma, which is like a polyp but may be closer to a cancer warning sign. Polyps and adenomas do *not* mean you have cancer. They mean it was a really good idea for you to have this procedure now. If your parents haven't done it yet, feel free to get on them about it.

After the test, you'll rest in a recovery area, where they are basically waiting for you to fart. One patient, not knowing that, tried her best to avoid making a sound. Finally the nurse told her what they wanted. She delivered. Once you do, they know that everything is moving normally, and you'll be able to go home soon.

Because you have been sedated, you will have to be picked up. *Do not drive.* A taxi or public transit doesn't count. You need someone you know who can drive you home and make sure you're safely settled in when you get there. If you find yourself unable to think of anyone who can pick you up, your first job after the colonoscopy is to make some reliable friends! To find a willing driver, try talking with acquaintances who are nice people and offering to take turns driving for colonoscopies or other medical tests. Don't have any acquaintances? A lot of churches will step in—call the ones in your neighborhood and most will be able to help you.

Double-Contrast Barium Enema

Sometimes you can have a double-contrast barium enema instead of the colonoscopy.

You don't need to do both. An enema of barium sulfate is given through the rectum to partially fill and open the colon. When the substance is removed, the colon is then partially inflated with air to expand the colon and increase the quality of the X-rays that are taken. What goes in must come out, of course, so expect plenty of gas.

Preventing Colon Cancer

Nobody knows exactly how to prevent cancer in everyone. Over the years of cancer study, however, we've noticed that some people with common habits are less likely to have cancer. It's not a guarantee, but it's a very good idea to follow these habits.

Foods to Fight Cancer

What foods give your body its best chance against colon cancer? We know that in countries where people eat a lot of fiber, the colon cancer rates are lower. There are many good reasons to increase your fiber, but the fiber itself doesn't prevent cancer—it's all the fruit and vegetables you eat that help.

Your diet makes a big difference. People who get 1,000 to 1,500 mg of calcium a day—the level that is currently recommended for healthy bones—have a decreased chance of getting colon cancer. Calcium regulates the growth of the cells that line the inside of your colon.

On the bad-news side, meat and **saturated fat** may be broken down in your body into **carcinogens**, which can increase colon cancer risk. Cooking meats with high heat generates **nitrosamines**, which may be carcinogenic. Many processed meats are preserved with nitrites that may be converted to nitrosamines in your body.

Fruits and vegetables are good protection. Remember the **free radicals** we talked about in chapter 4, Your Skin? Well, those free radicals don't just come from sunlight and oxygen. They are natural by-products of your body's metabolism. These free radicals may cause damage to your body, including colon cancer. Luckily, fruits and vegetables can help.

Exercise—Yet Another Reason to Do It

Your large intestine is a bit like a sewage treatment plant, recycling the food your body can use and storing the remainder as waste for disposal. The longer waste sits in your intestine, the more toxic materials from the food you eat go back into your body. Exercise stimulates peristalsis—the wavelike muscular contractions that push poop through your colon—and speeds up the process. Exercise can decrease colon cancer risk by up to 40 percent, although we don't exactly know why. Exercise also decreases the incidence of other risk factors for colon cancer, such as obesity and diabetes.

Smoking—Yet Another Reason Not to Do It

I keep repeating the advice not to smoke because it's associated with so many diseases, including colon cancer. Smoking may cause 12 percent of fatal colon and rectal cancers. Inhaled or swallowed tobacco smoke moves carcinogens to your colon. Tobacco use also appears to increase polyp size. In general, the bigger the polyp, the higher the chance it will become cancerous. So add this to your list of reasons to stop or never start smoking.

Obesity and the Bad Apple

Obesity, defined as having a BMI (body mass index) of 30 or greater (see page 116), increases your risk of developing colorectal cancer. Obese men seem to be more at risk for colon cancer than obese women. The difference may be related to body type. Certain body types seem to have more risk than others, and having extra fat around your middle (an apple shape; see page 112) increases colon cancer risk more than having extra fat in the thighs or hips (a pear shape).

REAL LIFE FACT: I Almost Had Cancer!

When you search for the cause of unexplained symptoms you're having and you come across lists of possibilities, you will often find cancer included. Handling this information calmly until you have actual test results is a good life lesson to learn. Cancer is almost always the least likely diagnosis when you're young, but you still might panic at the very thought of a cancer test.

Let's say your doctor thinks an early mammogram or an ultrasound is a good idea because you have a family history and you have lots of fibroids (harmless lumps) in your breasts. Lumpy breasts are hard to examine reliably, and your doctor is wise to be cautious. You go for the tests. Now you have to wait a few days or weeks for the results.

How will you spend that time?

The best use of your time and energy is, of course, to forget about it. Some people can do that. Many people can't. It's normal to worry. What's not so normal is long spells of crying, sleepless nights, and talking about nothing else. If you're experiencing all of these, you need to work on stress reduction. Again, worry is normal; high anxiety is not. Exercise it off, or see a therapist or your doctor. Learning to handle stress is one of the best things you can do for your life, for your body, for your relationships, and for your family.

Doctor's confession: Every medical student I know secretly believes they have dengue fever, bacterial meningitis, and leprosy, based on what they are reading in their medical books. Your doctor knows how you feel!

Exercise may lower colon cancer risk by decreasing abdominal fat. There appears to be a relationship between physical inactivity and **insulin resistance**, which leads to your body's making too much **insulin**.

Insulin is a hormone whose main job is to help your body regulate sugar (**glucose**) levels. It also affects cell growth. Scientists are beginning to think that high insulin levels, known as **hyperinsulinemia**, may be what connects a sedentary lifestyle to an increased risk for colon cancer. Also, a diet high in refined sugars and low in dietary fiber causes hyperinsulinemia. The male tendency toward abdominal distribution of fat and higher insulin levels may account for the stronger association between high body mass index and risk for colon cancer in men than in women.

So You Really *Are* What You Eat!

Give your body the best future it can have. Treat it well. Keep it moving. Have the tests your doctor recommends. Don't make your body work overtime by eating toxic waste. Fill your diet with fruits, vegetables, healthy fats, healthy **protein**, and whole grains. And remember: eat fiber, drink water, repeat.

Now we'll move from your bottom to your top, to take an inside look at your very important neck and spine.

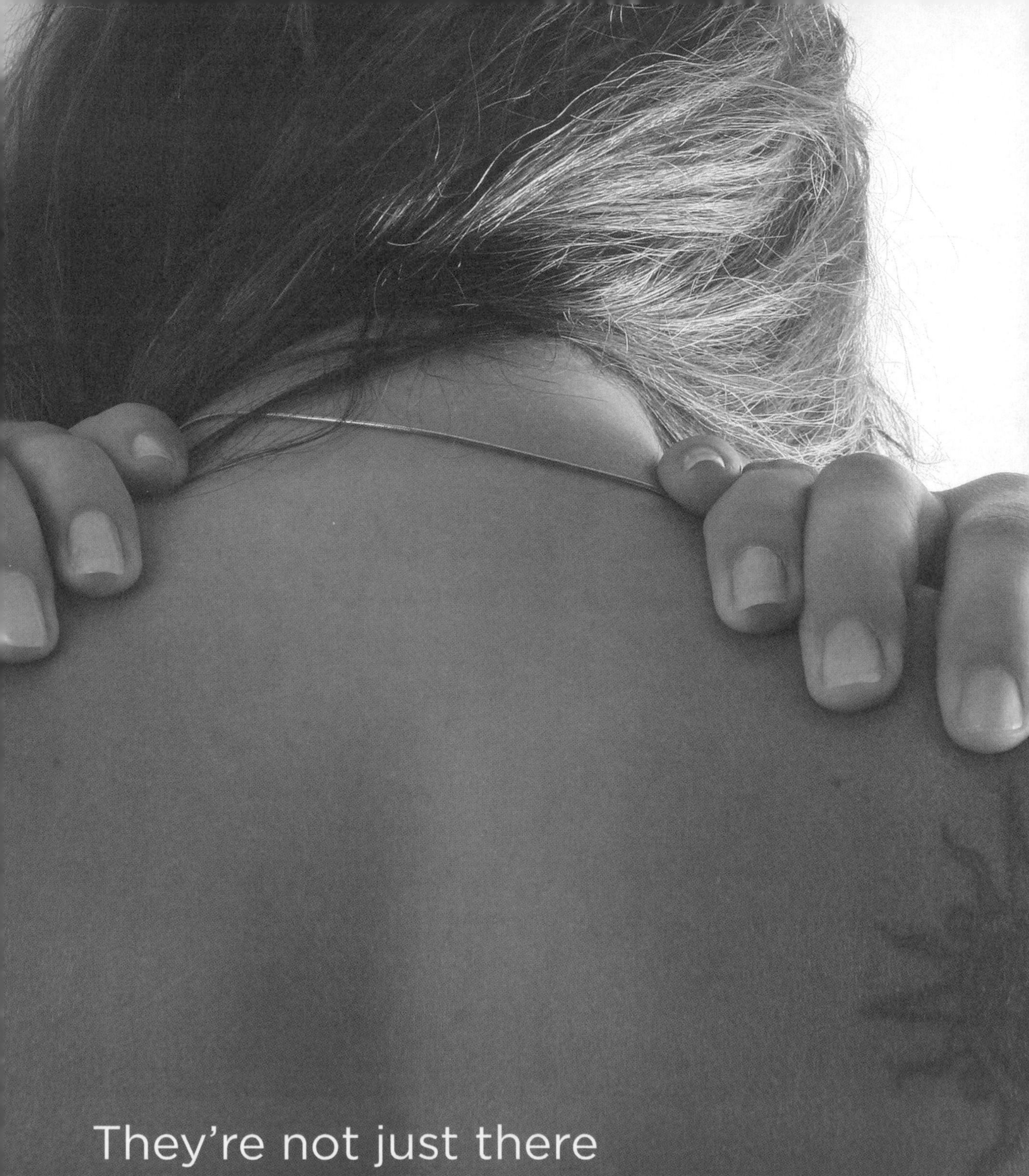
They're not just there
to hold up your head.

your neck and spine

How important is your neck? You can tell how essential it is by looking at the differences in species all over the planet. Something must be going on! The giraffe's long neck reaches the highest leaves without competition from other animals. Swans need a long neck to fish, and pelicans use theirs to carry food. Horses balance themselves with their necks like we do with our arms. Even an English bulldog benefits from his neck, which makes him look adorable despite his underbite and being a terrible snorer with a house-clearing gas problem. According to the American Kennel Club, this short-necked fellow is one of our top ten most popular dogs.

There is even great variety among human necks, from the think, muscled neck of a football player or a boxer to the long graceful neck of a ballerina. The rest of your spine is essential, too. Its most important job, other than keeping you upright, is to contain the spinal cord. The cord carries the brain's messages after they pass through the neck. If you're breathing, that's a spinal cord signal. Running? Reading? Coughing? All messages carried by the spinal cord.

The spine's structure is made up of a series of vertebrae (the plural form, pronounced *VER-te-bray*; the singular form is *vertebra*, pronounced *VER-te-bra*). These are groups of bones that protect the spinal cord. Believe it or not, a giraffe has only seven vertebrae in its neck—the same number as we short-necked humans have.

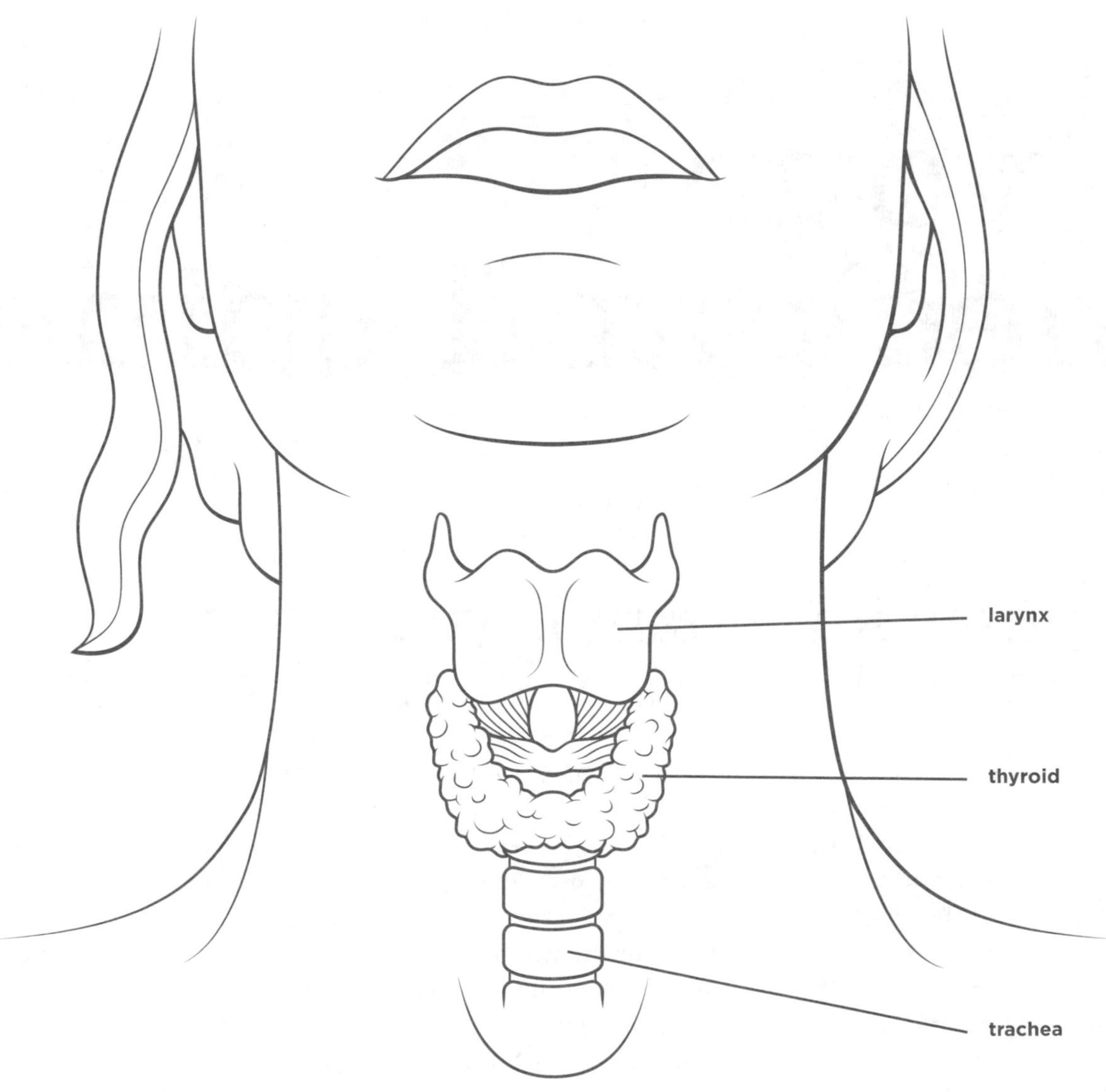

Your neck: It includes muscles, bones, nerves, blood vessels, your windpipe (trachea), your esophagus, your voice box (larynx and vocal cords), and your thyroid gland. The thyroid is a butterfly-shaped gland at the front of your neck that produces hormones.

The Neck: Your Body's Superhighway

Your neck is the only connection between your body, your head, and your brain. Traveling along this major road system are little trucks carrying the vital elements that keep your body alive: blood, hormones, oxygen, and food. Your neck includes muscles, bones, nerves, blood vessels, your windpipe (**trachea**), your **esophagus**, your voice box (larynx and vocal cords), and your **thyroid gland**.

Your blood vessels run through your neck from your heart to your brain and back, bringing nourishing oxygen and removing **carbon dioxide**. Food and oxygen pass through different tunnels on their way through your neck to your stomach and lungs.

Inside your neck there is one major part that does not extend into the body or the head: your thyroid gland. It produces hormones that work far from where they are made. It controls your body's hormones, energy, and metabolism.

The neck also acts like a telephone for your body: it's the central pathway for communication from command central (your brain) and the rest of your body.

Like any good highway, yours needs maintenance. Your spine and posture keep the road straight and give it structure. Mom was right: sit up straight! The nerves that travel through here are protected by the spinal cord, so keep it strong and healthy.

A Pain in the Neck and More: What Can Go Wrong?

Some neck pain is life threatening, such as pain from a heart attack or a major trauma. Fortunately, this type of neck pain is rare for young women. Simple strains and **musculoskeletal** pain is what's most likely causing any pain you have. This kind of neck pain is related to the ways you sit, stand, walk, move, work out, and nearly everything else. If you live at the computer or have a desk job, it's essential to keep your back and neck healthy so you don't develop **chronic** pain as you get older.

Our ancestors must be laughing. We took these desk jobs because we didn't want the hard life of the factory or the farm, and now it turns out we get chronic pain from sitting still! So, what can you do now to protect yourself later?

Posture: Walk Like You're on the Red Carpet

More good advice from Mom! Using good posture and body mechanics protects your back and neck when you are sitting, lying, standing, and lifting. Hold your head up, too, but make sure you are moving and not sitting stiffly. You'll just get tired otherwise.

Tension headaches can be caused by locking up your neck and back **joints**, as well as by mechanical factors that set you off balance. That can lead to stress and tension, which can cause neck and back muscle spasms, all of which can lead to neck pain. To avoid stress-induced neck and back pain, keep good posture and get up from your desk regularly to walk around. And practice these six ways to have a healthy body: exercise, eat healthy meals with plenty of calcium, control your weight, reduce stress, get enough sleep, and don't smoke. Having good posture is a good number seven.

Doesn't that sound easy? Nope. Posture alone is a difficult change for many people. So make changes one day at a time, sometimes even an hour at a time. For posture improvement, start at fifteen minutes with your back straight but not stiff, your head high but still flexible, and your joints loose. Do this until fifteen minutes is easy. Then add another fifteen minutes.

You probably think I'm trying to turn you into a finishing-school graduate walking around balancing books on your head. No, that's not what we're after. Watch actors walk down the red carpet on TV one night and you'll notice that all of the women and most of the men have improved the one thing a stylist and a surgeon can't help: their posture. Shoulders back, head high, stomach in, back straight.

Pillow Talk

Bed pillows should support your head, neck, and shoulders, keeping them lined up, which relieves pressure in your neck and shoulders. Pillows create a feeling of comfort and ease, which helps you to get a good night's sleep.

Choose a pillow that keeps your head and spine in natural alignment in your favorite sleeping position. The human neck curves slightly forward (to hold up your head in a balanced way), and it's important to maintain this natural curve when lying down. Based on your body size and personal preference, your pillow should be about four to six inches high.

Are you a back sleeper? Your pillow should properly support the natural curvature of the cervical spine (the section of spine in your neck). Putting a pillow beneath your knees helps ease back strain by relaxing your lower back. Side sleeper? The pillow should be a bit higher so that your spine maintains a straight and natural line. And putting a pillow between your knees in this position is good for your back. Stomach sleeper? To be honest, try to shift to your side if you can. It's better for your spine.

NOTE TO SELF

Sleeping on your side with a pillow between your knees is good for your back!

Monitor Management

The heights of your computer monitor and your keyboard are important for neck health because they determine your neck and back posture. Poor posture can cause pain in your neck and back, and headaches too.

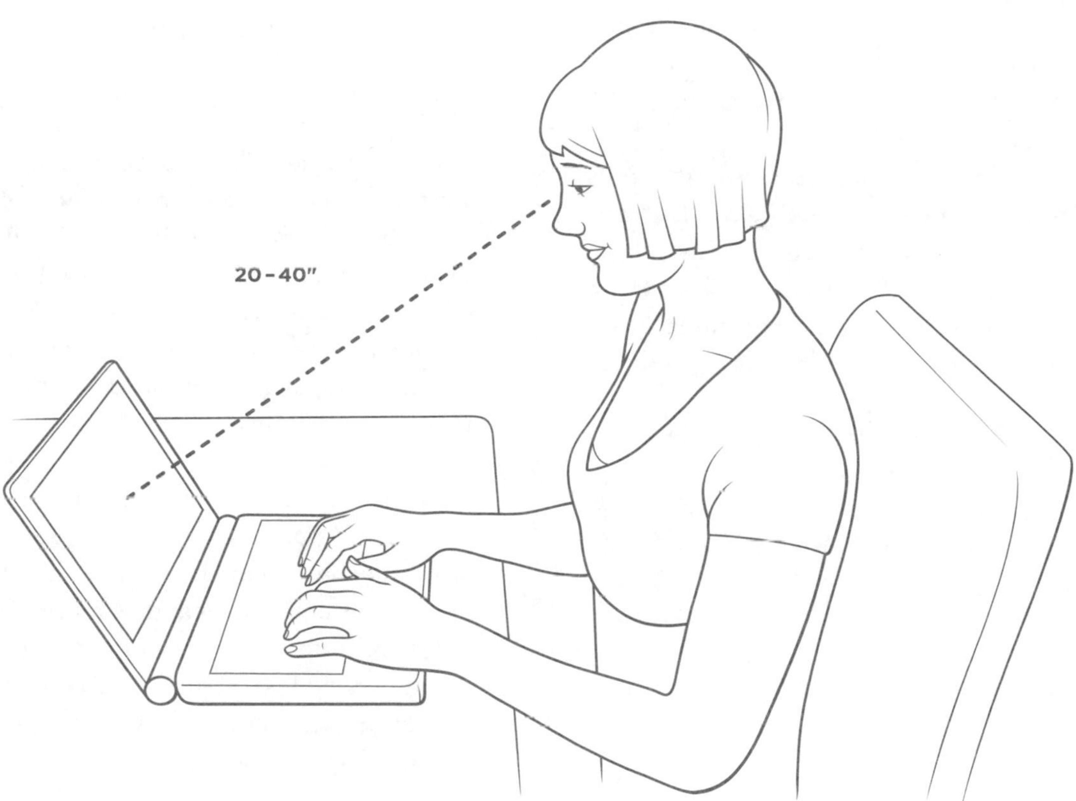

Your eyes naturally gaze at a downward angle, and you will feel more comfortable with a slight downward gaze when you are viewing close objects such as your computer screen. Straight-ahead and high monitor placements are linked with eyestrain, eye fatigue, and headaches.

Your shoulders and upper back will be happier with a lower monitor screen placement, too. Relaxation of the **trapezius** muscle (the muscle at the top of your shoulders) is improved with lower monitor placement. Studies also show that productivity and performance are improved by 10 percent with low screen placement compared with horizontal.

Your keyboard height is not easy to change unless you have an adjustable platform for it, but usually your chair height is. Adjust the height of your chair so that your shoulders are relaxed when using your keyboard. Your chair should be close enough to your desk that your upper arms are relaxed by your sides with your elbows bent at a 90-degree angle to use the keyboard. If raising your chair means your feet no longer touch the floor, invest in a foot rest or even use a shoe box so your knees don't feel strained.

It's not just computer use that puts strain on your neck. There's also PDA pain, iPOD injury, cell phone soreness, and Blackberry bruises! Bending over a tiny screen with shoulders hunched, fingers and thumbs flying, is not good for your neck or your posture. We call this "tech neck."

Use the same rules as for your computer monitor to minimize pain and suffering. Relax all those tense muscles and be good to your back. If you're feeling pain when you use your devices, make gradual changes in your position to find relief.

NOTE TO SELF

If possible, keep your computer screen just below eye level. It's good for your back and neck *and* improves your productivity!

Whiplash

Whiplash, an injury to the ligaments and muscles of the neck and shoulders, is caused by sudden acceleration or deceleration, such as in a car accident. Whiplash is most often caused by rear-end car collisions, in which the impact suddenly forces your head to snap back and forth. You can feel the effects from a low-force car crash at speeds as low as 5 miles per hour. Whiplash damages the surrounding tissues, including muscles, tendons, and ligaments.

Whiplash usually causes neck pain and stiffness, but you may also have back pain and headaches. Whiplash symptoms often don't appear until the next day or even later. Contact your doctor about whiplash for help in treatment and possible use of a cervical, or neck, collar. (Yes, people really do wear them outside of courtrooms!)

REAL LIFE INFO: Preventing Whiplash

- **Shop for a safer car when you buy a new one. Look for side and curtain air bags, safe head restraints, and antilock brakes.**
- **The headrest is a restraint meant to stop your head from snapping backward in a crash. Adjust your headrest to the right height for you! The widest point should be positioned behind your head, not below it.**
- **Wear your seat belt!**

Feel Tired Today? Ask Your Thyroid

The thyroid is a butterfly-shaped gland at the front of your neck, and you won't believe what that tiny gland does. First, it produces two thyroid hormones, triiodothyronine (T3) and thyroxine (T4), which circulate in the **bloodstream** to all tissues of the body. Thyroid hormones stimulate your metabolism by helping your body to break down food, release it as energy, or store it.

The thyroid is like one of those strong grannies who run the family. Thyroid hormones influence nearly every other organ system you have. They tell the organs how fast or slow they should work and tell the body systems when to use energy (like consuming oxygen and making heat). A deficiency in thyroid hormone can cause you to feel tired and cold, sleep badly, and have irregular periods.

The American Thyroid Association recommends that if you are thirty-five or older, you should have your thyroid tested at least every five years. Thyroid screening checks at least two hormones in your blood: thyroid-stimulating hormone (TSH) and free thyroxine. Early diagnosis can avoid worse conditions that result from untreated thyroid disease.

Thyroid Regulation 101

The thyroid is regulated by the pituitary gland, which is located at the base of the brain. The pituitary gland produces thyroid-stimulating hormone. TSH circulates in the bloodstream to the thyroid gland, where it tells the thyroid to produce more thyroid hormones.

Understanding how the thyroid gland works will help you understand how to interpret thyroid testing. The pituitary gland is stimulated to produce more TSH when thyroid hormone levels—T3 and T4—are low. When hormone levels are normal, TSH will be normal. When hormone levels are low, TSH will increase in an attempt to stimulate the thyroid gland to produce more thyroid hormone. When thyroid hormone levels are high, TSH production will be suppressed and very low.

Complicated? Yes. But it's really just like a checkout line where people keep inching up to make the line move. The pituitary gland is the cashier. In this case, the thyroid is the

THYROID TESTING

	TSH	Thyroid Hormone
Hyperthyroidism	Low	Elevated
Hypothyroidism	High	Low

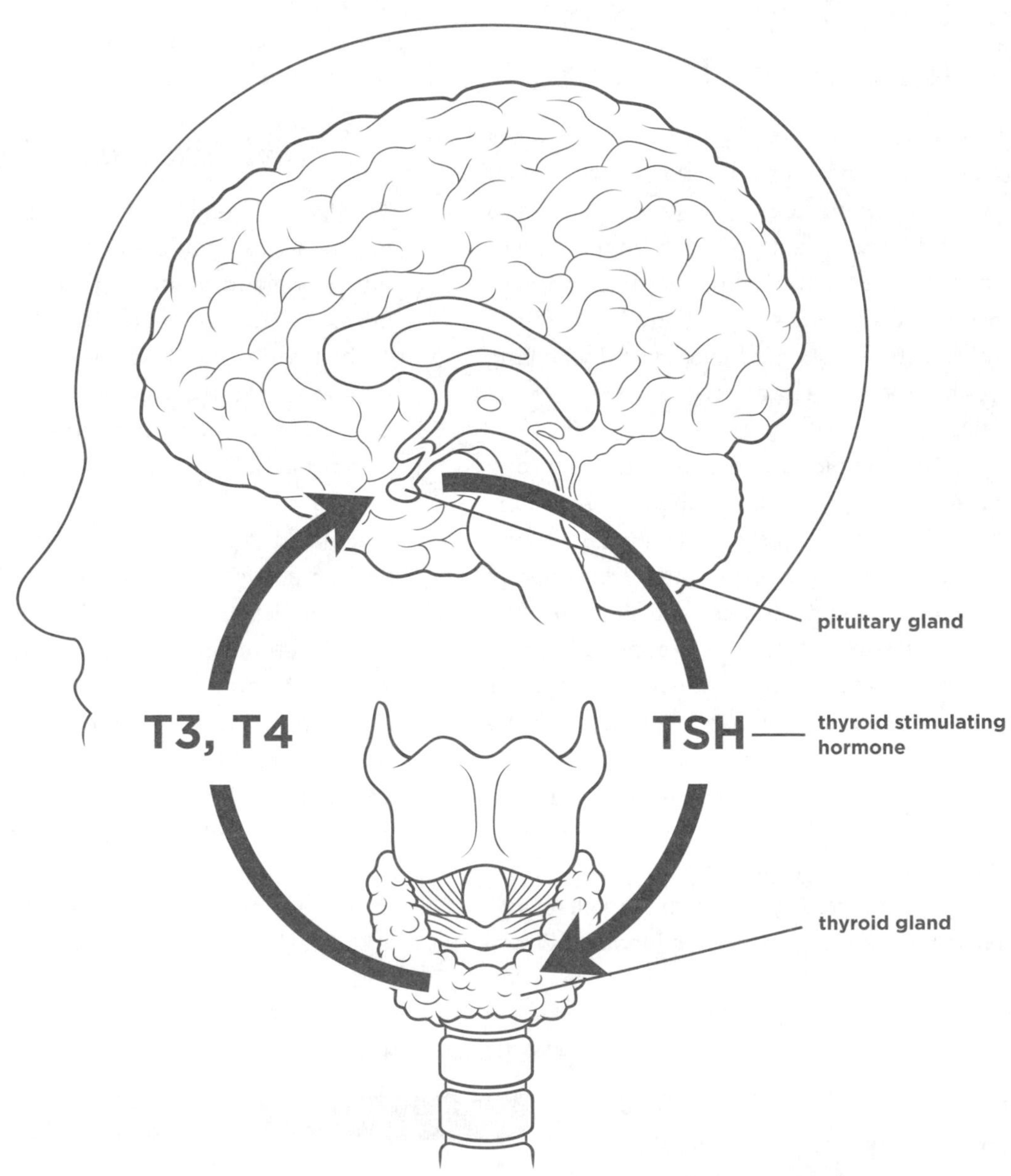

Your thyroid hormone production cycle: The pituitary gland produces TSH, which travels through the blood stream to tell the thyroid gland to produce thyroid hormones (T3 and T4). The pituitary gland is stimulated to produce TSH according to the levels of T3 and T4.

slowpoke paying by check and using fifty coupons, half of which have expired. The cashier does everything possible to keep things moving steadily.

Hyperthyroidism: Overactive Thyroid Gland

Too much thyroid hormone revs up the body's metabolism. Are you overweight and think that would be great? It's not; it's awful. Because the thyroid is producing too much hormone, the body develops an increased metabolic state, speeding up the functions of the body systems and producing too much body heat.

This condition affects women more often than men, but is still relatively rare, occurring in about 1 percent of women. One of the most common forms of hyperthyroidism is Graves' disease, which occurs when the immune system produces antibodies that attack the thyroid gland, stimulating it to produce hormones. This condition runs in families. In some patients with Graves' disease, the first sign noticed may be swelling behind the eyes that causes them to push forward or bulge. Or it could be anxiety or palpitations.

Other causes of hyperthyroidism include thyroiditis, an **inflammation** of the thyroid gland—sometimes caused by a virus—that typically causes neck discomfort or a sore throat. This sometimes happens in the postpartum (after childbirth) period. This condition can wax and wane, with the thyroid function cycling between too high, too low, and normal. This condition does not feel great, and I strongly urge you to call your doctor if you have these symptoms.

Hypothyroidism: Underactive Thyroid Gland

Too little thyroid hormone slows down the body's metabolism. An underactive thyroid gland can't make enough thyroid hormone.

REAL LIFE FACT: Symptoms of Hyperthyroidism

- **Anxiety**
- **Diarrhea**
- **Eye irritation**
- **Fatigue, trouble sleeping**
- **Infertility**
- **Irritability**
- **Feeling hot; hot flashes not associated with menopause**
- **Irregular periods**
- **Sweating**
- **Rapid heartbeat, palpitations**
- **Trembling**
- **Unexplained weight loss**
- **Weakness**

REAL LIFE FACT: Symptoms of Hypothyroidism

- **Constipation**
- **Dry skin**
- **Fatigue**
- **High cholesterol**
- **Hating the cold more than most people**
- **Menstrual irregularities**
- **Shortness of breath**
- **Slow heart rate**
- **Thin hair**
- **Weight gain**

Sometimes the cause of an underactive thyroid gland is a problem of the gland itself; other times it can be caused by the pituitary gland failing to produce thyroid-stimulating hormone and therefore not stimulating the thyroid to make thyroid hormone. That supermarket cashier just closed her station and told everybody to move to a different line.

Your body develops a decreased metabolic state, slowing down the functions of the body systems and producing too little heat and energy. You may feel sluggish and tired and gain weight more easily. Hypothyroidism, if not treated, can become a dangerous condition.

Why Am I Eating Iodine and What's a Goiter?

Your thyroid needs dietary iodine in order to produce thyroid hormone. Nowadays, many people don't know how important this is. Iodine deficiencies are rare in the United States since the 1920s, when the addition of iodine to salt became widespread, but such deficiencies used to cause terrible goiters. (Picture a baseball where your thyroid is.) In the developing world goiters are still a problem, but they are rare in the developed world.

However, with today's designer sea salts (many cooks prefer sea salt because of the

REAL LIFE QUESTION: How can I remember the meanings of "hyper" and "hypo"?

Hyper **means "overactive" and** ***hypo*** **means "underactive." You describe an overactive kid as "hyper." The "r" in hyper can help you remember "revved up" for** ***hyper. Hypo*** **is underactive, and a hypodermic needle goes under the skin.**

texture and taste) and restricted-salt diets, we are seeing a bit more iodine deficiency. Most people get plenty of salt in their diet from processed foods and seafood, so even if you don't used iodized salt, your levels may be fine. Be sure to add some iodized salt to your food to make sure you get iodine. Be aware that fast-food restaurants are not required to use iodized salt in cooking, and many of them don't.

Thyroid Nodules

Lumps in the thyroid are called thyroid nodules. They may be single or multiple; some are solid, others are cystic (collecting fluid). Although most of these nodules are **benign**, they need evaluation for these reasons:

- A small percentage may be cancerous.
- They may produce too much thyroid hormone (hyperthyroidism).
- They may become too large and press on adjacent organs.

Thyroid nodules are found in about 5 percent of people.

Thyroid Cancer

Only about 5 percent of thyroid nodules are cancerous. Unless it has spread, thyroid **cancer** is treated by surgically removing all or part of the thyroid gland, after which radioactive iodine therapy may be needed to destroy any remaining thyroid cells. If you have thyroid cancer, remember that most patients recover well from this type of cancer. As with all cancers, early detection is key. If you feel a lump, always call your doctor. Then quit worrying until you've got something to worry about, which I hope you never do.

A Straight-Up Look at Your Spine

If you were fifty, this would be a very different book. So many older people have back trouble that half the book would be about back pain. (The other half would be about **bowels** and peeing your pants.)

Lucky for you, it's not too late for you to have a different future. There are exceptions, of course. Young women can have back injuries or forms of **arthritis**. But for most of you, your job is to end up a vibrant old lady who never complains about her back unless she is skydiving.

First, let's check your posture with an oldie-but-goodie test. Stand against a wall with one hand in the small of your back. The small is where your spine curves in. Make sure that your head, shoulders, butt, calves, and heels are touching the wall. Oh, and make sure you have an even wall, top to bottom. One patient thought she must have curvature of the spine, but she really just had big baseboards. So stand against an even surface.

Now walk away. Relax. How much did your posture change? If it was a lot, you've got work to do. Most of us have work to do. Only a Marine can pass this test with an A+.

Remember, your goal is *not* to have stiff robot posture that will tire you out, but to have a strong, flexible posture that will help to protect your spine.

To understand your spine, imagine a train. The individual cars are connected to each other in a way that lets the train curve around a mountain or in a subway tunnel. In your spine, the cars are the vertebrae, or the bones of the spine. The vertebrae are connected by the disks, which make it possible for your spine to move. The disks also protect your vertebrae from everything you do to them, meaning any bouncy activity—particularly running on hard surfaces. The vertebrae protect the spinal cord—the bundle of nerves that sends messages to the muscles.

What Can Go Wrong at My Age?

It's a short yet painful list. It's most likely that the back pain you have as a young woman will come from injury, not health problems. Still, if you have back pain that does not go away, call your doctor.

Besides injuries from accidents or sports, a muscle spasm can happen when your body does an awkward twist. It might happen in sports—or emptying the dishwasher! It's very painful and makes you want to curl up into a little ball. Ice and rest will be prescribed, and possibly some muscle relaxants. If you take muscle relaxants, *do not drive*. And don't make any important decisions!

As you age, you face challenges that are much harder to treat. To be blunt, your spine may show signs of degeneration as early as middle age. My goal is to help you to prevent becoming the aunt at the bridal shower who can't stop talking about her aching back.

Herniated Disks

Between a pair of your vertebrae there is a disk that cushions and protects the bones. Sometimes that disk slips or herniates (due to injury and sometimes even just age) and touches sensitive nerves in the spine. (Some people also call this a ruptured disk or slipped disk.) Picture a hamburger, where the bun is the vertebrae and the meat is the disk. If you take a big ol' bite, sometimes the burger (disk) slips out from between the buns (vertebrae). This problem can start in your thirties.

Because the disk is touching your spinal nerves, it can be mildly painful or extremely so. The pain will probably convince you to call the doctor! It often starts in your back and sometimes seems to flow down your legs. Usually the first treatment is pain relief and rest for a few days, then you and your doctor can decide when it's time to try special exercises, stretches, and physical therapy. Some people are able to return to normal life in about a week, but others need a month or more. Today, nearly every doctor recommends a conserva-

REAL LIFE QUESTION: Do I use cold or heat to treat back pain?

At first, use a cold pack (either a first aid pack from your freezer or a bag of frozen peas) for about 20 minutes at a time. After a few days, heat will probably feel better. Use a heating pad where it hurts.

tive approach of pain relief and therapy. A few people will need surgery, but nearly everybody recovers long before that's even a question. Some people may also find relief by seeing a chiropractor or an acupuncturist.

To prevent a herniated disk, lift with your knees, not your back, when picking up heavy objects. And don't lift and twist. Hold objects you are lifting close to your body. Keep your posture strong, and follow my usual list of prescriptions, especially the advice about weight control and not smoking. Keep in mind that tall women are more prone to having herniated disks than short women. And some occupations, particularly those where you lift heavy things all day or night, also increase your risk.

Back Pain with Pregnancy

Oh, that blissful time of pregnancy! Your hormones cause your muscles and ligaments to relax, making it harder to keep your posture strong. The baby puts a strain on your back. Your center of gravity has changed so you walk funny. And your weight is going up. Result? Back pain.

Can you take pain relief medicine? No, except for mild doses of acetaminophen (Tylenol), and even then you should talk with your

REAL LIFE QUESTION: Why can't I drive while taking some medications?

You know the warning that says, "Do not operate heavy machinery"? Think of your car as heavy machinery, which it is. Medication can greatly reduce your response time and your judgment. As a surgeon told me, "Sure you can drive while you take pain meds, until a kid runs out in front of your car. Then you lose your house in the lawsuit and go to jail." Don't take chances.

doctor first. You might try acupuncture or chiropractic therapy with your doctor's consent, and a few of the ideas that follow.

First, you are pregnant and you shouldn't have to stand for a long time. If you're standing on the subway, learn to ask if anyone will give up their seat (hopefully you won't have to ask). Next, sleep on your side. Hug a body pillow or keep a pillow between your knees. Make sure your chair at work or wherever you sit most often supports your lower back, and add a pillow if it doesn't. Get up and take a walk every hour to relieve the tension in your back from sitting. Wear low heels. And don't lift heavy things. You need help and may have to learn how to ask for it.

Yoga Will Cure My Back Pain, Right?

Unfortunately, yoga is just as likely to cause back pain as to cure it. If you already have back pain, yoga exercises should only be done with a certified teacher. Even then, it's essential to follow the pain rule. If it hurts, stop. You know the difference between a good stretch and pain, don't you?

Never try to work through pain, especially when it's in your back. If you don't already have back pain, doing core exercises (those that strengthen your abdomen) are a great way to promote a healthy back and prevent pain.

How to Prevent Future Back Problems

You can't prevent everything that may happen to your back in your lifetime, but you can do a lot to avoid most problems:

- Maintain a healthy weight. Being overweight or obese is bad for your health *and* your back.
- Practice strong sitting and strong standing posture.
- Exercise to strengthen your abdominal core and your back muscles. Your doctor or physical therapist can recommend exercises that will be good for you. When exercising involves the back, be sure to get expert advice.
- Use your leg muscles when you lift a heavy object, not your back. Get down low, and hold heavy objects close to you as you rise.
- Get rid of your lumpy old mattress and buy one that doesn't keep you awake at night.
- Wear low-heeled shoes. Occasionally wearing high heels may not be harmful, but wearing them every day is.
- Quit smoking. Smoking causes **osteoporosis** (bone loss; see chapter 7, Your Bones and Joints). You knew that was coming, too!

- Get plenty of calcium, vitamin D, and magnesium in your diet or through supplements.
- Keep a good family health history. Tell your doctor if rheumatoid arthritis runs in your family because it can appear in younger women and runs in families.

Off to a Great Start

So, to keep your thyroid hormones, blood, nerve messages, oxygen, and all of the other vital body "traffic" flowing smoothly, take care of your neck and your spine. In fact, to remind yourself of the importance of your neck and spine—that superhighway that makes everything possible—maybe it's time to wear a new scarf or necklace that will remind you. (Yes, I know, you want to get a new tattoo instead.)

Follow my basic prescription to keep your posture strong, your weight and diet healthy, your body exercised, and your lungs free of smoke, and you'll give your back and neck a good head start.

Now we'll turn to another one of your body's essential systems: waste removal, or what I like to call your waterworks. To learn what it does, how it works, and what your body needs, read on.

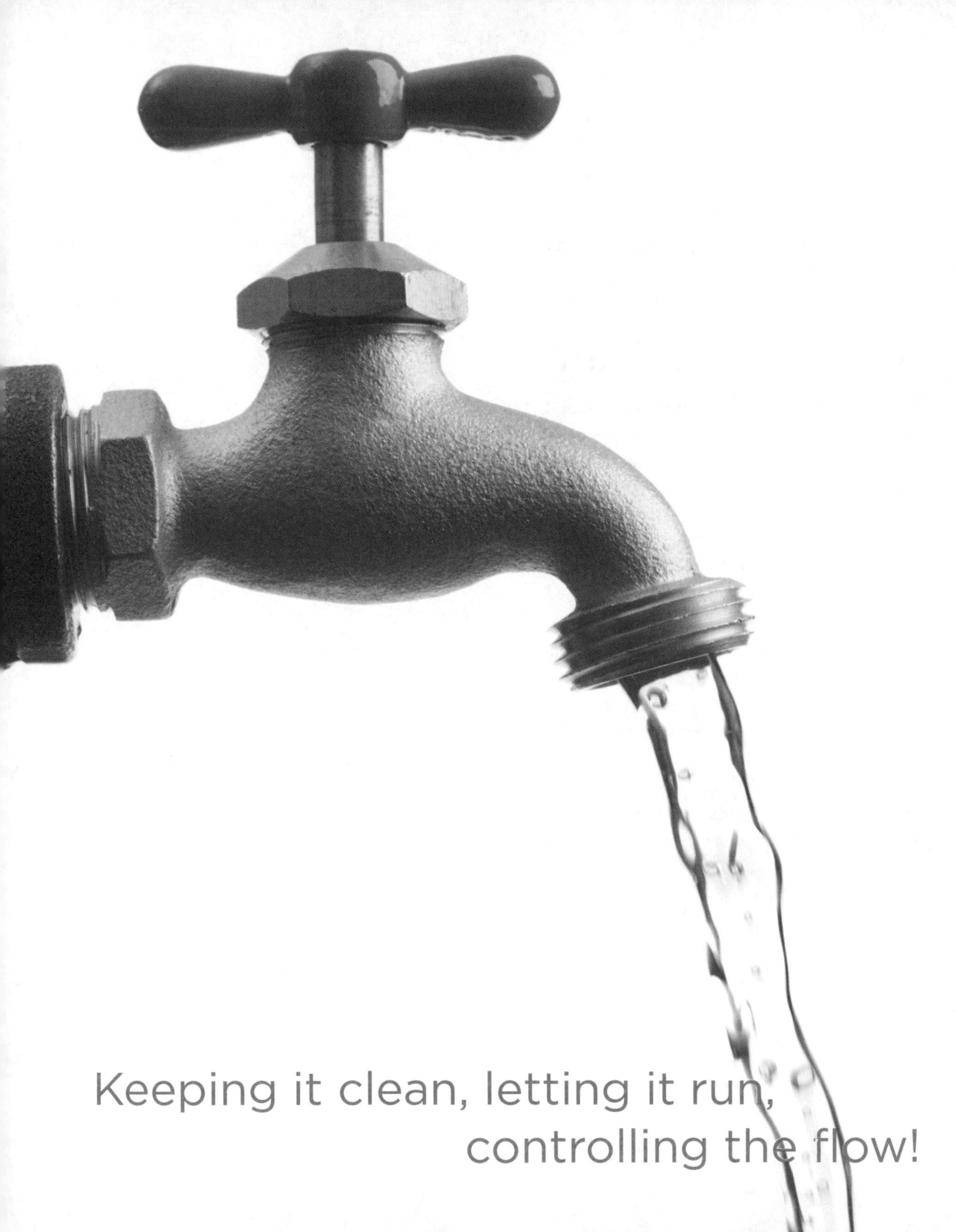
Keeping it clean, letting it run,
controlling the flow!

your waterworks

Your body is about 65 percent water. Depending on your lifestyle, you need about eight cups of water every day just to fill up your tank from what you used yesterday. Water works its way through your blood and through your **lymphatic system**. It carries oxygen and food to your cells, and it takes out the trash through sweat and pee. And your soft tissues and **joints** are softer and more supportive when you are well-hydrated. Your whole body depends on water to function well.

Our bodies are designed to get water even if we don't have a fresh water supply. Fruits and vegetables are full of water, as are meats and grains. But you still need to drink a lot of it, and you should drink according to your needs. If you exercise heavily, sweat heavily, or spend time in dry heat, you'll need to drink more than eight cups per day. (A menopausal woman in Arizona who's taking a jog and having hot flashes is going to be in serious trouble very quickly.)

If you are really drinking as much water as you should, you'll find yourself spending a lot of time in the bathroom. After racing to the ladies' room, desperate, you find a pregnant woman and an elderly woman already in line. Should you ask for frontsies? Perhaps not. If you do, that glowing woman-with-child and the sweet knitter may rip your **bladder** out so you don't need it anymore. (There's no cutting in line in the ladies' room.) All females over the age of five know that our bodies have a few design flaws. As one patient says, "Give me half the stomach and twice the bladder."

The Female Bladder

The bladder is where your pee is stored. In theory, it can hold about a pint (16 ounces) of urine. Some people have a bladder that could stretch out and hold as much as a quart. But the need to pee comes well before the bladder is full. The desire to pee (called the **micturition reflex**) can start as soon as you've got half a cup in there.

Besides being small, the bladder is located right near where you pee, and it's a short, straight line through the **urethra** to the toilet. Everything else in your body can lean on the bladder if it feels like it and make you want to pee. A baby, for instance. Plus, your muscles and **sphincters** become weaker as you age, but your micturition reflex keeps on ticking.

Some pregnant or elderly women . . . well, they may as well just stay in the bathroom all day. If you don't believe me, go to a baby shower. Wait until everyone is good and hydrated. Now tell a really good joke to make Grandma and the mother-to-be laugh. The hostess will be paging the upholstery cleaner the second the last guest leaves.

It doesn't have to be like this. There are steps you can take now, exercises that you can do now, that will keep you in control later. It's worth starting as soon as you read this, because the stronger you can make those muscles that keep your pee in, the better you will feel as an older woman about traveling or going to special events. Or sleeping through the night.

You probably don't think much about your bladder when it's empty. But when nature calls, it's *all* you can think about, right? Imagine that feeling of urgency all the time, or not being able to control your bladder. Well, there are things you can do to let the river run and to keep it dammed up when you don't want it to. There are even exercises you can do to improve your bladder's stamina.

Still, I have to be honest. If you gave birth last week and you just drank two glasses of

REAL LIFE FACT: Taking Out the Trash

Most of what we eat and drink gets used by the body, but there's always some waste left over. Gas, poop, urine, and sweat are the big ones. Your body takes what you eat from the colon and processes it into your bloodstream. Your blood is constantly being filtered by your kidneys. The kidneys catch salts, water, and toxins. Toxins are waste products such as urea, which is left over when your body breaks down proteins and ammonia.

water, plus something makes you sneeze and laugh at the same time, there's nothing you can do to protect your couch. Design flaw.

NOTE TO SELF

You can take a few steps now to avoid diapers later.

How Your Waterworks Works

The urinary tract includes the **kidneys**, **ureters**, bladder, and urethra. Everything you eat and drink goes through your digestive system (see chapter 8, Your Stomach and Intestines), where **nutrients** and water are absorbed into your **bloodstream**. After your kidneys filter waste products, tubes called the ureters drain from your kidneys into your bladder, which lies in the front part of your **pelvis**, just behind your pubic bone. The bladder has a muscular contraction to release the pee. It relaxes and opens a sphincter at the same time. The bladder then empties through the urethra.

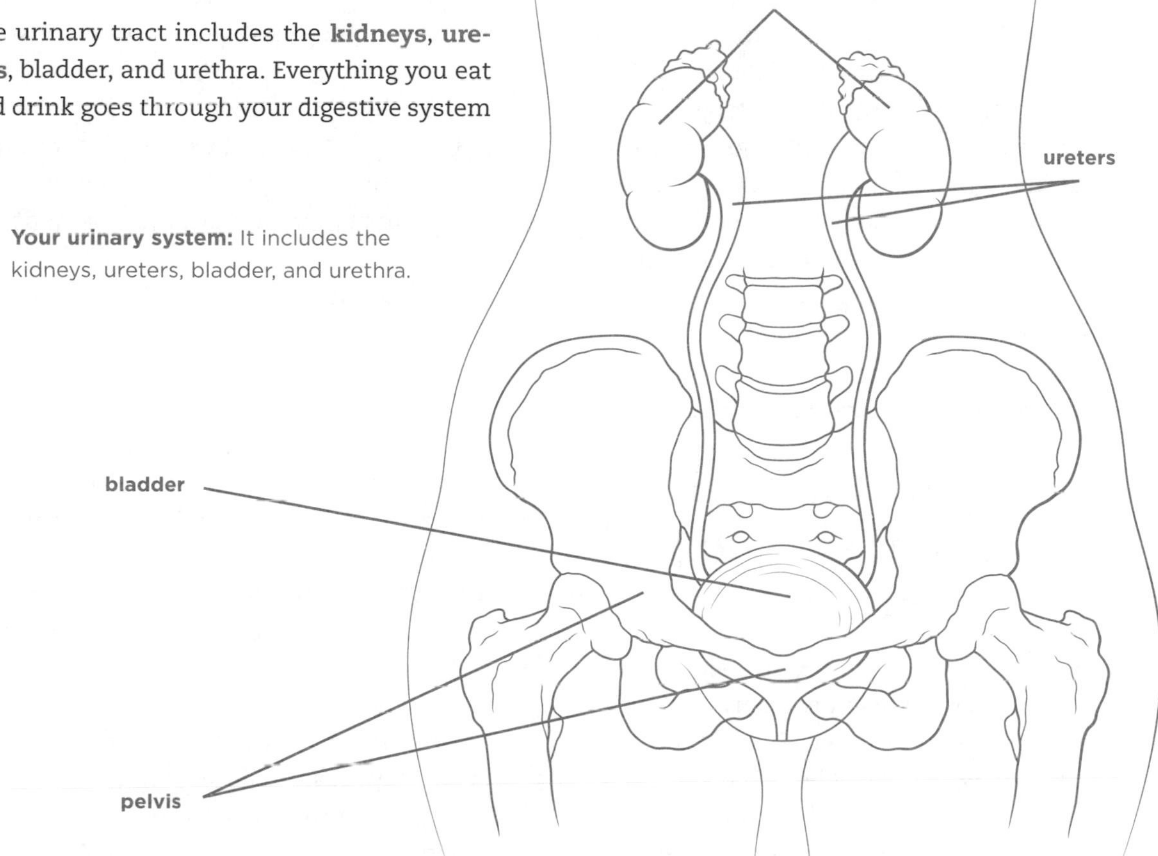

Your urinary system: It includes the kidneys, ureters, bladder, and urethra.

REAL LIFE FACT: Check Your Pee

If you are well-hydrated, your pee should be clear and as free of color as possible. It can be pale yellow, but should still be clear. Your first pee in the morning may be a little more concentrated and darker, but you should see it lighten during the day. Remember that many vitamin supplements, foods (especially asparagus), and medicines can change the color and odor of your pee. Before you panic when you see something green or bright yellow, ask the pharmacist about it! Or ask a guy. Seriously, they are proud experts on what makes their pee turn colors and smell.

Yes, your urethra is short. Men have a much longer urethra. Your urethral opening, your **vagina**, and your **rectum** are all close together in a line—close neighbors, in fact. This is not good neighborhood design. It's normal for your vagina and rectum to have **bacteria** living in them, but the nearby urethra and the urinary system are supposed to be sterile environments, with no bacteria living there. In this crowded neighborhood, bacteria from the vagina and rectum can be uninvited visitors to the urethra and urinary tract. We'll learn more about that as we explore what can go wrong.

What Can Go Wrong: Urinary Tract Infections

Most women will get a **urinary tract infection** (UTI) some day. Bladder infections, called **cystitis**, are the most common kind of UTI. As you know by now, it's a neighborhood problem.

A gang of germs, which normally hangs out in the vagina or the rectum, travels over to the urethra. If your body's Neighborhood Watch Group—your immune system—catches the germs, fine. If not, they become squatters in the urethra. I'm tempted to keep developing this neighborhood theme and say the germs buy a house and start having kids, but let's just say they multiply. When they multiply, they want to move to a bigger house and start an infection.

Again, the female urethra is a very short straight line to the bladder. If you were a man, the germs would have a long way to travel from the urethra to the bladder. The male urethra is way at the end of the penis. The male system is like an apartment building: a long hallway before you get home. The female system is a cottage: open the front door and you're in the living room. Men have a better chance of killing bacteria before it reaches the bladder. So UTIs are much more common in women than in men.

Bacteria from the rectal area cause most cases of cystitis. Think about how easy it is for that to happen as you wipe yourself on the toilet. The toilet paper carries and spreads whatever it picks up. It picks up germs, the normal germs from the vagina and rectum, and carries them to the urethra up there in the front seat. In case your mother never told you, this is important: Every time you wipe yourself—every time—wipe from front to back. Start where you pee, end where you poop. Never, ever, ever wipe your front with paper that has already got some poop on it. Never, even if you have not pooped, wipe yourself from back to front. You can still pick up germs from the rectum, and you will very likely pick up a few from the vagina. Those vaginal germs—wonderful in the vagina, useful and healthy—are not your friends when they get into the urethra.

"The Honeymoon Disease"

Wiping doesn't cause every infection. Some women develop cystitis after sex. The friction of sex can push bacteria from the vagina or rectum into the urethra, causing infection. Using a **diaphragm** can also lead to infections, because diaphragms push against the urethra and make it harder to empty the bladder completely. The urine that stays in the bladder is more likely to grow bacteria and cause infections.

Your grandmother called a UTI "the honeymoon disease." Couples were having sex for the first time and having a lot of it. The friction greatly increased the chances of a UTI. I have a patient who will never tell anyone that she has a UTI because "it makes her sound loose." Even though most cases of bladder infections or cystitis are actually caused by *Escherichia coli* or *E. coli*, a species of bacteria commonly found in the **gastrointestinal** tract, she still won't tell anyone.

Cystitis Symptoms

The symptoms of cystitis are different for everyone. Some people get mild symptoms, some will suffer with severe burning. UTIs must be treated, even if they are mild. It can get very serious if the infection spreads to your kidneys. Call your doctor today if you have any of these symptoms:

- Burning sensation when you pee
- Frequent and urgent need to pee

REAL LIFE QUESTION: Why do you keep saying "pee"?

Some doctors and nurses still say *void*, as in "Here's a cup. Please void your bladder," and *evacuate*, as in "We want you to evacuate your bowels." I might use those words with older patients, too. It used to be very vulgar to say pee and poop, and it probably still is, but I have three boys. I don't hear the difference anymore. And Monique has two girls, and she doesn't either.

- Feeling the urge to pee but not being able to, or going only a little
- Pain in the stomach, pelvic area, or lower back
- Leaking urine
- Increased need to get up at night to pee
- Cloudy, bad-smelling urine
- Blood in the urine
- Fever, including low-grade fever

NOTE TO SELF

Check out the appendix, Tools to Use, for help on deciding when it's time to call your doctor.

But let's say you were just in overdrive yesterday. You ran a race in hot weather in a dry climate. You didn't drink enough liquid or eat enough high-liquid foods. Then you ate a salad that had asparagus and strips of beets in it.

When you pee in the morning, you will run from the bathroom screaming. From your dehydrated state, your urine will be dark. From eating beets, it will look red—honest—and bloody. The asparagus gives urine an odor not found anywhere else on the planet. (Good tip for hostesses here: If you have house guests and one bathroom, don't serve asparagus.) These symptoms are normal after what you did yesterday. They mean that you're probably a little dehydrated, and the smelly and colorful urine is a result of your diet. You probably don't have a UTI (unless you have the other symptoms listed above).

Cystitis Diagnosis

We need a clean catch urine sample to test for cystitis. This means that you have to collect the sample carefully. If bacteria from your skin or the environment gets into the sample, it will just cause confusion about your diagnosis. It may give a false positive result. Let's say that bacteria is on your skin and gets into the sample. You actually don't have a bladder infection, but the germs will make it look like you do. You'll get the wrong diagnosis—and take medicine you don't need.

REAL LIFE QUESTION: What will increase my chances of getting a bladder infection?

- Wiping from back to front
- Being sexually active
- Using a diaphragm for birth control
- Medical procedures on the bladder, including having a catheter or being examined with a cystoscope
- Abnormalities of the urinary system
- Kidney stones

REAL LIFE FACT: The Clean Catch Urine Sample

The idea here is to collect some pee without getting any germs from the rest of you in it. You'll use wipes to clean yourself from front to back. Then you'll collect the middle of your pee stream—not the first drops. If you don't get this right the first time you do it, you're in good company. Your doctor thinks it's easy because she has done it eighty-five times. A few more times practicing and maybe she'll stop spraying her panty hose.

So it's important to follow these clean catch steps. The goal is to get the middle of your pee stream—not the very beginning—in a really clean way.

To give a clean catch urine sample, you'll be given some sterile wipes and a sterile urine sample cup.

1. Wash your hands first.
2. Open the cup to have it ready. Don't touch the inside of the cup.
3. Next, hold open the labia—the lips around your genitals—with one hand and wipe front to back with the sterile wipes with the other hand.
4. Pee a little bit in the toilet. This flushes out any bacteria that may be on the outside of your urethra.
5. Finally, pee into the sterile cup.
6. Put the cap back on. You'll either leave it there for collection or bring it back with you. Just ask what the procedure is.

This sample of your pee is tested for blood, **white blood cells**, and bacteria with a quick test called a **urinalysis**. Next, some of it is kept for twenty-four to forty-eight hours to see if any bacteria grow. If you have bacteria in your pee, you likely have cystitis.

Cystitis Treatment

Cystitis is treated with antibiotic drugs. **Antibiotics** will be prescribed for at least two to three days and maybe for as long as several weeks. The length of the treatment depends on the severity of the infection and on whether this is your first infection or a repeating problem. You will probably start to feel better after a day or two. However, it's important that you complete the entire course of medication. Otherwise the infection may easily come back.

Sometimes the quick urinalysis shows infection clearly. Your doctor may choose to start antibiotics even before the results come back. If the urinalysis is borderline, or even negative, then you need to wait for twenty-four to forty-eight hours until the urine culture is back before treatment.

In the laboratory, the bacteria are tested to see if common antibiotics will kill them. This is called a culture and sensitivity test. It's done because today, as we use antibiotics more and more often, some bacteria are becoming resistant to common antibiotics, and sometimes a stronger antibiotic must be used. This test for antibiotic sensitivity is important, especially if you have recurrent (repeated) cystitis, to make certain that we use the right antibiotic. It's why your doctor may ask you to come in and leave a urine sample, even if over the phone you report the classic symptoms of cystitis. It's also why you should be treated only if true cystitis is diagnosed by this urine test, as overtreatment with the wrong type or amount of antibiotic can promote the development of resistant bacteria. If you don't have bacteria, the antibiotic won't do you any good either.

If you experience repeat infections, your doctor may prescribe stronger antibiotics or have you take them longer. S/he may also recommend that you take low-dose antibiotics as a preventive measure, either daily or after sex. If you still have recurrent infections, you may be referred to a specialist to make certain there is no structural problem with your urinary tract that is making you prone to infections. You could, for example, have a urinary tract that doesn't empty completely because of a tight sphincter or too many twists and turns between the bladder and the urethra. These problems can usually be fixed with surgery. The good news: Today, surgeries like this are getting simpler and better.

Because urinary tract infections can be painful, you can take a medicine called phenazopyridine, which decreases the pain and bladder spasms. It will turn your urine and sometimes your sweat an orangey color, so you use pads to prevent staining your underwear. Brand names of the medicine include Azo and Uristat. It's usually available without a prescription and can relieve symptoms effectively while you wait for the medical treatment to work in the next day or two. It's important to realize that phenazopyridine won't treat the infection; it's a pain reliever that helps take the sting out of peeing while you wait for the infection to be fought off by the antibiotics. Many women start feeling better after only one dose of antibiotics (but finish the whole course so the infection doesn't come back).

NOTE TO SELF

Is this you? "I wish my doctor would give me some antibiotics." But wait, you've heard it all over TV: overuse of antibiotics has produced superbugs—germs that survive treatment with antibiotics. Also, many women develop yeast infections or diarrhea while taking antibiotics, because the drugs also kill the good germs in your digestive tract. And remember, if you don't have a bacterial infection or if you have a viral infection, no antibiotic is going to help.

Stop Those Unwelcome Visitors!

You can lessen your chance of getting cystitis and other urinary tract infections by preventing bacteria from entering the urinary tract. Talk with your doctor about which changes from the following list of suggestions would be helpful for you to make. Your doctor also may give you a low dose of medicine for several months or longer to prevent infections from coming back. If having sex seems to cause your infections, your doctor may suggest that you take a single antibiotic pill after you have sex.

Here are some other steps you can take:

- Drink plenty of liquids. Water and unsweetened cranberry juice are best. In fact, drinking unsweetened cranberry juice regularly seems to help lower the risk of developing UTIs. So now you know why Grandma had so much of it.
- Common bladder irritants to avoid are alcoholic beverages; caffeinated beverages, such as coffee, tea, and cola; acidic fruits and juices, such as citrus, pineapples, tomatoes, and tomato products (this is a doctor's way of saying avoid Bloody Marys); and carbonated beverages (even caffeine-free ones).
- Pee when you have the urge. Don't hold it.
- Pee after sex to help wash away bacteria.
- Use enough lubrication during sex. Try using a small amount of lubricant (such as Astroglide or K-Y Jelly) before sex if you're a little dry. Do *not* use petroleum jellies such as Vaseline if you use **condoms**! It weakens a latex condom.
- Always wipe from the front to the back, whether you have had a bowel movement or not.
- Avoid using douches and feminine hygiene sprays.
- Avoid bubble baths.
- If you get UTIs often, the diaphragm is not a good birth control choice for you.

REAL LIFE QUESTION : Does cranberry juice really help to prevent UTIs?

In many cases, yes! Several studies have proven that Grandma's right about cranberries. They're especially good for women who get recurrent infections. A substance in cranberries seems to keep germs from sticking to the walls of the bladder. Bacteria will wash away in your urine instead of hanging around to cause an infection. However, cranberry juice doesn't seem to help once a full-blown infection starts. It works best as a preventive measure.

How much cranberry juice do you need? Nobody really knows. I would try a cup (8 ounces) three times a day, or a tablet containing 300 or 400 mg of cranberry extract twice a day.

Interstitial Cystitis

Interstitial cystitis is one of the most puzzling and frequently misdiagnosed disorders. It's a **chronic inflammation** of the bladder wall that can cause chronic pelvic and bladder pain. It can also lead to scarring and stiffening of the bladder and reduced bladder capacity. Your bladder holds less urine, so you end up peeing more often.

No one knows what causes interstitial cystitis. It's different from plain cystitis, or urinary tract infections. The inflammation is not from a bacterial infection, so antibiotics are not a useful treatment. In rare cases, the inflammation can be so bad that **ulcers** form in the bladder lining.

Interstitial cystitis is much more common in women than in men, with 90 percent of cases occurring in women. Because it varies so much in symptoms and severity, most doctors believe that interstitial cystitis may actually be several diseases. One theory is that it's an **autoimmune response** that follows a bladder infection. Another theory is that there are substances in urine that irritate and damage the bladder in some people.

Scientists have not yet found a cure for interstitial cystitis, nor can they predict who will respond best to which treatment. Symptoms may go away for no apparent reason, and then return after days, weeks, months, or years. Because the causes are unknown, treatments are aimed at relieving symptoms.

Symptoms

The symptoms of interstitial cystitis include pelvic pain, pressure, tenderness, or intense pain in the bladder and surrounding pelvic area. You may have an urgent, frequent need to pee. Women with a severe case of interstitial cystitis may pee as many as sixty times a day.

Pain may change in intensity as the bladder fills with urine or as it empties. Symptoms often get worse during your period. Pain during sex is common.

Diagnosis

The first step in diagnosing interstitial cystitis is to rule out other conditions that may be causing the symptoms. We do tests to rule out bladder infections, **endometriosis**, **sexually transmitted diseases**, kidney **stones**, and (rarely) bladder **cancer**.

Cystoscopy is an important test. We look inside your bladder using a cystoscope. You'll be given anesthesia because otherwise the procedure hurts, especially if you have interstitial cystitis. We add liquid to your bladder using a **catheter**, which is a narrow tube inserted into the urethra. The liquid will stretch your bladder and allow us to view bladder wall inflammation, pinpoint bleeding, ulcers, small bladder capacity, or a thick, stiff bladder wall. (Pinpoint bleeding refers to small spots of bleeding under the bladder lining.)

Your doctor will review the recommended aftercare for you, which will depend on the extent of your cytoscope procedure. You may be uncomfortable for several days and may be advised to avoid exercise or sex until your doctor clears you.

Treatment

Medication has been shown to be helpful for some women with interstitial cystitis. Oral pentosan polysulfate (marketed as Elmiron) and other oral medicines, including aspirin, ibuprofen, stronger painkillers, antidepressants, and antihistamines work for some.

Your doctor will usually start with the least invasive treatments, such as medication and diet. Another option is bladder instillation, in which your bladder is filled with a liquid before being emptied at intervals. And transcutaneous electrical nerve stimulation (TENS) is a noninvasive treatment using electrodes to send small pulses to the bladder area. We don't know why TENS works, but it can provide relief from the pain and reduce the frequency of urination. Sacral nerve stimulation implants are also being studied as a way to relieve symptoms.

Interstitial Cystitis and Your Diet

Doctors and scientists don't agree on the role of diet in reducing the symptoms of interstitial cystitis. Many people report that alcohol, tomatoes, spices, chocolate, caffeinated and citrus beverages, and high-acid foods add to bladder irritation and inflammation. Others notice that their symptoms get worse after eating or drinking anything containing artificial sweeteners.

If certain foods or drinks make your symptoms worse, try avoiding them. Use the Digestion Journal (in the appendix, Tools to Use) to keep track of what you eat and what gives you symptoms. You can reintroduce foods one at a time to see which, if any, affect

REAL LIFE QUESTION: Why are the lines so long for the ladies' room and not the men's?

It happens whenever a large group of people go to the bathroom at the same time, such as at theaters and concerts. Women have smaller bladders and have to go a little more often. And women spend more time on the process because we always go into stalls (no urinals), we must partly undress and dress again, and we have to wipe. But smart architects are changing the restroom configuration. Movie theaters, for example, are being built with twice the number of stalls for women. That should meet about half the need.

you. As always, it's important to eat a well-balanced and varied diet, and be sure to keep your doctor informed.

Interstitial Cystitis and Pregnancy

Researchers have little information about pregnancy and interstitial cystitis, but believe that the disorder does not affect fertility or the baby's health. Some women find that their interstitial cystitis symptoms improve during pregnancy; others find that symptoms worsen.

The Family Stone

So, what are kidney stones? Well, the body sometimes makes stones—a buildup of salts and calcium—that get stuck in the urinary tract. These are usually small and pass through your pee unnoticed. If a stone gets big enough to block the kidney or the ureter tubes, you're in for pretty severe pain in the abdomen. Passing stones is painful, and in some cases the stones have to be removed surgically. Don't try to pass a stone on your own just because Aunt Milly did. And please don't turn to all of the "miracle cures" on the Internet. Kidney stones attract a lot of crazy ideas. Most of them don't work and some can be dangerous.

Symptoms: How Do I Know I Have a Stone?

The symptoms for kidney stones can be confused with serious problems such as **ectopic pregnancy** (an **embryo** that implants in a **fallopian tube** instead of the **uterus**). It's very important to call your doctor if you have these symptoms. Don't try to self-diagnose!

With tiny stones, you'll have no symptoms. They pass on their own. With larger stones, you'll have sudden pain that people say is the worst they've ever felt. The pain is usually in your back, your genital area, your abdomen, or your sides, and it can come and

REAL LIFE FACT: Another Good Reason to Have an Annual Physical

Your kidneys are essential for a healthy life. You can actually live a normal life with just one kidney, but not if both fail. It's very important to catch kidney problems early. At your annual physical, those blood tests your doctor orders may show the beginning of kidney trouble or of other conditions that may damage your kidneys. Serious kidney problems are major challenges, but finding a problem early can really limit the damage.

REAL LIFE INFO: Sign Up as an Organ Donor

Kidneys are another good reason to sign up as an organ donor. When kidney disease advances, patients have to undergo dialysis a few times a week. When that fails, the only option is a transplant. It's a terrible thing to see a young person with kidney failure unable to find a donor. Doctors look for living donors among relatives and volunteers, but chances are high that the patient's life will be saved by an organ donor.

There's no easy way to say this: when you sign up as a donor, you are agreeing to donate your organs when you die. Usually you can sign up when you renew your driver's license, but your most important step is to tell your family. Whether you have signed up or not, your family must know your wishes. If you should die unexpectedly, you don't want your family to deal with this issue while they are grieving. Tell them now to make it easier for them later. May it never happen to you, but if it does, give life to save someone else. (See the appendix, Tools to Use, for more information.)

go. You may feel sick to your stomach and may notice blood in your urine. Painful pee and frequent pee are common symptoms.

If you have more than one kidney stone or if you have a family history of them, you'll want to work with your doctor to prevent them in the future. Some stones can be minimized by diet changes and hydration. Others require medications. That's another good reason to work with your doctor on this issue—s/he can analyze the stones, determine which kind they are, and develop the plan that's right for you.

Should you call the doctor at two o'clock in the morning if you feel these symptoms? Yes. Although kidney stones are not a life-threatening emergency, the symptoms can be similar to other, more dangerous problems. They can also be extremely painful.

Controlling the Flow: Incontinence Can Be Treated and Often Cured

Urinary incontinence (peeing your pants) is not just Grandma's problem. About 22 percent of young women have some incontinence, and 8 percent have moderate to severe incontinence.

Incontinence means that you accidentally leak urine, especially when you laugh, cough, sneeze, or exercise. You can't wait to get to the bathroom. And sometimes you don't make it.

Among teens and young women, incontinence problems are often related to sports injuries. About 20 percent of college athletes report pee leaks during sports. Women in high-impact sports—such as parachuters, gymnasts, and runners—are at highest risk. In these sports, you're hitting the ground hard, which can damage pelvic muscles and connective tissue that supports the bladder. Weak pelvic muscles—and therefore incontinence—can also run in families, just like bad eyesight.

Incontinence can happen in both women and men of all ages, but women are twice as likely to have it. It's more common among women who have had a baby, and it gets more common as women age. As **estrogen** levels decrease during **menopause**, you can lose muscle tone in the pelvic floor, which supports the bladder, **bowels**, and uterus. Losing control of your bladder can affect your relationships, job, and social life. Some women are embarrassed by this condition, don't believe it can be treated, and never tell their doctor or their friends.

Why am I telling you this now? Because as a young woman, you don't need to resort to wearing granny diapers or to stop exercising. Incontinence can be treated and often cured.

Keep in mind that as a young woman, having an episode of incontinence doesn't always mean it will continue long-term. For example, temporary incontinence can happen during and just after pregnancy, and usually improves with **Kegel exercises** (more on this later in the chapter) and recovery from birth. Incontinence related to a bladder infection can happen at any age and is cured by treating the infection. Even if incontinence continues, it can be treated with pelvic exercises, lifestyle changes, medication, physical therapy techniques, or minimally invasive surgical procedures. Talking to your doctor is the first step to finding a solution that works for you.

So what causes the leaks in the first place? The most common causes are:

- Urinary tract or vaginal infections
- Weakened pelvic muscles due to pregnancy or childbirth
- Lack of estrogen due to menopause
- Pelvic surgery such as **hysterectomy**
- Injury to the pelvic area
- Side effect of certain medications

REAL LIFE FACT: Running the Numbers

In one study from England, surveys were sent to female medical, veterinary, dental, and nursing students. One-third of the women who had not yet had a baby admitted to occasional incontinence. Seven percent of these women had severe leakage that interfered with their social and physical activities.

- Straining due to constipation
- Chronic coughing
- **Diabetes**
- Heavy lifting

There are several different types of urinary incontinence. Women may have one or more types at the same time.

Physical Stress Incontinence

Stress incontinence often starts after you give birth. You head to your yoga class, ready to get back in shape, and in the middle of the workout . . . oops! You have an accident. Stress incontinence stems from weakness of or damage to the pelvic muscles or the sphincter muscles of the urethra. This damage allows urine to leak during exercise, coughing, sneezing, or other movements that stress the abdomen. This is the most common type of incontinence in younger women and is often related to pregnancy and childbirth.

The cause of stress incontinence is fairly easy to understand: pelvic floor muscles support your bladder. If these muscles weaken, your bladder can move downward. This prevents muscles that ordinarily force the urethra shut from squeezing as tightly as they should. Urine then leaks into the urethra during moments of physical stress. Stress incontinence also occurs if the muscles that do the squeezing weaken. If you are really concerned about leakage, you can wear a pad.

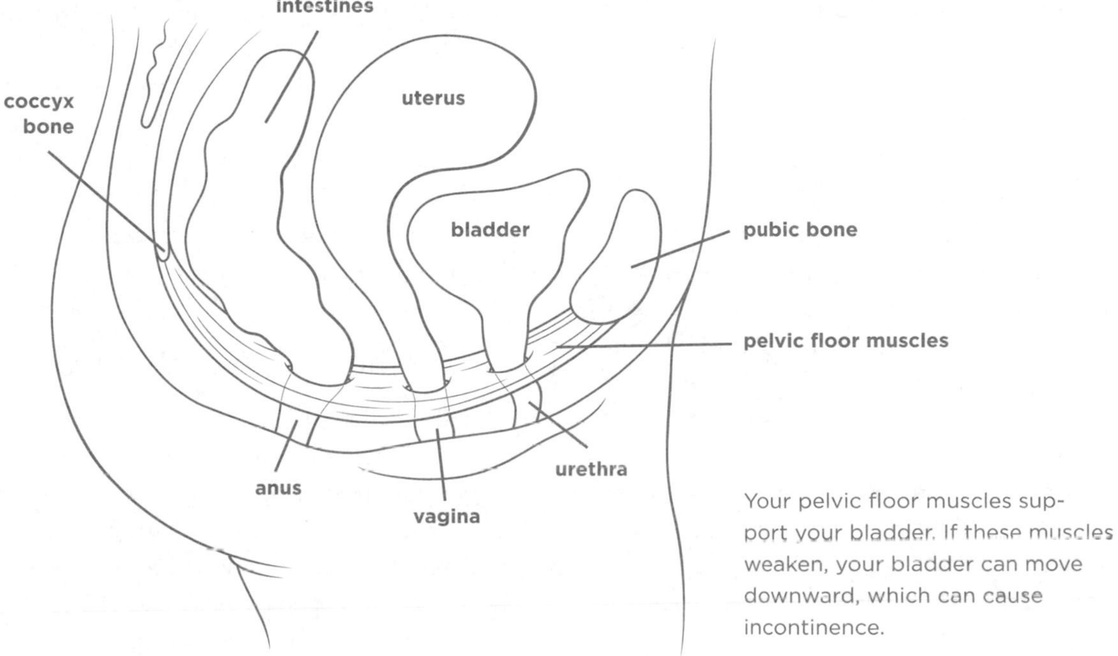

Your pelvic floor muscles support your bladder. If these muscles weaken, your bladder can move downward, which can cause incontinence.

REAL LIFE QUESTION: What's your worst bathroom story?

Everybody has one eventually. We start small—like forgetting to flush the toilet at the new boyfriend's house just before he goes in. Then we get pregnant, and by the time we give birth, we have desperately gone into men's rooms in every place on the planet. Men are terrified of pregnant women, so you could take over the men's room and rob everybody and they would never even look you in the eye.

Marathoner Uta Pippig takes the grand prize, for expelling all known bodily fluids in public during the 1996 Boston Marathon. She apparently got diarrhea and her period at the same time. She was the front-runner, so the truck of press cameras from around the world was right on her. Mile after mile. Think of Uta next time you feel awkward about a little leakage. Leakers are in very good company.

Urge Incontinence

Urge incontinence is caused by an overactive bladder that suddenly contracts and passes urine. It can make you wet the bed or pee after drinking a small amount or even when you touch water or hear it running.

An infection or damage to the nerves that control the bladder may be responsible. Caffeine, alcohol, and high-acid foods aggravate urge incontinence. Multiple sclerosis, Parkinson's disease, Alzheimer's disease, **stroke**, and injury—including injury that occurs during surgery—all can harm bladder nerves or muscles. Urge incontinence is more common in older women.

And remember—just because you wet the bed last night doesn't mean you have a dreaded disease. It can mean that you just forgot to pee before you went to bed and you are a sound sleeper!

Overflow Incontinence

When the amount of pee in your bladder is bigger than you have room for, it leaks. Weak bladder muscles or a blocked urethra can cause this type of incontinence. Nerve damage from diabetes or other diseases can lead to weak bladder muscles. Tumors and urinary stones can block the urethra. Overflow incontinence is actually rare in women and more common in men.

Functional Incontinence

Functional incontinence means that you can't get to the toilet in time, even when your urinary system is normal. People who have trouble planning and communicating might not make it. People with physical disabilities may be blocked from getting to a toilet in time. It's a common problem in nursing homes—another reminder to stay ahead of aging by practicing good habits now.

Diagnosing Incontinence

If you have incontinence, your doctor is going to ask a lot of questions about your pee habits. Your pattern for peeing and leaking can help him or her figure out what kind of incontinence you have. You'll be asked about your medical history, including any straining and discomfort, use of drugs, recent surgery, and illness. If your medical history doesn't define the problem, it will at least suggest which tests are needed.

Your doctor will also measure your bladder capacity and any urine left behind for evidence of poorly functioning bladder muscles. To do this test, you'll drink plenty of fluids and then pee into a measuring pan. The doctor will measure any pee remaining in the bladder. Your doctor may also recommend any of the following:

- **Stress test:** You relax, then cough vigorously as the doctor watches for loss of urine.
- **Urinalysis:** Urine is tested for evidence of infection or urinary stones.
- **Ultrasound:** Sound waves are used to evaluate your kidneys, ureters, bladder, and urethra.
- **Cystoscopy:** A thin tube with a tiny camera is inserted in the urethra and used to see the inside of the urethra and bladder.
- **Urodynamics:** Various measuring techniques are used to check pressure in the bladder and the flow of urine.

REAL LIFE QUESTION: Is there such a thing as too much water?

Yes! There is a rare but very serious danger of overhydration among athletes, called hyponatremia. Four female marathoners have died from it. In a study done of Boston Marathon runners, 13 percent were found to be overhydrated.

What does it mean? Too much water, and not enough sodium or electrolytes. Without enough electrolytes, the cells cannot absorb the water, which is particularly dangerous for the brain. The first symptoms are often behavioral, such as confusion, shouting, or dizziness. Runners with overhydration will often gain weight during a race from fluid retention.

Many runners now use sports drinks instead of plain water—but if you are an endurance athlete, don't rely on magazine articles or rumors. Talk with your doctor about a hydration plan. Overhydration is also a problem for people with disorders of the body's organs. So yes, doctors want you to drink more fluids, but don't drink a gallon a day of plain water.

Your doctor may ask you to keep a diary for a day or more, to record when you pee and how much. Thankfully, measuring your urine is easy. You'll be given a plastic pan that fits on the toilet seat. It has measurement lines on it. You pee, then you look at the measurement, write it down, and then empty the pan. Nurses call the pan a hat. Yes, they do.

Going Against the Flow: Treatment of Incontinence

Incontinence is a symptom with many possible causes, so treatment varies widely depending on the cause. It may include exercises to strengthen your pelvic muscles, medication, behavior modification, external collection devices, or surgery to restore support to the pelvic muscles or reconstruct the urinary sphincter.

Kegel Exercises

The good news is that doing pelvic floor exercises, called Kegels, which help strengthen the muscles that control urine flow, can strengthen pelvic floor muscles. Kegel (rhymes with *bagel*) exercises strengthen or retrain pelvic floor muscles and sphincter muscles. Doing them regularly can reduce or cure stress leakage.

Once you learn these exercises, you can practice them virtually anywhere. Kegels won't help muscles that are already stretched or torn, but they can strengthen pelvic muscle tone to prevent future stretching. Kegel exercises can also help your sex life, as you'll see in chapter 11, Your Best Sex. The stronger your pelvic muscles, the better. Keep your muscle tone around the pelvic area and bladder, and stress incontinence is less likely to become a major problem.

Is it hard for you to remember to do a daily exercise? Tie it to some daily downtime, like commuting, getting morning coffee, falling asleep. Be sure to tell your doctor if you are unable to do your Kegels for any reason.

To do Kegel exercises:

1. **Identify the correct muscles.** Place your pointer finger in your vagina and squeeze around your finger. If you feel pressure on your finger, then you are squeezing the right muscles: the perineal muscles. Another way to identify the proper muscle group is to pee and then stop the flow of urine. These are the same muscles.
2. **Isolate the muscle.** While doing Kegel exercises, be sure to keep your body relaxed so that you can isolate the pelvic floor muscles you are trying to strengthen. The most common error is to squeeze your buttock muscles.
3. **Do the exercise routine.** Squeeze and repeat. Squeeze your perineal muscle and hold the squeeze for five seconds. Then relax the muscle slowly for five seconds. Do as many repetitions as you can, working up to five-minute sessions twice a day. Don't hold your breath

while you squeeze. Breathe slowly and deeply.

4. **Get stronger.** Once the exercises become easy, squeeze for ten seconds and then relax for ten seconds. Do the repetitions for five minutes, twice a day.
5. **Be consistent.** It takes six to twelve weeks after starting a Kegel exercise routine for most women to notice an improvement in bladder control, and consistency is key. Some women find it useful to get into a routine of doing Kegels around the same time each day, such as before getting out of bed in the morning and before going to sleep at night.
6. **Stay toned.** Once you have developed improved bladder control, you can keep your perineal muscle toned by maintaining your Kegel exercise routine at five minutes, three days per week. If incontinence comes back, you may need to increase to five minutes, twice a day, or more.

Electrical Muscle Stimulation

Electrical muscle stimulation (EMS) of the pelvic floor is a noninvasive method of working the pelvic floor muscles. Brief doses of electrical stimulation can strengthen muscles in the lower pelvis in a way similar to exercising the muscles. Electrodes are temporarily placed in the vagina or rectum or on the skin to stimulate nearby muscles.

Side effects of EMS are small. Some people report some pain when a high level of electrical stimulation is applied, but most people notice only a tingling sensation. The improvements in incontinence may continue after treatment from a few weeks to as long as several years.

Biofeedback

Biofeedback uses measuring devices to help you become aware of your body's actions and functions. By using biofeedback to track when your bladder and urethral muscles contract during your Kegel exercises, you can do a better-quality exercise. Biofeedback can be used along with Kegel exercises and electrical stimulation to further decrease stress and urge incontinence. Your doctor may work with you to train you in biofeedback or refer you to a specialist.

Medications

Medications can be used to decrease many types of leakage. Some drugs stop the contractions of an overactive bladder. Others relax muscles, leading to more complete bladder emptying when you pee. Some drugs tighten muscles at the base of the bladder and urethra to prevent leaks. Not all types of incontinence can be improved with medications.

NOTE TO SELF

A spa has opened in New York that will teach you Kegels and check your pelvic strength. You can buy a gift certificate, too. Somehow I don't recommend this as an anniversary gift.

Surgery

Does the word *surgery* scare you? Well, most incontinence treatments today are minimally invasive. Don't let fear stop you from getting help for incontinence!

For example, stress incontinence is often caused by the bladder dropping down. The surgeon can make a tiny incision in the abdomen or vagina and raise the bladder, attaching it to a muscle, ligament, or bone. For some types of stress incontinence, the surgeon may secure the bladder with a sling. Slings can also change the shape of the bladder and urethra to prevent leaks. Sometimes collagen or other materials are injected into tissues around the urethra, providing pressure to limit leaks.

Bladder Boot Camp

If leaking is not a major problem for you and you're looking for a nonmedical, nonsurgical approach to minimize your mild symptoms, try these lifestyle adjustments, which may just do the trick. Watching the types of foods you eat and the timing of when you drink, and doing some simple exercises to strengthen the pelvic floor muscles can reduce mild incontinence.

NOTE TO SELF

Don't hate me because I'm continent. Everyone has a friend who never has to go. It's not as bad as having a friend who never gains weight, plus you never have to let her go first in the ladies' room. Be grateful.

- **Drawn-out drinking:** Drink slowly! Rather than drinking a big bottle of water at one time, which goes through your system as one big wave of fluid, drink it over the course of several hours. It's much easier for your bladder to handle.
- **Drink plenty:** Do you think that drinking less water will keep you from leaking? Nope—it's the opposite! If you don't drink enough, you irritate the lining of the urethra and the bladder, which may increase leakage. Drink two to three quarts of water a day.
- **The good pee diet:** Some foods and drinks can make incontinence worse, as they contain irritants that can contribute to frequency, urgency, and urge incontinence. Alcoholic drinks; caffeinated beverages, such as coffee, tea, and cola; acidic fruits and juices, such as citrus, pineapples, tomatoes, and tomato-based products; and carbonated beverages (even caffeine free) are common bladder irritants for many people.
- **Avoid irritants:** Spicy foods, sugar, chocolate, corn syrup, artificial sweeteners, vinegar, and vitamins B, C, and E are irritants. Eliminating them—one at a time—might help. To identify irritants to your system, keep a Digestion Journal (see the appendix, Tools to Use) of what you eat and drink. Choose fruits that are less irritating, such as pears, apricots, papaya, and watermelon. Instead of coffee or tea, try noncitrus herbal teas.

- **Timed tinkle:** Like any muscle, the muscles that control continence can be trained. By lengthening the time between trips to the bathroom, bladder training can help women with urge incontinence. You start by urinating frequently, every thirty minutes or so. You increase the time gradually until you're going only every two to four hours. The clock dictates your toilet visits, not your bladder. You take routine, planned bathroom trips. Doctors call this "timed voiding." To start, you fill in a chart of peeing and leaking. From the patterns that appear in your chart, you plan to empty your bladder before you would otherwise leak.
- **Exercise:** Be sure to use your muscle conditioning—your Kegels or bladder training—to help support your work. And if you can't make today's goal, don't let your urge to pee become an emergency! Go ahead and go, on schedule or not—but get right back on the plan.

What to Remember about Your Waterworks

You can start today to improve your life tomorrow. Leave your embarrassment home when you talk to your doctor about urinary problems, because untreated problems can get a whole lot worse. Drink water frequently and slowly, but be sure to drink enough. If you start having infections or chronic problems, making lifestyle changes such as cutting down on citrus juices can be helpful. Learn to do Kegel exercises and then make them a regular part of your day. And keep the area around your urethra clean to protect yourself from infection. This is all part of keeping your body in its best shape for lfie.

Now that your plumbing is healthy, it's time for the fun part. In the next chapter, it's all about sex.

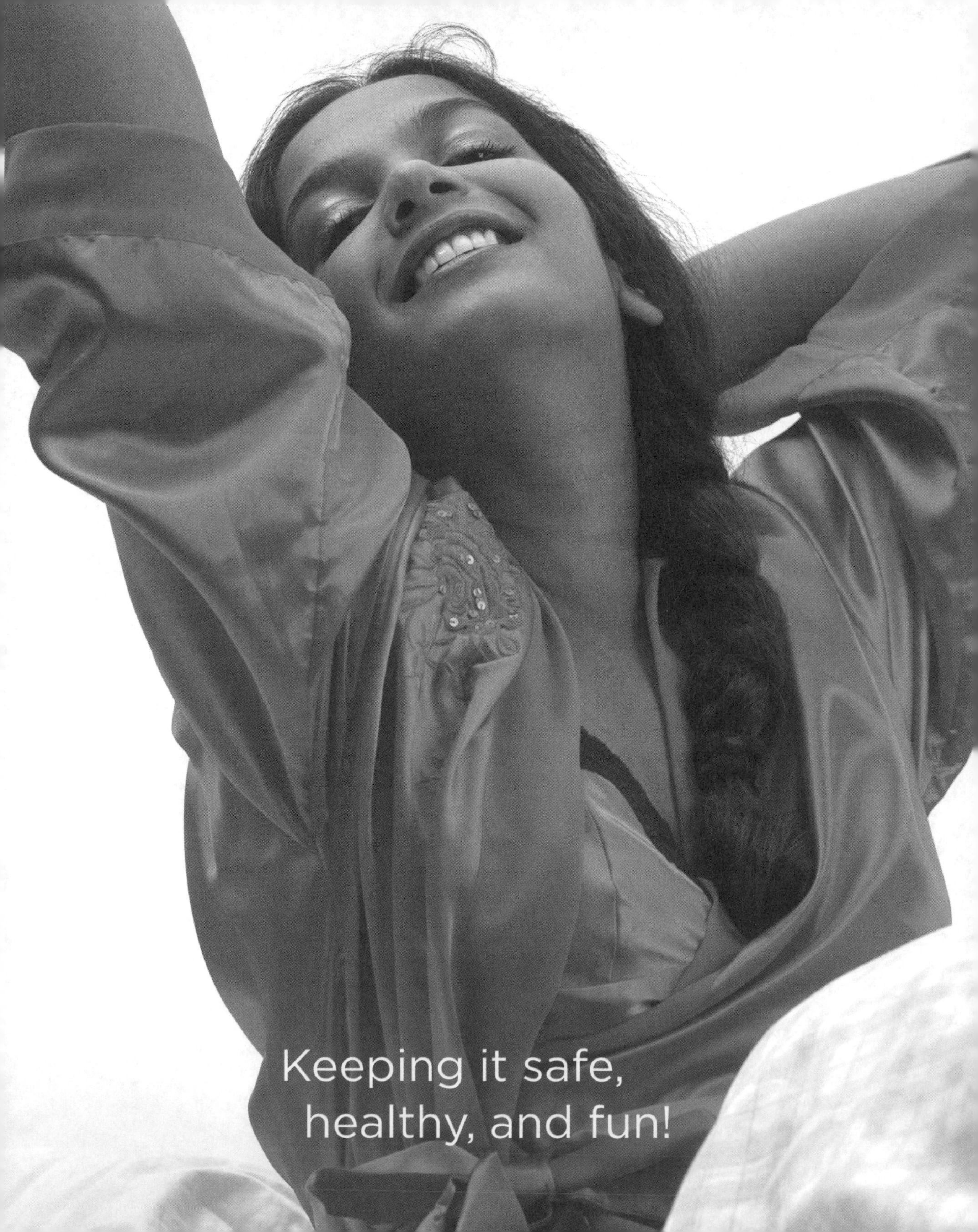
Keeping it safe,
healthy, and fun!

your best sex

Google the word *sex*. You'll find eight hundred million sites. Now Google *God*. God gets a measly fifty-four million. (In fairness, both *Jesus* and *Allah* beat *God* by a mile too.)

So here we are at last, on the big topic for humans. What I'd like to do is have an honest talk about it, because the world you live in screams *sex*! at you 24-7.

Try to picture your parents' coming of age. They might have snuck into a James Bond movie. They were thrilled to see cleavage and "necking." They would have argued about whether the actors were really French kissing or just pretending to.

Your life is *a little* different. There's more cleavage in a bridal magazine than your parents ever saw in a 007 movie. Turn on the TV and there's Hugh Hefner pretending to satisfy the needs of a dozen women in their twenties. They are almost begging for his attention. On MTV you watch young girls writhing around a rap star, also begging for his attention. And if the shows you watch are not sex filled, the commercials are! Oddly, it's not the Viagra commercials that show a lot of sex. It's the ones for trucks and lipstick.

That's prime-time, mainstream media. Venture into the world of pornography and you'll learn that men who fix photocopy machines are apparently offered sex daily by gorgeous women. He

REAL LIFE QUESTION: What is great sex?

You both enjoyed it. That's it!

may be hairy with a mullet and a moustache, but the woman is dazzled. She undresses the man, and they have seven different kinds of sex on the office equipment.

Is this what sex is about in real life? No, of course not. All sex on TV is fictional—as it was fictional in the 1960s for all TV couples to sleep in twin beds. Back then we knew it was fiction because some TV characters had magic powers but didn't do the obvious, which would be to use them to do the housework.

A world in which sex is a freely discussed subject and not something repressed is a good thing. But the flood of information about it is mostly wrong, and I think it's as harmful to girls and women as the skinny models are. So let's start with the basics about your sexual body and explore a healthy sex life.

By the way, now Google *love*. Depending on the day—two billion sites!

NOTE TO SELF

Sex is different for everyone. One patient said, "I was terrified the first time I had sex. The first minute was painful and I bled a lot. It got better after this. After the first time it was fine."

A Note Before We Start: It's Your Call

So what does sex mean to you? It's part of every woman's life at some level. Some of us love it and some of us don't, for many reasons. Your feelings about sex will change over the course of your life like a roller coaster ride—up, down, and back again! Some women choose never to have sex, but most women make it a part of their lives.

Knowledge about your body is the first step to a healthy sex life. This chapter will help you to learn about how your sexual body works. As a doctor, my job doesn't stop there—knowledge about the health of your sexual relationship comes next. A woman's sexual health is holistic: physical, emotional, and social health are all important to us. Unhealthy sexual relationships can erode your mental and emotional health and, in the case of abusive relationships, even put you in physical danger. A current or past experience with violence can also have a significant effect on your sexual and emotional health. And getting a **sexually transmitted infection** hurts both emotionally and physically.

How Does It Work? The Nuts and Bolts of Sex

Many people think that sex begins and ends with the genitals, but it's important to know that your whole body is involved in great sex. When you are kissing and your partner strokes your hair or rubs your back, it's all part of the hundreds of small sensations that cause and sustain arousal. When your partner looks into your eyes across a crowded room, makes a sexy phone call, or writes you an actual letter, all of these background incidents can contribute to great sex. Massage is another great arouser for nearly everybody. You may not be in the mood when you start out, but a nice oily massage may get you there. Or, as one patient says, "Skip the massage. Do the laundry, and I'm yours."

So although we're going to focus on understanding your sexual anatomy, please remember that all of your anatomy is important, especially what goes on in your brain!

Anatomy 101

Your **vulva** is central headquarters. Starting from the outside, your vulva is made up of the **clitoris**, outer **labia**, inner labia, vestibule, **hymen**, and vaginal opening. The hymen is different in every woman, but for all it's a thin fold of **mucous membrane** around the vaginal opening. It *can* break and cause a little bleeding when you first have sex—but not necessarily. The size of the opening of the hymen varies from one woman to another, so it doesn't always break with first sex if your opening happens to be a little larger. Don't think of it as a marker of whether or not you've had sex. You really can't tell anything by looking at it.

As you look at pictures of your anatomy throughout this book, remember that real people don't actually look like this. We're trying to show you clearly where everything is, so the vulva looks very organized. Many people have much wider labia, or much narrower. In real life everything will look a good bit more wrinkly, too.

But the clitoris is always located up front. It likes a lot of attention. During **foreplay**, your breasts and the clitoris are usually important

REAL LIFE QUESTION: Can I have sex while I have my period?

Yes, but be sure to put some towels underneath you! Some people, male and female, don't like to have sex at this time. It's a personal preference.

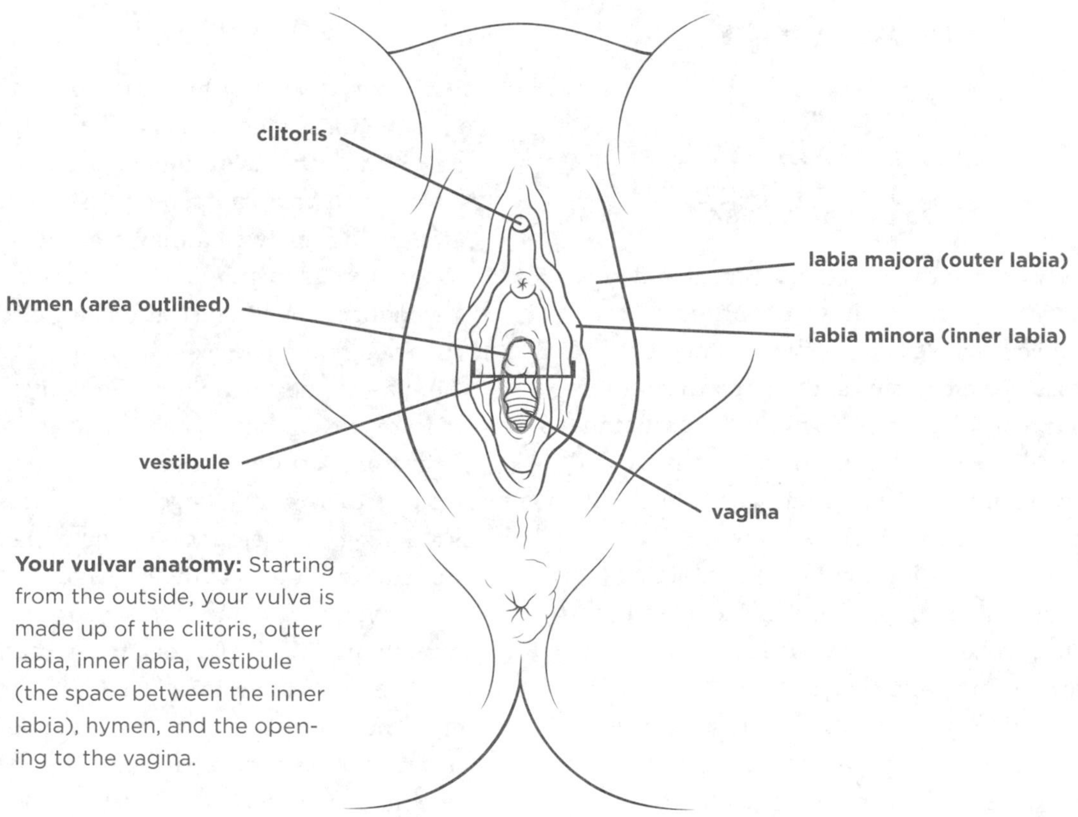

Your vulvar anatomy: Starting from the outside, your vulva is made up of the clitoris, outer labia, inner labia, vestibule (the space between the inner labia), hymen, and the opening to the vagina.

places for stroking. In fact, a woman can have an orgasm without anything going on in her **vagina**, from stroking of the clitoris alone.

Throughout history, many scientists and cultures have believed that women did not (and should not) enjoy sex. There's the oft-repeated motherly advice from Victorian times to perform sex as a duty to have children for your country: "I lie back, open my legs, and think of England." Amazingly, people have been studying the female orgasm for centuries now! Even Freud got involved. For some reason, people care a lot about whether your orgasm happens from stimulation of the vagina (as it happens in standard intercourse) or stimulation of the clitoris (which won't necessarily happen in standard intercourse). Mountains of books have been written about this issue, and then mountains of books were written wondering why.

The G-Spot

In 1950, Dr. Ernest Grafenberg, one of endless scientists studying the orgasm, announced that he had found a spot, where the **urethra**

REAL LIFE QUESTION: Will having sex during my period keep me from getting pregnant?

It's rare, but not impossible, to conceive during your period. The sperm can survive four to five days inside you, so if you have sex late in your menstrual cycle and ovulate early, yes, you could get pregnant.

backs up to the vagina, that would give women heightened enjoyment. Men have been trying to find it ever since. In 1981, his theory was named after him: the **G-spot**.

You have a lot more nerve endings in your clitoris than you do in your vagina, which supports the school of thought that says orgasms are clitoris based. Grafenberg's theory was that the G-spot is a part of your vagina that is near the urethra and that the urethra is involved in arousal. He said that it was in this spongy area on the front wall of the vagina that a vaginal orgasm would happen. I think that would work if you could find a man whose penis has a 90-degree bend to it!

Grafenberg, in fact, recommended "doggy-style"—penetration of the woman from behind—as the best position for reaching the G-spot. In 1953, Grafenberg edited his paper, taking out a lot of the emphasis on the G-spot. Some people say he changed his mind; others say he didn't like the criticism that came his way. Nobody's told *Cosmo*, which likes to run a cover story on it every month.

So what's true? I'm pretty sure the G-spot does not exist. Rather, your whole body and your whole relationship combined make one big G-spot. The clitoris is a lot of fun on its own, but it's an even richer experience when it's combined with vaginal sex. Parts of your vagina wall may give *you* more pleasure, and if you and your partner move around a bit or even try different positions, you'll find sex more satisfying. If you use your fingers to explore the inside front of your vagina, you will find a spongy area. It's not, however, a magic button!

Why am I telling you all this? Because at some point in your life a magazine article is going to talk about G-spots, and I wanted you to know the whole story. At some point you may also meet a man who is on an endless quest for the G-spot. You can tell him that there's no ignition button in your vagina, or you can let him continue his quest if you want to.

How You Get Turned On

Let's move on to something a little less exciting for a moment: what happens to the body's systems during sex. Medically, the female sexual response cycle consists of four stages of arousal, each one with its own specific mind and body changes.

- **Excitement:** The first stage is excitement, which is triggered by mind, body, or emotional stimulation. Your blood starts flowing to the genital area and your whole body picks up speed; your heart rate increases, your vagina swells, your respiration increases, and the vagina is lubricated.
- **Plateau:** The second stage is sustained excitement called the plateau. Your breasts get bigger, your nipples harden, and your **uterus** drops lower in your **pelvis**. Vaginal swelling, heart rate, and muscle tension may increase as long as stimulation continues. You need constant stimulation during this stage to have an orgasm.
- **Orgasm:** The third stage is orgasm, with vaginal, anal, and abdominal muscle contractions and intense pleasure.
- **Resolution:** The blood rushes away from the vagina. Your breasts and nipples go back to their normal size. Your heart rate, respiration, and blood pressure all slow down.
- **Refractory period:** After resolution, there is a refractory period, in which your body has to recover before another orgasm can happen.

How long is each stage? Everyone's different, and each time you have sex is different. Some women move from excitement to orgasm rapidly, some seem to take all day. And others alternate between plateau and orgasm several times. Women and men are quite different too. On average, women's time to orgasm is thirty minutes, with little or no refractory period. Remember that to come up with an average number we include everybody—of all extremes. The refractory period is the amount of rest time after an orgasm before a person is physically ready to orgasm again. It takes men, on average, between five and ten minutes to reach orgasm, with a refractory period that can last from five minutes to several days.

What's with that twenty-minute gap between men and women?! Remember that these are average numbers, so you may take more or less time, but most couples do have a gap between the man's path to orgasm and the woman's. How do couples handle this? Practice.

REAL LIFE FACT: La Petite Mort

Somebody named the feeling you have right after orgasm *la petite mort*, which is French for "the little death."

Practice helps you to understand your body, what works for you and what doesn't. The first time you have sex with a man, he is relying on his previous experience about what works. He may be a talker, for example, when you are not. He may be focused for so long on your breasts that he skips the clitoris entirely.

When you learn your own body, you can guide him. You can say something, especially to the talker, or you can slide his hand where you want it to go. Self-pleasuring gives you a road map for what you like and don't like and can help you guide your partner. I wish we had another word for *masturbate*. The word still has a bad image, but it's generally considered a good idea for young women to try their bodies out on their own.

In pornography, men and women often have their orgasms at the same time. In real life, they rarely do. If you meet a woman who says she has a mutual orgasm every single time she and her husband have sex, well, you know you've met a liar, who probably answered the survey you'll read about a little later in the chapter.

Well, What about Him?

So you've learned a little bit more about your body and sex now. If your partner is female, I hope this information will be valuable to you as a couple. If your partner is a man, this section looks at his mechanics. I'm not going to go into the whole biological reproductive part, though. Let's just do the naughty bits!

Page 228 shows what a guy's penis looks like when it's unaroused, or flaccid. Remember that illustrations can't show you the wide variety of what's normal. Some guys have flaccid penises that look like little prairie dogs peeking out from underground. Others look like they've been lifting weights. Penises come in many different sizes, and you can't tell from the flaccid view how big it's going to be when it's erect.

This penis appears rather big. Your partner may be smaller, but he also might be a grower, not a show-er. Just think of all that time he wasted comparing himself to the other boys in the locker room, when it's the erect size that matters to us!

Page 228 also shows the aroused penis. Now, let's stop and take a look at circumcision, the biggest basic difference you'll see in penises around the world. Circumcision is the process of removing the foreskin from the penis, and it usually happens when boys are infants. It's very common in the United States. Many men from other cultures, however, are not circumcised. Their flaccid penis always looks like it's wearing a little hood. When it's erect, it looks a lot like a circumcised penis, but the foreskin will move up and down during—there's no other way to say it—a hand job.

Circumcision can be a religious ritual (called a *bris* in Judaism) or a common practice without ritual (as in Islam). It's less common to see circumcision among Hindus and Buddhists. In the United States, circumcision has become a popular way to keep the penis clean.

The choice to have a child circumcised can be complex, and the medical evidence is

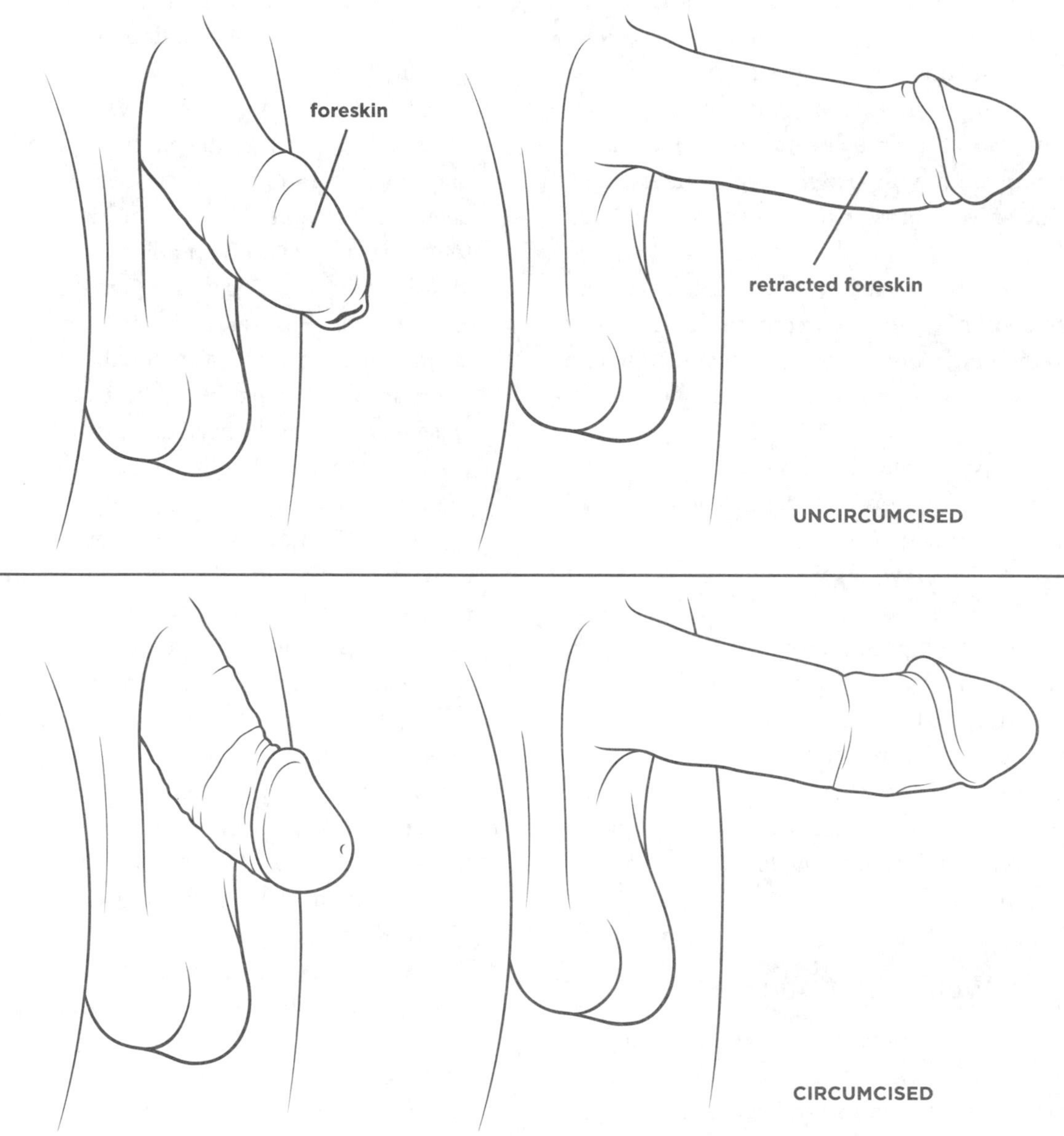

The male mechanics: The uncircumcised penis (top left) looks similar to the circumcised penis (bottom left) when erect (top and bottom right, respectively) because the foreskin is retracted.

ever changing, so you are likely to encounter men of both types. There are many websites dedicated to the subject to help parents decide which way to go.

If you are used to one style, the other may look odd before you get to know it. You will get used to either one, but I thought I'd get you ready for the differences. Asking him "What's that?" during foreplay is not on *Cosmo*'s Top Ten Sexy Things to Say to Drive Him Wild.

As you read through the stages of the female orgasm above, you probably realized that it's all pretty complicated, isn't it? Well, as you become more sexually experienced, you'll also notice that your orgasm is really different from your partner's. Anthroplogists and biologists love to create theories about the gender orgasm, just like the G-spot, but we really only know that they are different. We could have a long discussion about this, and I think it's an interesting thing to study, but you're looking for more practical information, so let's track the basic male sex experience.

First, you should know that because the male orgasm can happen quickly, most men are trying to slow themselves down when they're having sex. Yes, they really do think about baseball as a way to delay the climax. They want to please you, and a flaccid, post-orgasm penis is not good at sex. So start slowly.

You'll be kissing and fondling each other. Stroke his back, play with his nipples, stroke his inner thighs, whisper in his ear. He'll be touching and kissing your breasts and playing with your nipples with his tongue or fingers. He'll start to touch your genitals—but wait awhile before you touch his penis. You want to enjoy this lovely period of arousal, and if you go for the penis right away, you'll end it quickly.

When you want to go for penetration, you can move from stroking his inner thighs to stroking his balls. Be gentle here—and then move up to the penis, touching softly from bottom to top with your fingertips, and back again. Eventually, you'll want to grab it gently and start to stroke up and down. When you do, he'll be wanting penetration soon.

When a man reaches climax, it's because of a stroking stimulation—no matter what kind of sex you have. When he comes, he'll produce a small spoonful or so of milky white semen, which carries the sperm that will seek the egg in your body. Remember, to protect yourself from pregnancy and STIs, always use a **condom** every time you have sex unless you are in a long-term, committed relationship with a partner who has been tested and cleared for sexually transmitted diseases and you are using another form of birth control.

NOTE TO SELF

Remember that every woman likes different things about sex. One patient said, "I don't mind oral sex, but please don't kiss me afterward. For at least a day."

Is Oral Sex Sex?

If you want to get a group of teenagers' parents really hopping mad, tell them you don't think **oral sex** is sex. The generation gap in the

1960s and '70s was about the war in Vietnam. Today, it's about oral sex.

Oral sex is when one person stimulates another person's genitals with the mouth or tongue. For men, this means a woman (or a man) takes the penis in the mouth and stimulates it for foreplay or until he reaches orgasm (or to use the more common term, until he comes). The female version is to have the clitoris and/or vagina stimulated with the partner's tongue. Although you can't get pregnant from oral sex, you can spread sexually transmitted infections this way.

Doctors—and afternoon talk shows—are seeing a major rise in stories about teenagers giving and having oral sex, especially young teenagers. It's the biggest surge ever reported. Some studies estimate that 40 percent of teenagers have had oral sex, many with more than one person. The attitude about oral sex seems to be that oral sex won't give them a bad reputation or negatively affect how they think about themselves, or make them pregnant. To them, oral sex is simply "no big deal." Many teens think there are no health risks to oral sex. But STIs are skyrocketing in this age group. If a teenager believes that oral sex isn't sex, she won't protect herself. My message to her: Please don't be fooled!

NOTE TO SELF

Oral sex is sex. So be sure to protect yourself against STIs!

Herpes is probably the biggest STI risk from oral sex. Two strains of herpes—herpes simplex virus types 1 and 2—can live in the mouth or the genitals. They are spread, especially during outbreaks, by direct contact with the sore. Having oral herpes, also known as a cold sore, is usually a pain for about a week. Genital herpes, however, can be much more complicated and uncomfortable. It's not a good idea to have unprotected oral sex when you have any lesions, either oral or genital, because the virus can be transmitted from mouth to genitals and from genitals to mouth.

Other oral sex STIs? **Chlamydia** and **gonorrhea** can infect your throat. **HIV** can be passed through unprotected oral sex but is more likely to be passed during unprotected intercourse. The infected semen or vaginal fluid enters the body through a cut or sore in the mouth

REAL LIFE QUESTION: If we practice withdrawal before orgasm, am I safe from STIs when having oral sex?

Not completely, even though you have a slightly better chance. The problem is that fluids from the body leak long before climax. Herpes is spread from the actual herpes lesion, so withdrawal does not lower the risk of herpes at all. The safest protection is a condom or a dental dam.

or **esophagus** to cause infection. The virus is unlikely to be passed from a person's mouth to another person's genitals. Syphilis can also be transmitted through oral sex.

How to Use a Dental Dam

A **dental dam** is a sheet of latex that you use as a barrier during oral sex so you don't come in direct contact with body fluids or lesions. Many people make them out of condoms by cutting off the condom tip and then cutting down the side of the condom so you are left with a rectangular barrier. (And yes, they are used in dentistry.) Some people also make dental dams out of plastic wrap, but the material that condoms are made from is better than plastic wrap because it does a better job of preventing germs from passing through.

Remember that the purpose of a dental dam is to prevent the spread of disease during oral sex. To use one, make a mark with permanent marker (in advance) on the side of the dam that will face your partner (so you don't accidentally switch sides in the moment). Spread the dam over the vagina or anus, being sure to cover the entire area (because you may decide to do more than you originally planned). Use your tongue as you normally would during oral sex to arouse your partner or bring him or her to climax. If the area you need to cover is large, use a piece of plastic wrap instead of a condom, especially if both the vagina and anus will be involved. Even if the anus won't be stimulated, many women find the perineum to be an arousing destination. Keep the whole area covered—and never, ever reuse a dam.

How to Use a Condom

Using a condom the right way can prevent pregnancy and protect you and your partner from STIs. Put a male or female condom on *before* sex, not during. A male condom should be put on an erect penis.

To use a male condom (see illustration on page 232), place the rolled-up condom over the tip of the erect penis. Hold the end of the condom to allow a little extra space at the tip. With the other hand, unroll the condom down over the penis. Right after ejaculation, hold the condom against the base of the penis as it's withdrawn from the vagina, to avoid spilling any semen. Then throw the condom away. When the condom is off, it's not safe to resume sex. There are plenty of sperm left behind.

To use a female condom (see illustration on page 233), squeeze the inner ring between your fingers and insert it into the vagina (like a tampon). Push the inner ring into the vagina as far as it can go. Let the outer ring hang about an inch outside your body. Guide the penis through the outer ring. Right after ejaculation, squeeze and twist the outer ring and pull the pouch out gently. Like the male condom, it should be thrown away. Never use it again.

Do not use the male and female condom at the same time! This makes both condoms more likely to break.

NOTE TO SELF

One of my patients told me, "My definition of marriage is that for once you are hoping the pregnancy test is positive."

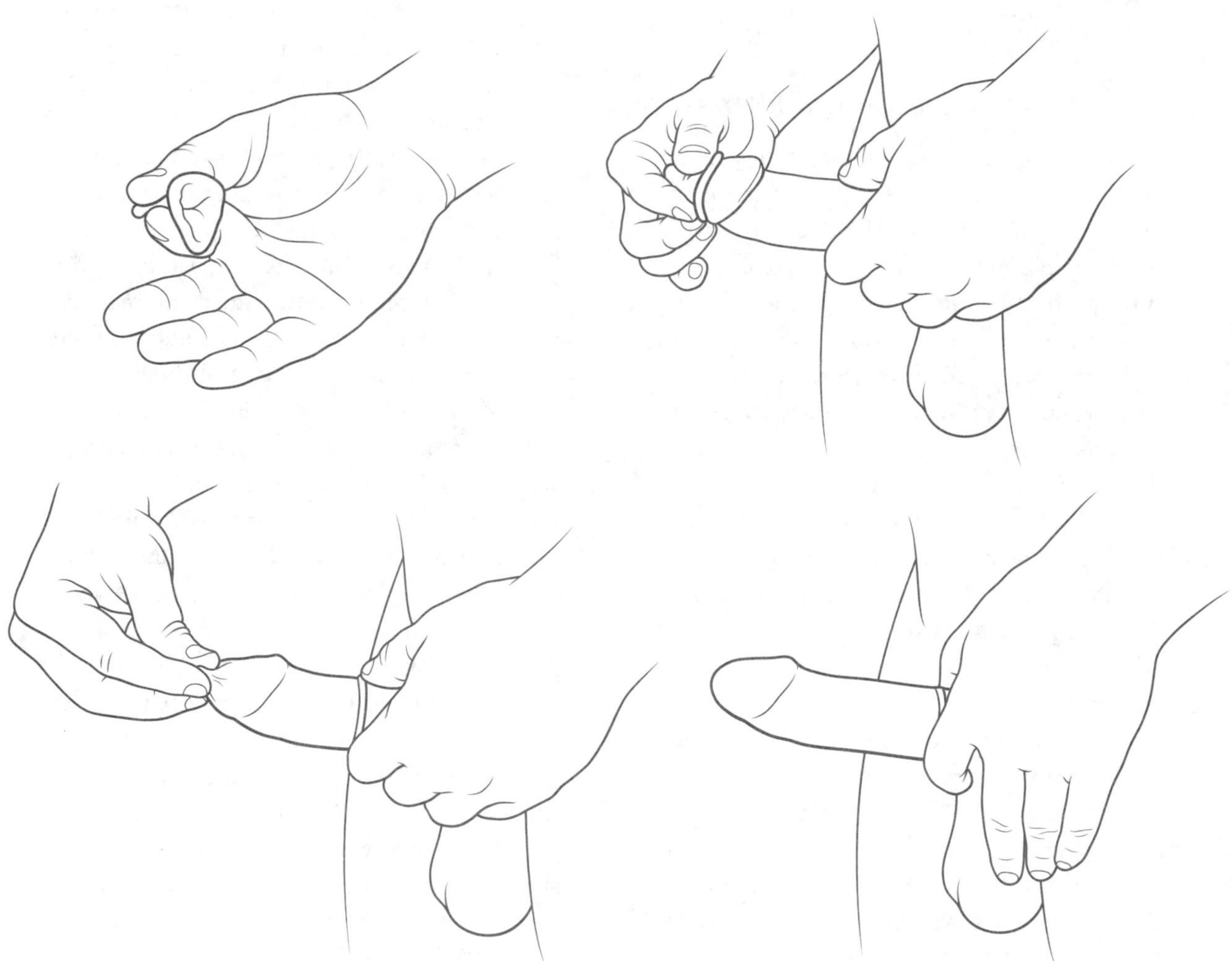

To use a male condom, place the rolled-up condom over the tip of the erect penis. Hold the end of the condom to allow a little extra space at the tip. With the other hand, unroll the condom down over the penis.

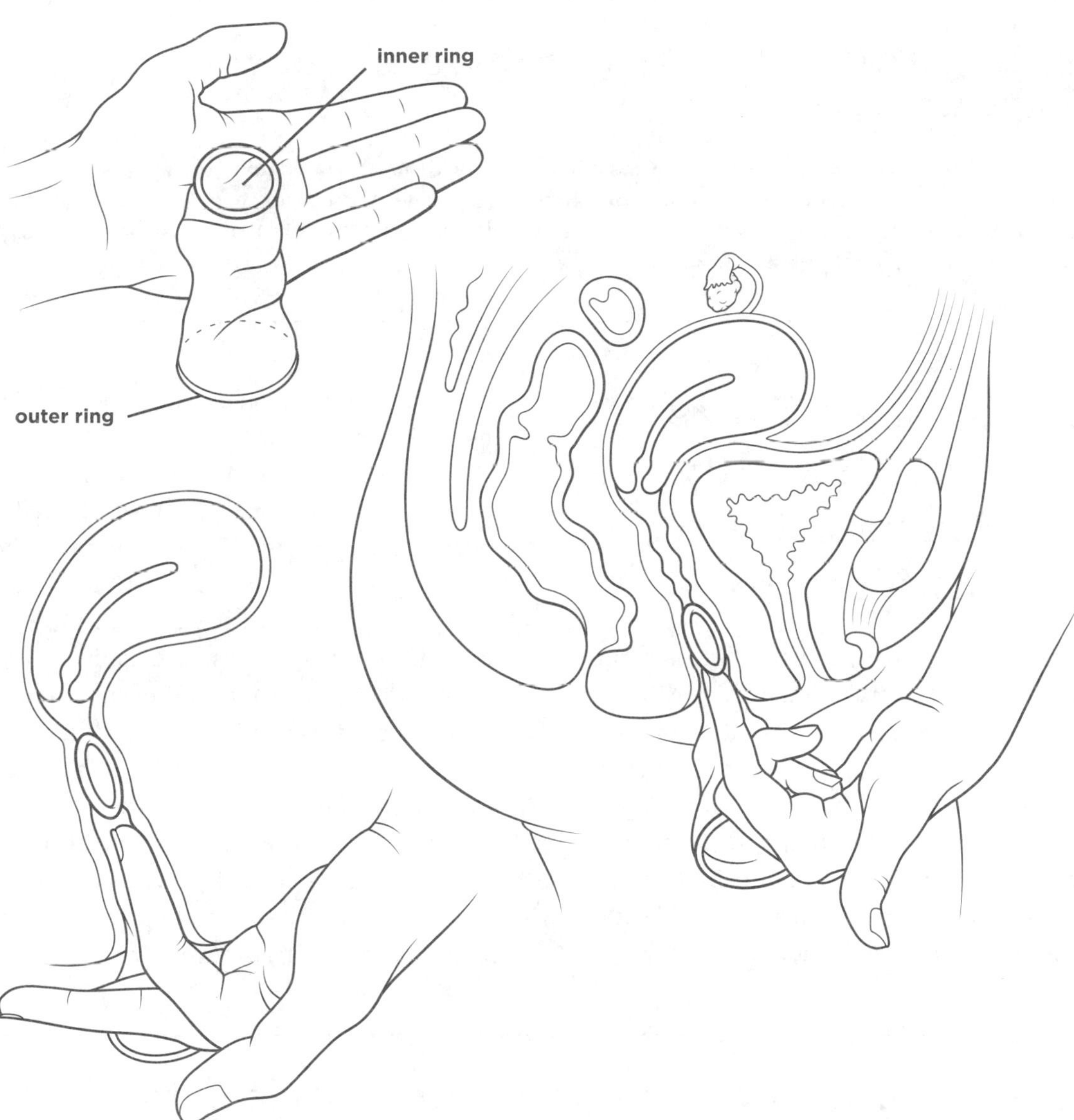

To use a female condom, squeeze the inner ring between your fingers and insert it into the vagina (like a tampon). Push the inner ring into the vagina as far as it will go. Let the outer ring hang about an inch outside your body. Guide the penis through the outer ring and into the vagina.

REAL LIFE QUESTION: Does having a cold sore mean I have an STI?

Not necessarily. Most cold sores on your lips are spread by kissing. You usually get your first case in childhood when someone with a cold sore kisses you. It's very common for Mom and Dad to pass on sores to their little ones. Cold sores are very contagious, though. Don't kiss any part of your partner when you have a cold sore.

Protecting Yourself from Sexually Transmitted Infections

Worries about sexually transmitted infections will put a damper on your sex drive. STIs are diseases that are spread by sexual contact—by having oral, anal, or vaginal sex with someone who has an STI (see chapter 13, Your Vagina and Cervix, for details). Some STIs can damage your potential to have a baby later on. Some are painful, and HIV can even kill you if it results in acquired immunodeficiency syndrome (**AIDS**) and you don't get a timely diagnosis and treatment.

Some STIs, like gonorrhea, can be cured. Others, like herpes and HIV, can be treated but not cured. Anyone who has sex, even one time, can get pregnant or get an STI. Use a condom every time you have sex until you are in a committed, long-term relationship and you have both been tested and cleared. It's the only effective way, other than abstinence, to reduce the risk of infection. Use a dental dam made from condoms for oral sex.

The human papillomavirus (**HPV**), believed to cause certain cervical **cancers**, is sexually transmitted. Condoms can give you a little protection, but you are still at risk

REAL LIFE QUESTION : As a lesbian, do I need to practice safe sex?

Absolutely yes. STIs don't know you are a lesbian. They travel via human skin and genital contact. Use protection, such as a dental dam, until you are in a long-term, committed relationship and both of you have been tested for STIs. If you use sex toys, do not share them outside the relationship.

because HPV can spread from contact with the areas not covered by the condom, such as the scrotum, vulva, or **anus** or the skin between those areas. If you qualify for the HPV vaccination, make sure you get it.

How Often Is Everyone Else Doing It?

Everybody wants to know what other people are doing. Your friends aren't a large enough group to give you the dirt you want, because you want to know about *everybody*.

Search the Internet for sex surveys, and more than a million results come back because like you, everyone is curious. Now turn on the news. If it's sweeps week, the investigative news team will have conducted a shocking in-depth study of American sex habits. The problem with these reports? People, including you and me, lie to pollsters. You remember high school and the boys who said they had had sex with thirty girls when there were only three girls who had had sex at all? We tell more lies about sex than about anything else.

There's a condom company, Durex, that regularly surveys the world about sex. It's entertaining, because they announce how often people in each country have sex, and then the media in those countries goes wild. Here's an excerpt.

DUREX GLOBAL SEX SURVEY: How many times a year do people say they have sex?

Top Six		Bottom Six	
Greece	138	Malaysia	83
Croatia	134	Hong Kong	78
Serbia and Montenegro	128	Indonesia	77
Bulgaria	127	India	75
Czech Republic	120	Singapore	73
France	120	Japan	45

The United States is eleventh, at 113 times a year. I'm sure you noticed that the top six are all more or less neighbors, and so are the bottom six. I don't know what that means, but I'm sure it means something. Here's what else people said about themselves:

- The most common place to have sex outside of the bedroom is the car.
- Worldwide, the average age to have sex for the first time is 17.3 years.
- The average number of sexual partners is nine. (We'll never really know, because men tend to exaggerate the number and women tend to lower it.)
- About half of all adults in the world have had unprotected sex.
- About 13 percent of adults have had a sexually transmitted infection.

How Often Should I Be Doing It?

So what is a normal sex "schedule"? I think it works like this: You find somebody incredibly attractive. You want to have sex all the time. Your weekends are spent in bed. Eventually, one of you will suggest going to a movie. You go to the theater, then race back to have sex. Next time, you linger over coffee and just talk. Slowly, your sex drive slows down, over weeks, maybe months. That's a natural pattern. So now sex isn't the only thing you do. Being together is just as important.

At this point, you'll either stay together because you actually love this person and feel loved, or you'll break up and look for the next partner who gives you that same excitement. I've noticed that people who are divorced many times often can't tell the difference between excitement and love. When the sexual excitement cools down, they think they're not in love anymore.

That excitement is what keeps us reproducing. But love is different. Over the course of a marriage, there will be sexual hills and valleys even when love is strong. A newborn in the house is a definite downer for sex, but great for love. The toddler years are exhausting, and by the end of a day you feel that if one more person touches you, you'll smack them. By the time the kids are in school, you become more comfortable getting a sitter, going out on a date, and having sex when you get home. Oops, now they are teenagers. They are out of the house and you could be having sex all evening, except that you are sitting home in terror because they have the car. Then someday the kids move out, and hopefully you have an increase in your sex life again.

As you grow older, your hormones don't give you the same urge for sex. But your brain does! Nobody believes that Grammy and Pop-Pop do it, but you'd be surprised. Sex is just different at every stage of your life. There's an old saying that if you put a penny in a jar every time you have sex in your first year of marriage, and then you take a penny from the jar every time you have sex after that, you'll never empty the jar.

Well, I don't believe it. Someday we're going to find the guy who made this up and realize that he didn't have much sex after his first year of marriage because that's when his wife kicked him out. And then I hope we discover that *her* penny jar is . . . empty.

Because people lie on all of these surveys, women get the idea that if they're not having sex morning, noon, and night, then they are below average. Just think for a moment: What would you and your partner say if a pollster asked you how often you have sex?

"Oh, all the time."

Sexual practices and beliefs vary. Defining *normal* is challenging. Some couples like to have sex daily. For others, once a month is enough. Many people see oral sex as a normal

NOTE TO SELF

One patient told me, "I was so tired from law school I used to tell my husband, 'Honey, just cover me when you're done.'"

REAL LIFE FACT: Don't Believe What You See in the Movies or on TV

Since the 1960s, the media has exploded with sexual images and information. Sexual freedom has been good for many people, but there's one big problem: Everybody thinks they should perform like Mullet Man and Busty Girl. Men believe they are expected to have instant erections. Women feel inferior if they fail to reach orgasm at least once in every session of sex. If you find yourself feeling inadequate, remember that the only true measure of your worth as a lover is the pleasure you and your partner find together. Sexuality is just one part of our need for closeness, touch, playfulness, caring, and pleasure.

part of foreplay, but some can't stand it. Here's my definition: if you hear a sexual idea and think "Hmm, that sounds fun," then it's normal. If you think "Eew, that's disgusting," then it's abnormal. Normal for you and your partner is whatever gives you pleasure together. Both partners should agree on how to make their sex life happy.

Making a Decision to Have Sex

With all the sex being shown on television, in movies, and in music videos, it's easy to think that everyone is doing it. Not true.

What your feelings about sex? Are you ready for it in this relationship? Do you really know how your partner feels about sex? Make up your own mind about when is the right time to have sex. If you are not ready for sex, say so. Anyone who truly cares about you will respect your decision. If someone tries to pressure you into having sex when you don't want to, keep saying no. The person who won't respect your refusal is giving you a very clear picture of his or her character. Kick this bully to the curb.

Waiting for marriage before having sex has become less common today. I don't believe it's simply a moral issue. Remember that a hundred years ago, girls could marry at sixteen. A young woman today is more likely to be twenty-six when she gets married. That's a very long time to abstain.

Other Sexual Acts You May Have Heard About

This is not a book about sex, and there are plenty of them out there. But I want to give you a short description of sexual styles, positions, and practices that you may hear about—and wonder about.

- The *Kama Sutra* is a nearly-two-thousand-year-old Indian text with a big section about sex. It shows drawings of sexual positions that are anatomically and geometrically impossible. Do your back a favor and don't try them at home!
- Tantric sex is apparently different depending on the teacher, but it appears to be a school of thought about slowing down, doing a lot of breathing, and operating on a spiritual plane.
- Anal sex means inserting the penis into the anus. More widely known among gay men, it also happens among heterosexual couples. One patient had it happen by accident while she and her husband were trying "doggy-style" sex—true story—and said it was "worse than constipation." Because anal sex comes with a very high risk for STIs, a condom is essential. Anal sex can cause tiny tears in the **rectum**, creating the perfect entrance for STIs, including HIV.
- "Doggy-style" is not anal sex. It is inserting the penis into the vagina from behind you instead of in the man-on-top position, which is also called the missionary position. Some couples love this, some don't, and not everybody can actually do it. A lot depends on the angles of your bodies, inside and out.
- Cunnilingus and fellatio are the official names for oral sex. Cunnilingus is using the mouth and tongue to stimulate the clitoris, as foreplay or to climax. Fellatio is using the mouth and tongue to stimulate the penis (also known as a blow job).
- Analingus is using the tongue on and in the anus. This is also called a rim job. To be blunt, I can't think of a faster way to spread **bacteria**. If your partner is interested and you are too, well, you're lucky to find each other. But seriously, this is going to make one of you sick. Please use a dental dam.
- Scissoring is when two women open their legs and join together at the vulva, each forming the shape of a pair of scissors. The friction of rubbing against the genitalia leads to orgasm. This is also called tribadism or tribbing.
- Fisting is a technique using the fist to arouse a woman and give her an orgasm. The idea is that the hand can fit into a truly relaxed vagina, where it will naturally form a fist. For this not to be painful, the woman must be extremely aroused already and highly lubricated. Many women cannot tolerate fisting.
- Dildos are fake penises some women use in sex or masturbation, sometimes with a vibrator. Many dildos have a little extension on the front to stimulate the clitoris.
- Sex toys range from sexy outfits to vibrators to bizarre things you can't figure out. Most people who use sex toys do so when they have been married a long time and want to spice things up,

but young couples sometimes try them too. Some people even give sex toys as gifts at bridal showers. Word of advice: Think that through carefully.

- Fetishes are sexual obsessions with objects that are not normally considered sexual, such as feet and shoes. Fetishes are usually harmless. Only you can decide whether your partner's fetish is tolerable.
- Autoerotic asphyxia is a truly crazy idea that your orgasm will be better if you are strangled. Don't try it, under any circumstances. It kills people. If anyone ever suggests trying this, remember how it started: people noticed that when you hang a man, his penis hardens before he dies. I guarantee this didn't happen because he was excited.
- Sadism is hurting, controlling, and humiliating your partner. Masochism is wanting your partner to hurt, control, and humiliate you. Bondage is being tied up for sex. Some people try "bondage lite," meaning your hands are tied together with a ribbon or some such. Hard-core bondage is a much more intense, harsh activity. If you or your partner wants to make the hard-core version of these activities a regular habit, my personal view is that you should see a therapist first. You may find a therapist who will tell you that "everything is normal;" just make sure the kids never find out.

The Top Ten Questions I've Been Asked about Sex

As a female doctor, I get asked lots of questions about sex by my young female patients. Here are their top ten questions. I bet you've been wondering some of these things, too.

1. Can you avoid pregnancy using withdrawal?
   No. I repeat, no.
2. Do birth control pills make you fat?
   The Pill has changed! Scientific evidence says the Pill does not cause weight gain.
3. If you give oral sex and swallow the semen, can it make you pregnant?
   No.
4. Can it give you an STI?
   Yes. I repeat, yes.
5. How do I ask a man to use a condom?
   If you can't ask that, you don't know him well enough to have sex. In the meantime, follow this practical advice: Pack your own condoms. Hand him one or put it on him yourself.
6. How do I teach my partner what I like?
   Keep responding positively when you like something your partner does. Then have a conversation about it when you're not in the middle of sex: "I love it when you . . . "
7. How can I get my partner to be more adventurous?
   Ask him or her to, with specific suggestions. Nobody has the same definition of adventurous. You might be thinking, "sex while

bungee jumping," whereas your partner thinks, "sex with the lights on."

8. It hurts to have sex. Should it?
   No. Good time to call for an appointment with your gynecologist. In the meantime, see if you need extra lubrication; there are many good brands available. Try different positions.
9. Why does my partner insist on turning out the lights? I want us to see each other.
   Some people are very uncomfortable unless the room is dark. You can try taking turns. A candle might be a compromise. One patient of mine has not undressed in front of her husband ever, in forty years of marriage.
10. Should I fake an orgasm?
   Only if you are late for work.

What Can Go Wrong: When Sex Isn't Good

Sex is not always perfect. Sometimes it's far from perfect. If your sex life is not satisfying you, you're not alone. Problems with sexuality that bother you are what doctors call sexual dysfunction. Sexual dysfunction is defined based on personal dissatisfaction with either the amount of sex or its quality. There's no universal definition, for example, of too much sex or too little sex.

Some women have no sexual desire. Some feel pain with sexual intercourse, which quickly snuffs out any desire they may have had. Others feel desire, but then their bodies don't seem to respond. Still others have bodies that respond, but they don't reach orgasm.

REAL LIFE FACT: Faking Orgasms

Everyone has done it. What are your reasons?

- **I don't want to hurt my partner's feelings, but I just want to stop and go to sleep.**
- **I want my partner to think I'm a sexy woman who has multiple orgasms.**
- **I never have orgasms during sex, so I fake it. I'm too embarrassed to tell my partner what I really want, or that I need more foreplay.**
- **It's my first time having sex with this partner, who turns out to be not so great, and I want to get it over with.**

So should you or shouldn't you? Faking an orgasm is a white lie—but it's a bad habit to get into. It lets your partner get lazy, for one thing. But mainly, you deserve to enjoy sex and to do it in a way that satisfies you.

There is no single age group for which sexual problems become more of an issue. Women report problems with sexuality when they are in their late teens to their elderly years. Problems with sexuality can arise from medical problems, emotional issues, and often a combination of both. Doctors divide problems related to female sexuality into four classifications of female sexual dysfunction to help understand and treat them, but there is a great deal of overlap across the groups.

NOTE TO SELF

About 40 percent of women are dissatisfied with their sex lives.

Hypoactive Sexual Desire Disorder

Hypoactive sexual desire disorder is a low sex drive—defined by you, not by anyone else. It's not really accurate to call this a disorder, given that it happens to everyone at some point in life. You may notice that you've stopped having sexual thoughts, fantasies, or desires. More often, a woman's interest in sex diminishes because of lifestyle factors or problems in the relationship with communication, anger, trust, and intimacy. A low sex drive can be part of depression and often is one of the earlier signs of being depressed. When people are depressed, they usually lose interest in things that used to give them pleasure, including sex.

There is a big difference between low libido caused by a medical issue and low libido caused by a husband who scratches his balls at the dinner table and won't change a diaper. Raising children and running an overly busy life won't help your libido either.

There's no easy fix for low libido, but most people find that lifestyle changes and partners counseling are helpful. There *are* some simple steps that you can try on your own. Look at your lifestyle first: How much sleep are you getting? How healthy is your diet? A healthy body tends to be more interested in sex.

Next, practice arousal when you are alone. Rent a movie that you find arousing. Explore your body. To take the pressure off of you, tell your partner that you'd like to be the one who initiates sex for a while. Then be sure to do so sometimes, so your partner doesn't fear this is your way of ending sexual contact for good.

Sexual Arousal Disorder

Step one of sex is excitement, and step two is arousal. If sex is what your mind wants and your body doesn't respond, doctors call it **sexual arousal disorder**.

During arousal, your body normally produces genital lubrication, swelling, and nipple sensitivity. Lubrication depends on the swelling of blood vessels in the genitals. Any condition that cuts blood flow to this area can cause problems with sexual arousal. Conditions that can cause blood flow problems include pelvic surgery, such as hysterectomy;

childbirth; breastfeeding; and certain medical disorders.

We're not positive that surgery is a cause. Although some studies show sex improving after pelvic surgery (such as **hysterectomy**), others show difficulty with vaginal lubrication and a loss of genital sensation. Some experts believe that the removal of the **cervix** and injury to the nerves during surgery can compromise blood flow and sensation to the genitals. This is controversial. Vaginal tearing from childbirth sometimes causes nerve and vascular damage and problems with vaginal and clitoral sensation. Usually the tissues heal and women feel just fine after childbirth.

Other medical diseases that can affect blood flow to the pelvic region include **heart disease**, high blood pressure, **diabetes**, and high **cholesterol**. No blood flow? No arousal.

NOTE TO SELF

There is more to sex than orgasms!

Orgasmic Disorder

Difficulty reaching orgasm, or climax, after sufficient sexual stimulation is called **orgasmic disorder**. Orgasmic disorders include premature ejaculation in men. Premature ejaculation is a very common sex problem, especially among younger men. As with most sex-related problems, it affects both partners—some studies suggest that nearly 30 percent of couples report premature ejaculation as the biggest sexual problem in their relationship.

How do we define premature ejaculation? Realistically, I would define premature ejaculation as male orgasm that happens shortly after sex begins. If a woman takes an hour to achieve orgasm and the man can last forty minutes, that's technically premature ejaculation for that couple! At the other extreme, one minute is too little time for most couples, as very few women are going to climax within a minute. But remember that you can still have plenty of fun and reach a climax through touching or oral sex.

REAL LIFE FACT: Breastfeeding and Dryness

Breastfeeding can cause your lubrication to slow down, a problem many women experience. This happens because your prolactin hormone levels (the ones that cause your breasts to produce milk) have increased and your estrogen levels have decreased. This reverses once ovulation resumes, your estrogen levels return to normal, and your period restarts. For some women, periods return even while breastfeeding. For others, periods, lubrication, and estrogen increases won't happen until the baby is completely weaned. For most women, sex feels fine once they feel like their body is their own and their hormones are back to normal.

REAL LIFE QUESTION: I think I peed while having an orgasm—is that possible?

Most likely you are a woman who ejaculates liquid during sex. Many people have never heard of that, but it's real, so you can assure your partner that you did not just wet the bed.

If one or both of you is having a constant problem with achieving an orgasm, or with premature ejaculation, start by checking your thoughts. Because the mind is a major part of sex, attitude can make or break your satisfaction. Is orgasm a goal? If so, a goal-oriented person may be very bothered by the effort to have one and any failure to achieve one. Sexuality can be very satisfying even when orgasm is not the end result. People who are pleasure-oriented can find any sexual activity to be an end in itself; it doesn't have to lead to something else. Sometimes it's very satisfying just being close or touching each other. There's a great deal of pleasure in the process of sexuality, and sometimes it helps to focus on that.

It's important for women to remember that there is much more to sex than orgasm. Exploration, sensuality, and connection can be lost when the sex act becomes goal-oriented, focusing on orgasm as the ultimate experience. At the same time, you may just need a minute of clitoral stimulation to bring you over the top—and you, or your partner, or you and your partner together could do that.

Sexual Pain Disorder

Recurrent or persistent genital pain associated with sexual intercourse is called sexual pain disorder. It's perfectly natural and normal to find sex painful occasionally, especially in certain positions. A vaginal **yeast infection** can make the vagina and external genitalia very sore and tender. It's only a sexual pain disorder if the pain is keeps coming back or won't get better.

Sometimes pain comes from incomplete arousal and lack of vaginal lubrication. You can help this by taking more time with foreplay or using a vaginal lubricant. Pain can also be caused by **vaginismus**, an involuntary tensing of the vaginal muscles causing severe pain with any vaginal penetration. Sometimes vaginismus is the result of psychological trauma, often from a past history of sexual abuse or trauma. It requires help from a trained specialist to uncover the cause and help develop treatment strategies.

Pain during or after sexual intercourse is known as **dyspareunia**. Although this problem can affect men, it's more common in women.

Women with dyspareunia may have pain in the vagina, clitoris, or labia. **Endometriosis**, an often painful condition in which tissue similar to the uterine lining grows abnormally inside the pelvis (see chapter 13, Your Vagina and Cervix), can cause pain with intercourse. **Inflammation** of the area surrounding the vaginal opening, called vulvar vestibulitis, can also cause pain. And skin diseases, such as lichen planus and lichen sclerosis, that affect the vaginal and vulvar area can cause pain.

NOTE TO SELF

No time for sex? Make an appointment this weekend!

Other Reasons for a Not-So-Great Sex Life

I've covered the medical reasons for dips in your sex life, but there are plenty of other causes. Nearly everybody has them at some point, so remember that these issues often come and go.

Busy Lives

Some women find that their to-do lists and busy lives leave them exhausted and without a sex drive. You have choices: change your lifestyle, set aside appointments for intimacy, schedule in a date night. A good question to ask yourself is "If I were alone with my partner on a remote island, would I have a sex drive?" If the answer is yes, then the answer to your issues with sexuality lies in making changes in your lifestyle.

Relationship Bumps

A relationship that's not satisfying or fulfilling is very unlikely to offer a sex life that's satisfying or fulfilling. One of the very first things to examine when your sex life is not going well is the relationship. Are you communicating with each other? Are you connecting emotionally? Are your emotional needs being met? Are you giving equally to each other? Sometimes a third party, such as a therapist, can help find the answer when relationship issues are the root cause of sexual dysfunction.

Choose therapists carefully. Get recommendations from people you trust. Move on to a new one if you are not satisfied. Sometimes it can take a few tries to find a therapist you connect with and whose style works for you.

Babyhood, Toddlerhood, Teenagerhood

Women who provide hands-on mothering much of the day may well be "touched out" by the end of the day and just want to be left alone. Some are exhausted. Some completely lose themselves in mothering until it swallows up their lives, their identities, and their self-worth. Not a great environment for sex.

Even a woman in love with her partner may not want sex under these circumstances. The answer? Help, help, help, patience, and time. Be sure that you look carefully at the division of labor in your home. I look at it this way: You and your partner both work all day, whether that's inside or outside the home. Once you're both home, the labor should be divided equally. Give your workload a little review and see how it could be shared. And remember, nobody ever volunteers to do anything if you just keep doing it all the time. If your partner is responsible for laundry, step away from those machines. Resist the temptation to do it yourself!

Medications That Trash Your Libido

Many common drugs—including medications for blood pressure, **migraines**, antidepressants, and birth control pills—can interfere with sex drive, arousal, and orgasm. Drugs used to treat high blood pressure and migraines, known as beta-blockers, can cause sexual dysfunction. Antihistamines can impair vaginal lubrication.

If you are having difficulty with sex drive, ask your doctor if there are other options for these medicines that might cause fewer sexual side effects. Some women who take birth control pills notice a diminished sex drive and vaginal dryness. Switching to a different pill or a different method of birth control can usually help. The antidepressants known as **selective serotonin reuptake inhibitors** (SSRIs) such as Prozac, Paxil, and Zoloft can cause loss of libido in as many as 60 percent of patients. Talk to your doctor about switching to medications known to have less effect on sexual function or trying lower doses. Therapy for depression instead of an antidepressant medication may work well for some women. As noted in chapter 2, Your Head, some couples, working with the prescribing doctor, schedule short breaks from drugs to have a romantic weekend.

Depression

Which comes first, the loss of libido or the depression? Depression means loss of interest in activities that used to bring pleasure, including sex. Losing interest in sex can be an early sign of depression. The first thing to do when you notice a low libido is to check in on your mental health. Be sure to read chapter 2, Your Head, for help.

Alcohol

Alcohol can ruin sexual enjoyment. It gets some people in the mood, but it can interfere with arousal and orgasm. Being drunk also gives you very poor judgment about having sex! As Mom says, "Everything in moderation."

Sexual Abuse

If you've experienced sexual abuse in the past, it could be affecting your current sex life. Counseling is recommended for survivors of sexual abuse. The treatment process is long and challenging, but it can help you to reclaim your sexuality. It can also help you to keep an otherwise healthy relationship—but do it for yourself.

Again, try to get referrals for therapists from your doctor as well as recommendations from people you trust.

A Few Ways to Turn Up the Heat (Including Some Bad Ideas)

Does that sound like a story on a magazine cover? It is. You'll hear lots of ideas in magazines about heating up your sex drive and sex life. Some are very good and good for you, and some are not. Let's start with a great idea.

Kegel Exercises

You know from chapter 10, Your Waterworks, that **Kegel exercises** can be magically effective. I'm going to repeat the directions here in case you only read this sex chapter.

Kegel exercises work the muscles around your vagina and pelvic floor, and working them can improve your sex life. Kegels improve blood circulation to the genitals, increase vaginal responsiveness, and can make you more aroused.

To find your pelvic floor muscles, practice when you go to the bathroom. Start the flow of urine, then try to stop your urine stream. Now slowly tighten the same muscles for ten seconds. Then slowly relax for ten seconds. Repeat this ten times.

NOTE TO SELF

Kegel exercises increase your sexual pleasure (and no one has to know you're doing them).

Next, try a quicker squeeze and release of the same muscles. This is a faster move that works slightly different muscle fibers. Squeeze and release in rapid succession ten times. Do one set of fast and one set of slow Kegels each day, working up to three sets of both daily. It's also possible to buy little exercise balls to place in the vagina, sold in "sex toy" shops and online.

REAL LIFE FACT: Sweetness Is a Turn-On

One of my patient's libido was down to zero. Her smart husband did not express any frustration or anger. Instead, he went out and rented her favorite romantic movie. The libido definitely went up a few points.

Your Kegels will help you now and later in life (with urinary control); they can also be pleasing to a male partner. Slow squeezes on his penis can be very arousing for both of you. Experiment—try squeezing as he thrusts in and then when he is moving out.

Viagra for Women?

A women's version of Viagra has been disappointing. The studies of the effects of Viagra on women found that it increases blood flow to genitalia and thereby facilitates sex, but provides little in the way of arousal. In short, women's bodies may be ready, but their minds are not.

Viagra appears to relax the clitoral and vaginal smooth muscle and to increase blood flow to the genital area. Viagra helps to engorge the vagina with blood, causing it to become lubricated, much the same way it causes the blood vessels in a man's penis to become engorged, which produces an erection. Viagra seems to help only the subset of women who have physical arousal problems, not those with a low sex drive.

Erotica

Reading an erotic book or watching an erotic movie can help to get you in the mood. If you decide to watch a movie as a couple, be sure that *you* choose the movie. Women are more aroused by soft-core productions that might include some character development and plot, whereas many men might choose Mullet Man.

If you find that erotica can arouse you, try it out before you get into bed.

Some people also find that role-playing can help the libido. The many books and magazines on the subject offer endless ideas. Take whatever bit of information you can use—and discard the rest. Anything that requires a lot of work on your part isn't going to help if you have a busy life. You know the kind of ideas I mean: "Dress yourself in a French maid costume and dress your partner as the man of the household. Decorate your bedroom to look like an eighteenth-century chateau. On the next day, switch the scene to the stables."

Testosterone—Not a Proven Idea

Some researchers have theorized that a woman's libido is linked to her **testosterone** level. When this was first reported, interest in the idea exploded. Unfortunately, there's not much scientific data to support it. One major problem is that most published studies have evaluated women whose ovaries were removed and who were therefore testosterone-deficient. Other studies have used very high levels (supraphysiologic levels; that is, larger or more potent than would naturally occur in the body) of testosterone.

Testosterone therapy in women has not been studied enough to determine if it's safe or effective for improving sexuality. Following are some known dangers.

REAL LIFE FACT: Testosterone Therapy

Testosterone and DHEA are unproven supplements and their safety is also unproven. Take a pass until much more is known.

- It's hard to regulate how much testosterone is delivered to the body with current medications.
- Testosterone can increase the risk of heart disease because it can change the ratio of **HDL** ("good" cholesterol) to **LDL** ("bad" cholesterol). Your body converts some percentage of testosterone to **estrogen**, which can fuel estrogen-dependent cancers, such as many breast cancers.
- Testosterone can cause **liver** damage.
- Testosterone can cause facial hair and voice changes. The voice change cannot be reversed.

What about DHEA?

DHEA, short for **dehydroepiandrosterone**, is quickly becoming the next big nutritional supplement craze. DHEA is a steroid hormone produced by the **adrenal glands**, which are located above the kidneys of both males and females. Males make slightly more than females. The body converts DHEA into the steroid sex hormones—testosterone, in particular, and estrogen. This supplement gives me the same concerns as medically prescribed testosterone replacement therapy.

Could these supplements be helpful with little risk? Possibly. As a doctor, I can't advise you to take anything without knowing what the impact on your body will be in the future.

NOTE TO SELF

A healthy lifestyle can lead to a healthy sex life.

Lifestyle Matters: Explore All Your Options

Low libido is probably neither all in your head nor all in your body. It's a good idea to cover your bases by visiting your doctor to address any potential medical issues. A good therapist can help you sort out whether lifestyle or relationship issues may be part of the problem and help you develop strategies to manage these.

Two practical reasons to look at a healthy lifestyle? Too much alcohol blunts your sexual responsiveness. And cigarette smoking restricts blood flow. Decreased blood flow to your sexual organs lowers sexual arousal.

Make holistic changes. Avoid drinking excessive amounts of alcohol, stop smoking, of course, and make time for leisure and relaxation. All are as important for your sexual health as for your overall health. Learning to relax despite the stresses of your daily life can give you the ability to focus on the sexual experience and get better arousal and orgasm.

Make changes in your life gradually and remember this tried-and-true healthy way of life: exercise regularly and eat a healthful and varied diet. That's a safe method to boost energy, improve self-image, elevate mood, and enhance sex drive. Regular aerobic exercise can increase your stamina, improve your body self-image, and make you feel happy.

Aim for Connection, Not Perfection

If you and your partner feel overwhelmed, busy, and stressed by life, one approach for improving your sex life is to aim for connection and not perfection. This piece of advice, one of the most useful I've heard when it comes to sexual issues, comes from a very smart and practical therapist, Dr. Aline Zoldbrod.

She instructs couples to set time aside for some kind of emotional and physical connection and wait to see what happens. Be open to many possibilities. Not every interlude in a couple's life has to look like the fireworks you see on television. Put on some music, give each other a massage, and even if you just fall fast asleep in each other's arms, this experience is likely to be wonderful. The more you get caught up in goals of sexual perfection, the more daunting it becomes to make an intimate connection. Getting caught up in the drive for perfectionism is not great for lots of areas of your life, and your sex life is no exception. Perfection is overrated.

Real Sexual Freedom

Only you can decide how important sex is to you, what you like or don't like, what you can compromise on or not. As a woman, understanding sexuality and your body is a good first step. If you're in a long-term relationship, try to talk about your sex life together. It's hard at first for many, many couples but worth it, for healthy and hot sex.

Your breasts have a starring role in sex, but there's a lot more to them! In the next chapter, we'll take an in-depth look at how to keep your girls healthy.

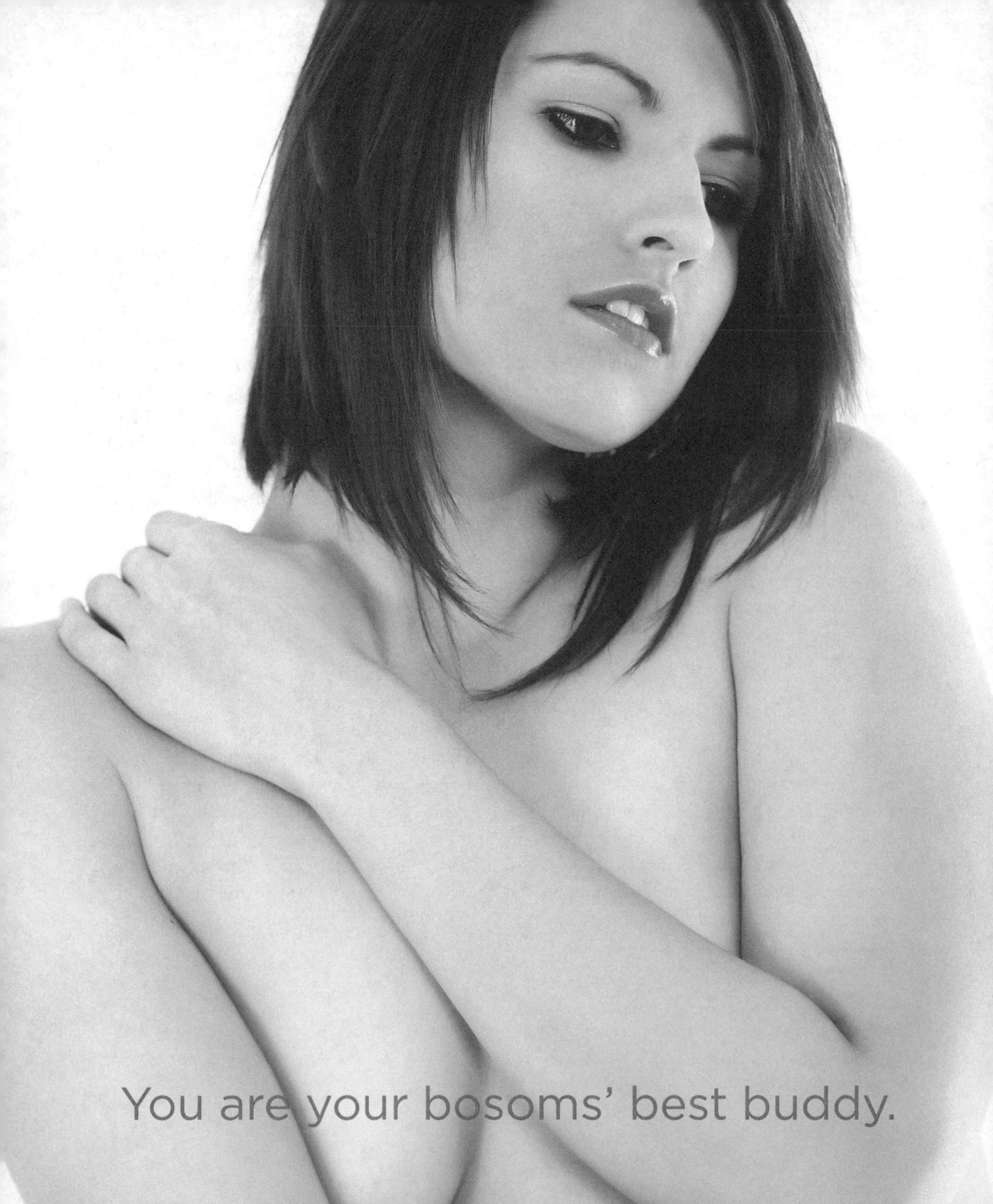
You are your bosoms' best buddy.

your breasts

Is there anything new to be said about breasts? In poetry they're shining, silken glories. In magazines, they're a sex object. Touching them arouses both men and women, which is a reaction you don't seem to see in any other lactating mammal. And if you were at war and could somehow implant a breast on one of the male generals, you would win because he would stay home and play with it all day.

But really, most of us only know what we read about breasts in magazines. Magazines are fun, but they aren't always the best source of the solid information you need for your health. In this chapter, I'll cover everything you need to know to have healthy, beautiful breasts for a lifetime.

In recent decades there's been a big change in women's breast health. A generation ago, the subject of breast **cancer** was never discussed. A woman was suddenly in the hospital because she had a lump. She would wake up from surgery to find that her breast and all of her **lymph nodes** were gone. There was no reconstruction, and she wore a prosthesis (a fake breast) for the rest of her life. Many women credit Betty Ford (first lady from 1974 to 1977) for going public with her breast cancer and educating the world.

NOTE TO SELF

"Being a lady does not require silence."
—Betty Ford

The downside: When you educate the world, it's a bit like playing Operator—the facts get jumbled. You will hear, for example, that your chances of getting breast cancer are one in eight. That's completely true—if you are eighty-five. If you are thirty, your chances of having breast cancer are 1 in 2,525. So as you read about breast cancer in this chapter, remember how unlikely it is that you will have it anytime soon, no matter how much of an epidemic there appears to be.

Yes, if you have a lump, you have to go to the doctor. Just do it calmly and keep your anxiety level down. The doctor may decide to do some tests or may want to watch it closely by having you come back from time to time. If the doctor feels nothing but you are pretty sure something is there, insist that the lump be evaluated. This is an important message—take charge of your health, and if you are not comfortable with the doctor's recommendations, find a new one.

Breast Basics

Let's start with a few facts. Breasts have two functions: producing milk to feed our young and providing sexual arousal for men and women alike.

What makes a breast big? Fat does.

How? Your breasts consist of fatty and connective tissue. Each breast contains fifteen to twenty lobes. A lobe is a rounded mass of tissue; think of a group of earlobes arranged in a circular fashion. Each lobe has many lobules (small lobes) in it, with ducts (tubes) leading to the nipple. The lobules produce milk. These ducts deliver milk to openings in the nipple where milk comes out during breastfeeding. (More about nipples later.)

The spaces around the lobes and ducts are filled with fat. The amount of fat determines how large or small your breasts are. But the lobules and ducts are just about the same size in everyone, and that's why breast size does not make a difference in your ability to breastfeed.

Your breasts have many other tubes, called lymphatic channels, which lead to the lymph nodes. These channels drain lymphatic fluid from your breast to be filtered in the lymph nodes under your armpit, breastbone, and collarbone. From here, the filtered lymphatic fluid is returned to your blood circulation. The **lymphatic system**, along with your **white blood cells**, is important in fighting off infection and cancer in your body. Cancer can also spread through the lymphatic system.

REAL LIFE FACT: Three Things That Don't Increase the Chance of Getting Breast Cancer

- Large breasts
- Underwire bras
- Antiperspirants

Your breasts change (in size and in other ways) with your menstrual cycle, pregnancy, and breastfeeding, and as you grow older. Hormones cause the breasts to develop and enlarge and, in pregnancy, cause the glandular cells in the ducts to produce milk. The three major hormones that affect breast development and function are **estrogen**, **progesterone**, and **prolactin**, all of which cause glandular tissue in the breast to change. Through any of these changes, there may be soreness and lumps—harmless lumps that go away as the cycle continues.

I want you to know about healthy breasts and the changes they go through to help you avoid anxiety over each little change and lump you may have. And if you learn what you can do to keep your breasts healthy now, it can make a difference later in life.

NOTE TO SELF

Small-breasted women make just as much breast milk as large-breasted women. Large-breasted women simply have more breast fat, not more milk-producing tissue.

Your breasts consist of fatty and connective tissues. Within these tissues lie the milk-producing lobules and ducts. Throughout the breasts run lymphatic channels, which drain into lymph nodes under the armpit, breast bone, and collar bone.

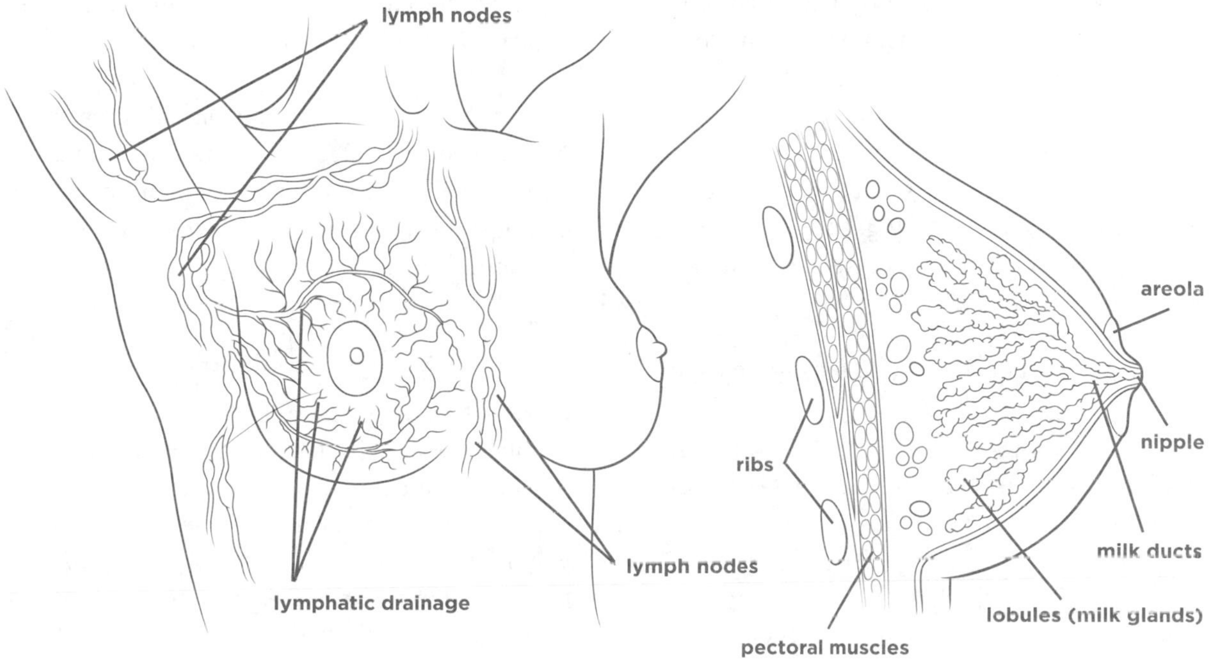

What about firmness? Younger women have more fibrous tissue and less fat in their breasts. Fibrous tissue usually functions like a strong piece of flexible fabric. Older women tend to have the opposite—more fat and less fibrous tissue. Fibrous tissue feels lumpier and harder than fat. That's one reason why younger women's breasts often appear firmer than older women's breasts, and why mammograms are sometimes more difficult to read in younger women. (Please see the section on mammograms on page 270.)

Nipples

Nipples, like breasts, come in many different shapes and sizes—flat, round, standing up, sitting down. The nipple is surrounded by the areola, a ring of skin slightly lighter-colored than the nipple itself. The areola often darkens during pregnancy and breastfeeding.

You may notice small pimplelike bumps on your areola. These bumps, known as Montgomery gland tubercles (see illustration, right), lubricate the areola. They get larger in pregnancy. Don't be tempted to squeeze them—they can get infected if you do.

The nipple can be very sensitive, as it contains many nerve endings. The nipple and areola contain muscle fibers that contract, which means to pull in tight. Cold weather and sexual arousal make the areola pucker and the nipples become hard.

One patient told me there was an awful time after Dr. David Reuben's book *Everything You Ever Wanted to Know about Sex* came out.

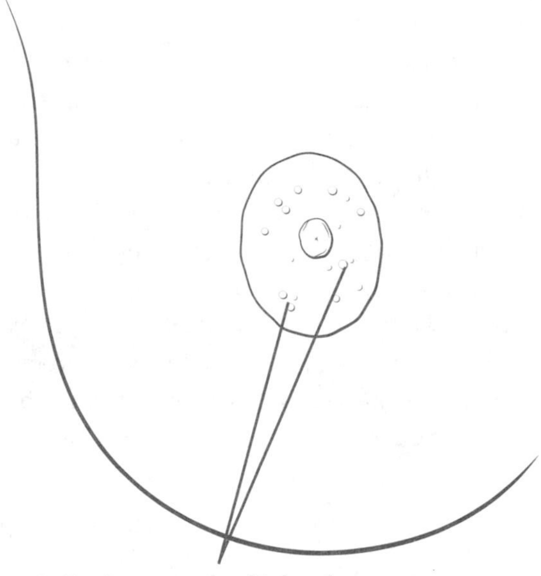

Montgomery gland tubercles

It claimed that a woman had not had an orgasm if her nipples weren't erect. Millions of American men reportedly started reaching for the nipple after the woman's orgasm "to make sure." So let's clarify that this often happens—but it doesn't always. Man's never-ending quest to prove our orgasms must wait for more studies.

Inverted Nipples

Nipples that don't stick out are called inverted nipples. Some nipples are mobile—which means they are inverted some of the time and sticking out at other times. If one (or both) of your nipples is always inverted, that's nothing to worry about. If, however, your nipple suddenly becomes inverted and isn't the mobile type, it may be abnormal. **Inflammation**, or, much more rarely, breast cancer can pull on the ligaments, which in turn can pull the nipple in. Your doctor should check a newly inverted nipple that used to stick out.

If you are planning to breastfeed, show your doctor your nipples if you think they are inverted. S/he can give you a few ways to make it easier to bring the nipples out.

Accessory Nipples and Breast Tissue—Too Much of a Good Thing

You wouldn't believe how many people I see who have extra nipples and, less often, an extra breast. Extra nipples are known as accessory nipples, and they can appear anywhere from your armpits to your groin. Many times they are not particularly noticeable, and you might not even realize you have an extra nipple.

Another variation on too much of a good thing is extra breast tissue, usually found between the typical breast location and the armpit. Extra breast tissue can appear with or without an extra nipple and can enlarge and change with your menstrual cycle and pregnancy, just like normal breast tissue. It can be tender before menstruation, it can develop breast cancer, and it can enlarge and produce milk when you are breastfeeding. Some women notice this extra breast tissue for the first time during or just after pregnancy, when the breasts enlarge and the tissue becomes enlarged and engorged with milk. The extra breast tissue may go away after weaning. Other women have an extra breast all the time.

Extra breast tissue is not a health risk, but it may be uncomfortable if it is big enough to show when you wear a tank top or bathing suit. A good plastic surgeon can easily fix this problem. Confirm with your health insurance company that the surgery will be covered. It usually is. And be sure that your doctor doesn't mark it "cosmetic" surgery on the forms.

Distressing Discharge

Although nipple discharge tends to be normal, any discharge should be evaluated by your doctor. In young women in particular, nipple discharge is usually the result of a **benign** process. About half of young women are able to produce a very small amount of nipple discharge by squeezing on their nipples. But in very rare cases (less than 1 percent in young women), nipple discharge can be caused by cancer.

The most common cause of nipple discharge in young women is examining your breasts and stimulating your nipples too often, which can cause you to make some milk, as the stimulation from your own exams can cause the breast to produce milk. A milky discharge during pregnancy or breastfeeding is also normal and is caused by the normal stimulation from the hormones. Benign discharge (called galactorrhea) can be the result of medications or **thyroid** disorders, or from the use of oral contraceptives that act like the hormones of pregnancy and breastfeeding.

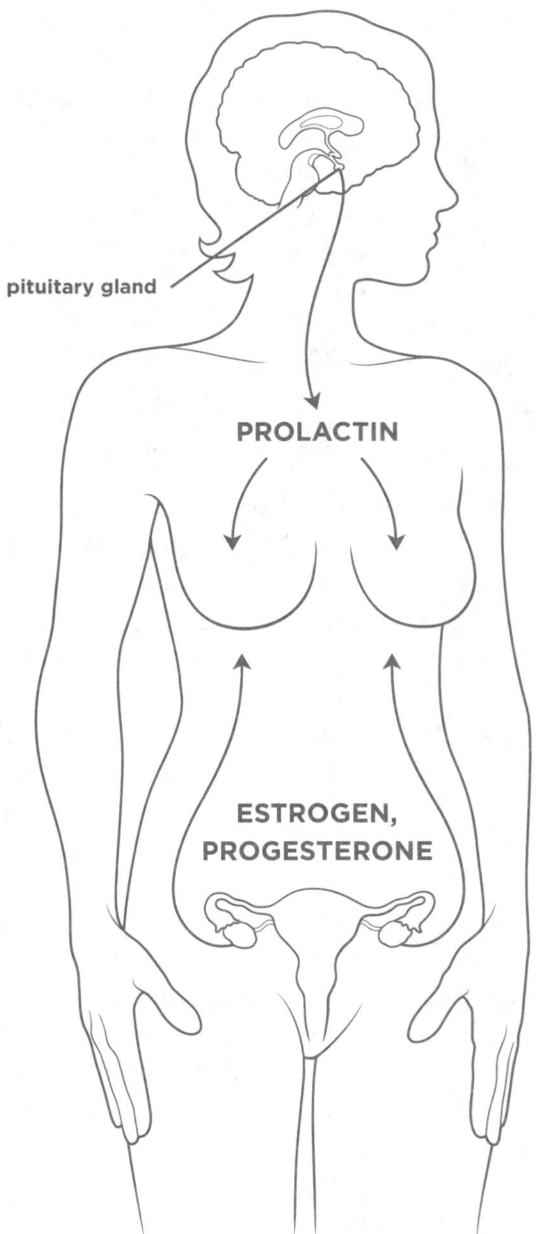

The three major hormones that affect breast development and function are estrogen, progesterone, and prolactin.

If you have a milky discharge, you should be evaluated by a doctor, because you might have an underlying hormonal problem or trouble with your pituitary **gland**. Your pituitary gland, located in your brain, produces hormones that allow you to breastfeed, and a fairly common benign tumor called a prolactinoma can cause abnormally high levels of prolactin, which can cause your breasts to make a bit of milk. Benign tumors of the milk ducts (and in rare cases cancerous tumors) can also cause discharge. This discharge comes in many different colors and consistencies. It may be white, yellow, pink, red, or green. It may be creamy, watery, or bloody. In general, green is good, as green discharge often indicates benign fibrocystic changes in the breast. (See more later on fibrocystic changes.) To sum up: Any discharge—whether clear, a color, or milky—requires a look by your doctor.

Breast Pain

Don't worry too much about "diffuse" breast pain, which is soreness over most or all of both breasts. Diffuse soreness in your breasts goes with the hormones of your menstrual cycle. The tenderness and pain usually increase from midcycle and continue through your period, and both the size and nodularity (lumpiness) of your breasts increase too. After your period, pain usually decreases or goes away entirely. Some women find that their breasts are so engorged and sensitive before menstruation that they can hardly be touched, and even putting on a bra is impossible. Usually, the swelling and tenderness go away quickly within a day or so after your period starts.

There are other types of breast pain that don't seem to vary with your period. Pain that is in one spot usually has a different cause. Duct ectasia is one such common benign problem. It's an inflammation of the breast ducts, which can lead to scarring and localized breast pain. It tends to worsen in cold weather. Usually the pain comes on suddenly, and some women report a burning sensation behind the nipple. Often there is a sticky, green nipple discharge. Sometimes the nipples invert or there is an lump in the areolar area around the nipple.

A less common cause of breast pain is Tietze's syndrome, an inflammation of the cartilage where the rib cage meets the breastbone. With this condition, you might have pain between the breasts. Breast cysts, which are benign, can also cause pain in one place in the breast. Often these can be felt as a tender, smooth, mobile lump.

Pain in one specific place in your breast should always be checked by your doctor.

Breast Pain and Cancer

Breast pain is rarely caused by breast cancer, especially in young women. But you shouldn't ignore pain, especially if it's in one place. It's important to realize that breast cancer can be associated with pain, despite the old adage you may have heard that if it hurts, it can't be breast cancer.

About 15 to 20 percent of breast cancer is associated with some discomfort. Cyclical pain that comes with your period and diffuse pain throughout your breasts are much less likely to be serious problems. The vast majority of breast pain in young women comes from benign causes, but don't hesitate to have it checked by your doctor to be certain. (For more on breast cancer, please see page 264.)

Caffeine Concerns

For years we believed that caffeine and breast pain were connected. More recent scientific studies don't prove that. In trials in which women were randomly given caffeine tablets or a **placebo** (sugar pills), there was no association between caffeine and breast pain. If you are troubled by breast pain, giving up caffeine is not likely to make much of a difference, so go ahead and have the mocha java.

What's a Woman to Do?

Some women have found that wearing a supportive bra, such as a sports bra, even at night, can help reduce breast pain. Others have had success by reducing salt intake, maintaining a low-fat diet, going on birth control pills, and losing weight if they are overweight. Evening primrose oil has been found in small trials to relieve breast pain in women with moderate to severe pain.

What *Not* to Worry About

The majority of lumps in the breasts of young women are benign. If you find one, don't waste your time panicking. Instead, show your doctor so you get proper reassurance or treatment. Like many women, I've heard horror stories about doctors who ignored a lump in a young woman. They do that because they are so used to finding the problem to be cancer free in this low-risk age group. So if you're concerned, push your doctor to run tests—or find another doctor.

It also helps to understand some of the more common benign breast issues in young women. Here they are.

Fibrocystic Misinformation

The normal texture of the breast in young women is lumpy and bumpy. This irregular texture is often overdiagnosed as fibrocystic breast disease. In the past, many physicians applied this name to fibrocystic, or lumpy, breasts. Fibrocystic breast changes are not a disease at all. Fibrocystic breasts are a common, noncancerous breast condition in which the normally lumpy, bumpy breast texture is extra lumpy.

A better name is fibrocystic breast changes. Having fibrocystic breasts is not a risk factor for breast cancer, just for discomfort and occasional anxiety. However, fibrocystic breasts can sometimes make it more difficult to detect a hidden breast cancer. Like all women, women with fibrocystic breasts tend to get their worst symptoms in the second half of the menstrual cycle, when their breasts may feel swollen, painful, tender, or even lumpier than usual. Studies show that women who take birth control pills get relief from the pain and symptoms of fibrocystic breast changes. And a well-fitted, supportive bra helps too.

Breast Cysts

Breast cysts—benign, fluid-filled sacs—are very common in young women. They are more often found in the second half of the menstrual cycle. If you find a lump that you think might be a cyst, an ultrasound should be done to confirm that it is a benign fluid-filled sac.

On an ultrasound, a cyst is categorized as simple if it is a round sac with no solid material. If a cyst is large or causes pain, it can be deflated by having a physician insert a needle and drain out the fluid so that it collapses. But simple cysts that cause no pain can be left alone. If a cyst is called complex, it means that there is a solid part. These need more study, such as mammography and **biopsy**, as there can be a risk of malignancy.

Fibroadenomas

Okay, so you've found a lump, and the ultrasound shows it's solid, not a cyst. It's a smooth, round marble in your breast. Don't panic. You have to have it looked at, but if you are a young

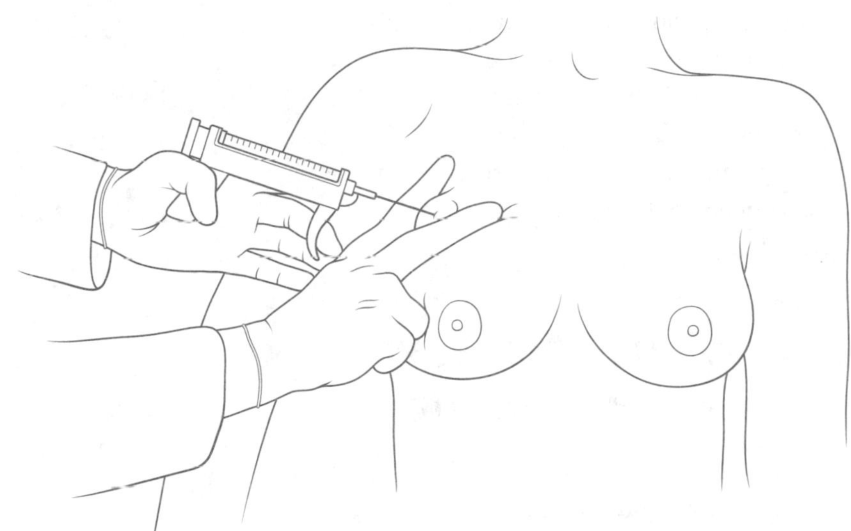

Fine needle aspiration is a technique to evaluate breast lumps. The procedure involves insertion of a very thin needle attached to a syringe into the lump. A small sample of cells is removed for examination.

woman, it's almost never breast cancer. In women under thirty-five, the most likely diagnosis fitting this description is fibroadenoma.

Fibroadenomas are benign solid lumps made up of fibrous tissue and glandular cells, and are usually singular (sometimes there can be a few), smooth, round, and mostly painless. They can get tender just before your period. Fibroadenomas often grow larger over time, but they are not precancerous growths, and they do not increase your risk of developing breast cancer later on.

The diagnosis of a fibroadenoma starts with a physical examination of your breasts by your doctor. If the typical finding of a smooth, round, and mobile marble is felt, the next step is an ultrasound. If the lump is solid, usually you'll have a mammogram, which is better for evaluating solid lumps. If this confirms a round or oval and well-defined lump that has a smooth surface (a cancerous lump is usually irregular), you may be told that the fibroadenoma can be followed up with physical exams. Or your doctor may decide to do a simple procedure called a fine needle aspiration. This procedure involves inserting a very thin needle attached to a syringe into the lump. The area is numbed up with an injection ahead of time, so it is not painful—except for the numbing part. A small sample of cells will be removed and examined under a microscope to rule out the possibility of a cancerous tumor. Fine needle aspiration is a very useful technique to evaluate breast lumps. Usually, you won't be seeing your regular doctor for these tests. You should be referred to a breast care specialist.

If fibroadenomas are painful, large, growing, or causing you anxiety, they can be removed. In some cases, they can grow very large, up to four inches. They are removed because of their size, not because they are cancerous or might become cancerous, or because they make examining your breasts difficult. Although any woman may find it scary to have surgery on her breast, remember that it's a benign lump, not cancer.

Your Breasts and Pregnancy

During pregnancy and breastfeeding, your breasts grow and change quite a bit. If you weren't a large-breasted woman already, suddenly you are. You'll develop more ducts and lobules, and your breasts will start to grow and become plump. The blood flow to your breasts at the end of pregnancy increases a startling 250 percent, and your breasts can double in weight! When you buy a nursing bra, you'll look for E, F, and G instead of A, B, and C cups. Your nipples and areolar area may darken during pregnancy and breastfeeding, too.

After you stop breastfeeding, your breasts' appearance will likely change. You can develop stretch marks and a bit of sagging. Even women who don't breastfeed have these changes after giving birth, although they tend not to be quite as noticeable.

Your breasts naturally start to show changes of aging at about age forty. So if you have children in your late thirties or forties, you may see changes in your breasts that are caused by both age and the hormone shifts of pregnancy and lactation.

To "B" or Not to Be "B": Enlarging, Reducing, or Otherwise Changing Your Breasts

Elective breast surgeries are now as common as nose jobs. Although they're growing more popular, the impact of these procedures on future health is often not fully understood by the young women who choose to have them.

Cosmetic breast surgery includes breast augmentations, lifts, symmetries (to make uneven breasts the same size and shape), reductions, and inverted nipple corrections. All of these procedures include surgical manipulation of the breast tissue and have possible implications for your later ability to breastfeed. The impact varies depending on the procedure. You should educate yourself about all issues that may affect your future health before making a decision about elective breast surgery.

Is Bigger Really Better?

The most common elective breast procedure is breast augmentation (implants). Breast augmentation is the procedure in which an implant is inserted into the breast to produce a larger breast size. It is usually done under general anesthesia in an operating room setting. The implant is inserted through a small incision in the lower crease area of the breast, under the nipple, or in the armpit. The fatty layer and muscle wall are pulled away from the chest and the implant is placed underneath. Breast enhancement is so common that some young women today get breast implants as graduation presents! Celebrities and models have created an illusion that normal breasts are huge, firm, and gravity defying.

Healthy breasts come in many different shapes and sizes. Breasts can be big or small, perky or sagging, symmetrical or asymmetrical—and everything in between. And with the help of a Hollywood stylist's secrets and some push-up devices, anyone can show cleavage if that is her life's goal.

My concern is about the whole you. If you feel that new breasts would make you happy, I want you to be happy *first*, and then decide if you really need bigger ones. Personally, I think many of the world's most beautiful women have small breasts, because they look so great in clothes! As always, surgery done for reasons of comfort or to repair some disfiguration are a different story.

In breast augmentation, an implant is inserted through a small incision under the breast, nipple, or armpit. The fatty layer and walls of the pectoralis muscles are pulled away and the implant is placed underneath.

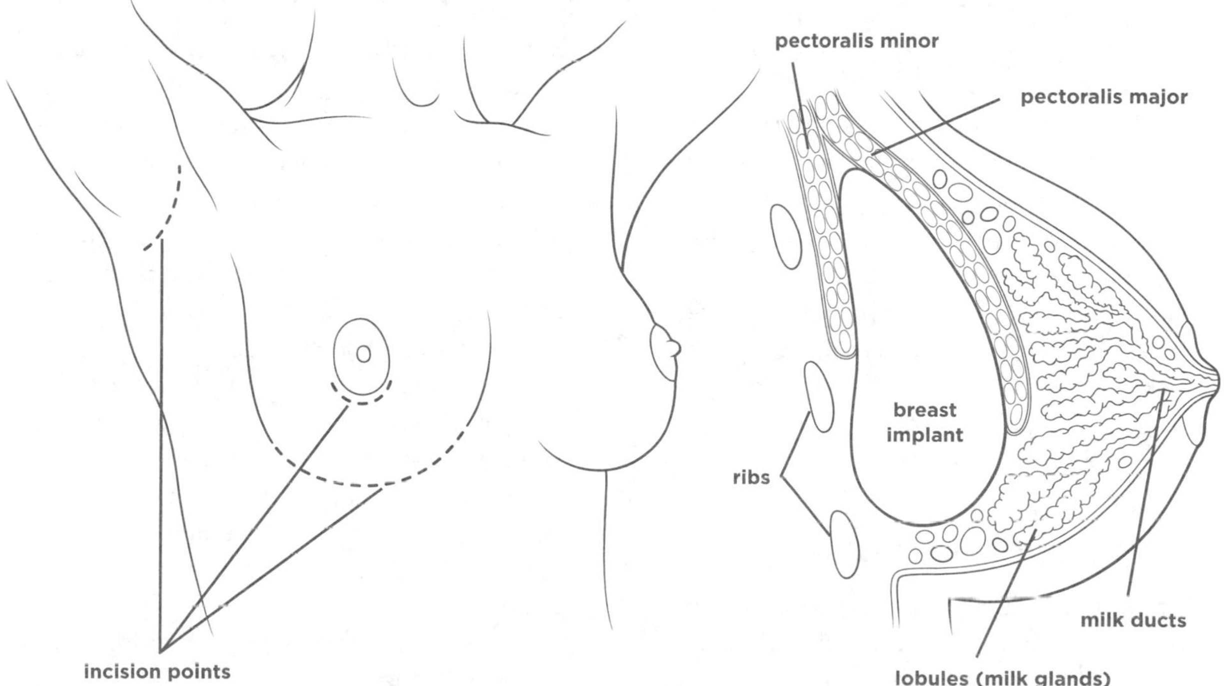

Silicone or Saline?

There are two types of breast implants: silicone or saline filled. Breast implants today are usually filled with saline. The U.S. Food and Drug Administration (FDA) banned the use of silicone implants for breast enlargements in 1992 because there were questions about their long-term safety. Connective tissue disease, cancer, neurological diseases, and other bad reactions were believed to be more common in women who had silicone breast implants. The FDA reversed the ban in 2006, so silicone implants are coming back. Some women prefer silicone over saline because they see them as more natural-feeling.

Health Risks of Implants—Fact or Fiction?

Studies of women with breast implants done for cosmetic reasons have found no major health risks to having implants, other than the small but very real operative risks of bleeding, infection, or complications of anesthesia. Most studies find no association between breast implants and increased breast cancer risk or death. There have been some reports of general health risks that are slightly higher in women with implants.

Breastfeeding and Implants

Of the three incision types used for implants, those made in lower parts of the breast tend be best for successful breastfeeding. That's because the ducts that carry milk from the glands to the nipple are not severed. Breastfeeding is less likely to work well when an incision under the nipple is used for implant placement, because the cut is made at the border of the areola and the surrounding breast skin. The breast ducts are in this area and are cut with this incision, increasing the chance of decreasing the milk supply or damaging the nerves so that breastfeeding may not work as well.

It's so important to tell your surgeon what your wishes are. You may really want to breastfeed your babies, but the surgeon has no way of knowing that unless you speak up!

Breast Reduction

Small-breasted women can't imagine wanting or needing to have their breasts reduced. Large-breasted women can't imagine making them bigger. It's a bit like the curly versus straight hair envy, except that large-breasted women can be subjected to considerable back, shoulder, and neck pain; posture problems; and difficulty with physical activity.

Breast reduction is used for women with large breasts that cause such problems, or for women who want them reduced for cosmetic reasons. Breast reduction removes tissue from the breast to create a smaller one. Reduction may interfere with a woman's ability to breastfeed, depending on the type of procedure done.

There are two breast reduction procedures. While nobody can guarantee that

REAL LIFE QUESTION: What's gaposis?

When your blouse keeps gapping open and you have to safety-pin it from the inside. Just ask a large-breasted woman.

you'll be able to breastfeed after having this surgery, talk to your doctor about choosing option one.

Option one leaves the nipple attached to the underlying breast tissue at one point. A portion of the breast tissue is removed so that the size of the breast is reduced. The remaining tissue is then repositioned and the outer skin rejoined. Option one keeps the glands in your breast tissue attached to your ducts in the nipple, but some glands are removed. Your milk volume may be lower, and you may have to add formula to your baby's diet. Some women make enough milk that, even after breast reduction, they can breastfeed exclusively. Basically, you won't know until you try. Talk to your pediatrician or a lactation consultant for help.

Option two, used in women with very large breasts, makes breastfeeding success much less likely. The nipple and areolar area are completely detached. The breast tissue is reduced and the nipple and areolar area are then reattached as a skin graft. This procedure severs all glandular ducts. Most women who use option two will not make breast milk after they have a baby. However, even after the severance of all glandular ducts, some women can still produce a small amount of breast milk and can breastfeed for some of the baby's feedings.

How do you know if option one or two is best for you? It depends on the size and shape of your breasts. If your breasts are extremely large and they lie quite low, you'll most likely want the nipple moved up higher, which requires option two. Otherwise, you'll have nice small breasts, but with the nipples oddly located on the bottom.

The risk of being unable to breastfeed may loom large for some women, but the benefits of breast reduction are fantastic for the majority of the women who consider it. I have met very few women who regret having it done. Once recovered from surgery, they say it feels absolutely great to be relieved of the weight and bulk, and they love buying clothes that don't gap open in the front.

Breast Lift

Another procedure gaining popularity is a mastopexy, or a breast lift. This procedure tightens the skin over the breasts, giving them a more perky appearance. The breast lift only tightens the skin, without changing the underlying tissue of the breast in which the milk ducts are found.

Unless there are complications from the procedure, there is no decrease in a woman's ability to breastfeed after having a breast lift procedure. Sometimes a breast lift is combined with breast implants. Breast lifts do not last forever, and with time the breast may again begin to sag as the skin and tissues age.

Breast Tattoos and Nipple Piercing

Tattoos and piercings are increasingly popular. Keep in mind that nipple piercings can interfere with your ability to breastfeed. Tattoos, although less invasive than piercing, can still do damage, although that's rare. Tattoos are created using a needle to inject colored dye into the superficial layer of skin, which carries with it a risk of infection to both the skin and underlying tissue. If the underlying tissue becomes infected, it could alter the amount of milk produced. An uncomplicated tattoo, though, should not interfere with breastfeeding.

When designing your tattoo, just remember that you will probably take pictures of yourself breastfeeding, so think about what images you want next to baby's sweet little face. And remember that your breasts change as you age and will usually do some sagging. Try to picture your tattoo stretched out before committing to anything!

Nipple piercing is done by running a piercing stud lengthwise through the nipple and out the opposite side. Like tattoos, nipple piercing carries a risk of infection. Plus, any penetrating trauma to the nipple can cause scarring. As the scarring is in only one small area, usually there are still plenty of working ducts to allow successful breastfeeding. In rare cases this scarring can stop up enough of the milk ducts in the nipple to interfere with breastfeeding. You'll need to remove the piercing in order to breastfeed, and often the hole closes up so that you can't use it in the future. (See chapter 4, Your Skin, for more info about tattoos and piercings.)

Breast Cancer

Many of us live in fear of having breast cancer. It is constantly in the media and often the topic of conversations with family and friends. It is particularly scary because it seems to strike just about anyone—even women who seem to have no risk factors.

Fortunately, breast cancer in young women is rare. Many people mistakenly believe that breast cancer rates among young women have been increasing, but that's not true. In fact, since 1985 the rate of breast cancer in women under age forty has declined 1.3 percent per year. However, this doesn't mean that young women don't get breast cancer, so risk reduction and early detection are still very important.

Can you prevent breast cancer? Do mammograms help in young women? What about the Pill or an occasional gin and tonic—are they bad? There's a lot of confusion, so let's go through the basics. The answers to these questions may surprise you.

Breast Cancer Myths

There are many myths about breast cancer. Let's take a look at a few of the more common myths and get the facts.

MYTH: Larger-breasted women develop breast cancer more often than smaller-breasted women.

FACT: Large-breasted women have the same risk of breast cancer as do small-breasted women.

MYTH: Underwire bras increase breast cancer risk.

FACT: An underwire bra, or any bra for that matter, does not increase breast cancer risk. Lymphatic fluid from the breast drains directly back toward the chest wall and the armpit—not underneath the breast where the bra might press against your chest.

MYTH: Antiperspirants and deodorants increase breast cancer risk.

FACT: The theory that using an antiperspirant or deodorant to block sweat stops your body from sweating out toxins, or that the antiperspirants and deodorants contain toxins that increase breast cancer risk, is false. There is no evidence that antiperspirants or deodorants are toxic, and recent studies confirm that breast cancer rates are the same in women whether or not they use antiperspirants or deodorants. The reason you are told not to use them before a mammogram is that most antiperspirants contain aluminum, which shows up as little specks on a mammogram and can cause confusion when the doctor studies your test.

Statistical Soup—What Are the Risk Factors for Breast Cancer?

It may feel like breast cancer is something that you are going to get no matter what you do. Don't believe it, and try not to feel helpless and hopeless about the risks. It helps to have a basic understanding of all those statistics that are constantly being tossed around.

The most common scary one is that your cumulative lifetime risk of breast cancer is one in eight. This is a statistically derived number that means if all women live to reach the age of eighty-five, then one in eight of us will develop breast cancer. This statistic applies only when you have reached the age of eighty-five. If you are under forty, in your age group there are fewer than fifty cases of breast cancer per hundred thousand women. This means that fewer than .05 percent of women in this age group get breast cancer. So although it definitely pays to take measures to decrease your breast cancer risk, the worry of one in eight over a lifetime is not a statistic for young women to worry about too much.

Everyone knows a young woman with breast cancer, and I have seen too many. So remember, please pay attention and take care of yourself—just reduce the panic level and save yourself some damaging stress.

REAL LIFE QUESTION: What increases my risk of getting breast cancer?

- **Family history.** A woman is considered at higher risk for breast cancer if she has a mother, sister, or daughter who has been diagnosed with breast cancer. She is at higher risk if detectable gene mutations run in her family. These include the BRCA1 and BRCA2 mutations, which can be found with a blood test.
- **Atypical hyperplasia.** This is a precancerous breast condition. Young women with a biopsy-confirmed diagnosis of atypical hyperplasia are at increased risk for developing invasive breast cancer later in life. (Biopsies are usually done because of a breast lump or an abnormal mammogram.)
- **Pregnancy factors.** A woman who has her first child after age thirty or who has no children has a slightly increased risk of breast cancer in her lifetime.
- **Menstrual history.** Women who start their periods before age twelve or go through menopause after age fifty-five have a slightly increased risk.
- **Alcohol use.** The risk of breast cancer rises with alcohol intake. The more you drink, the higher the risk.
- **Radiation therapy for Hodgkin's disease.** Young women treated with radiation for lymphomas (like Hodgkin's disease) have an increased risk of developing breast cancer.

Genetic Gibberish

The genetic inheritance of breast cancer can be confusing. The bottom line is that all women are at risk for developing breast cancer by virtue of being female. So on the one hand, don't despair if you have a family history of breast cancer, and on the other hand, don't feel overconfident that you are immune to developing breast cancer if you have no family history.

Only 5 to 10 percent of all breast cancer cases are estimated to be truly genetic and caused by a breast cancer gene. All family histories of breast cancer are not the same, and some are less risky than others. For example, a woman whose mother was diagnosed with breast cancer at age forty is more at risk of developing breast cancer than is a woman whose mother was diagnosed at age sixty-five.

Understanding Estrogen

Estrogen, a female hormone made in your ovaries and in your fatty tissue, stimulates your breast tissue to increase cell divisions. Cell division is a process that can have errors in it, and some of those errors can result in cancer. The more estrogen your breasts are exposed to over your lifetime, the more the cells divide, and the higher the risk of breast cancer. This basic underlying fact will help you understand the number of seemingly unrelated factors that can increase your risk of breast cancer later in life.

During each monthly cycle, you are exposed to higher estrogen levels at the time of **ovulation**. So the more menstrual cycles you have in your lifetime, the higher the risk of breast cancer. Both an early start of your periods and a late **menopause** increase breast cancer risk, because both will increase the number of menstrual cycles you have.

Obesity and Breast Cancer Risk

Do you keep hearing obesity is a factor? In young women, obesity can cause hormonal changes that decrease estrogen production by the ovaries, decrease ovulation, and can even result in infertility. So premenopausal obesity does not increase breast cancer risk, because it is associated with a lower number of ovulations.

After menopause, though, obesity increases breast cancer risk by increasing your level of estrogen. Fatty tissue is where the majority of estrogen is produced at this time of life, when the ovaries are no longer producing estrogen. The more body fat you have after menopause, the higher your estrogen level. Obesity in your younger years, because of its association with a decrease in ovulation, actually lowers your risk. (But I'm not recommending it!)

Food and Breast Cancer

How do you know what to eat to prevent cancer when the news seems to change every day? The issue of diet and breast cancer risk is confusing and controversial, and in general the connection between diet and breast cancer risk is not strong. Newer scientific studies show that a diet low in **saturated fat** and animal fat may reduce breast cancer risk. Not all fat appears to be bad, though. There is no proven connection between breast cancer and unsaturated fats, and heart-healthy omega-3 fatty acids even appear to offer some protection.

Diets that are in high in fiber, antioxidants, and fruits and vegetables are well proven to reduce the risk of **diabetes** and **heart disease** and are good for your overall health. Soy is somewhat controversial. Some researchers believe that in large amounts it is harmful for postmenopausal women. Some studies show that consumption of soy foods in your premenopausal years may be protective. My advice? Think about your heart first. A diet that is good for your heart and your whole body is also good for your breasts!

Alcohol and Breast Cancer

Drinking alcohol increases your risk of developing breast cancer. We don't know how, but one theory is that alcohol tends to increase levels of estrogen in the **bloodstream**. Alcohol, which is high in **carbohydrates**, may also work by raising blood levels of insulin-like growth factors (IGFs), which, like estrogen, can promote abnormal growth of breast cells.

Do you need to give up that glass of wine with dinner? Is there a safe level of alcohol that you can drink? Scientists have calculated that a woman's risk of breast cancer rises by 6 to 10 percent for each alcoholic drink she has on a daily basis. Although this may seem like a small increase, young women today are drinking more. Since 1984, the proportion of young women drinking more than three drinks per day has doubled, from 9 percent to 18 percent. So while one drink a day (defined as 12 ounces of beer, 5 ounces of wine, or 1.5 ounces of spirits) increases breast cancer risk by only about 10 percent, two to five drinks a day can increase it by as much as 50 percent.

No, most of you don't have to give up that glass of wine. Four or five drinks a week shouldn't have a measurable affect on your risk, so if you drink a moderate amount of alcohol, your risk still remains low. If you have a strong family history of breast cancer, you might want to be even more moderate. Trim it down to as low as one or two a week to keep risks lowest.

Cancer Protection and Pregnancy

Going through a full-term pregnancy can protect you against breast cancer. This seems contradictory because of the estrogen factor. Here's what we think happens: the breast goes through hormonally induced cellular changes, making it more resistant to **carcinogens**. Some scientists think the changes are genetic, and that genes that code for cancer may be shut off by the early exposure to hormones. Other scientists think that pregnancy might actually immunize against future breast cancer. These ideas are currently being investigated.

What we do know is this: if you wait to have children until you are older, your risk is increased compared to women who have babies in their twenties, because their breasts will be put into a more resistant state earlier in life. But pregnancy is protective at any age. If you breastfeed, you gain even more protection. You get both the maturing of breast tissue and the very low estrogen levels in your body while you are breastfeeding. The more children you breastfeed and the longer you nurse them, the better your protection.

But please don't have more babies just to decrease your breast cancer risk!

Abortion, Miscarriage, and Cancer Risk

A major international research collaboration investigating the relationship between abortion and breast cancer found that having an abortion or miscarriage does not increase a woman's risk of developing breast cancer. The number of abortions a woman had was found not to be associated with an increase or decrease in breast cancer risk. Earlier, smaller, and less well-designed studies had found an increased risk.

The Pill and Breast Cancer

There are a lot of myths and confusion out there about the Pill and its relationship to breast cancer risk. Fears about breast cancer and the Pill have diminished now that several well-respected scientific studies have been consistent in finding little to no increased risk. Even if you have a family history of breast cancer, this seems to hold true. So go ahead and include the Pill in your discussions with your doctor about the best birth control option for you.

The Breast Self-Exam Controversy

You may have already heard conflicting advice about examining your breasts for cancer. "Do this exam carefully once a month," your doctor says. Now you read in the papers that doing the exam doesn't make a difference. What's the truth?

First of all, there's nothing *harmful* about doing breast exams. A major study simply came out that found no statistical difference between the survival rates of women who do it and women who don't. The only risk the study identified is that women who do more self-exams find more benign lumps and have more invasive biopsies.

But what if you have little or no regular health care? What if you live far from your doctor or are uninsured, underinsured, or can't afford your copayment and go only for your annual visit? You are a good candidate for self-exam.

Doctors will tell you that most women find their lumps in the shower. Whether you are a good candidate for self-exam or not, know your body. Give yourself time to learn the normal shapes of your breasts at each point in

REAL LIFE QUESTION: If early detection is so important, how come I have to wait two weeks for an appointment after finding a lump?

Breast cancer is typically slow-growing. In the United States, a new lump patient will typically wait at least two weeks for the first appointment. This is tough on your mental outlook, but not on your breast. Your chances of having cancer are small, it's not going to grow in two weeks, and every breast care office in the country is swamped. Try to be patient, but if your breast is red or the skin is puckering, ask the receptionist to tell the breast surgeon what symptoms you have and that you need to be seen sooner. Or ask your own doctor for help in getting an earlier appointment.

your cycle. If a lump arises, you'll notice that something is different.

The controversy about breast self-exams does not mean that young women should not pay attention to their breasts—they should. Physician breast exams have been shown to make a difference in your breast health, and it is important that you have an annual breast exam by your physician to discuss lumps, pain, or anything that concerns you. If you or your physician do find a lump, you should have a mammogram and an ultrasound. That's because even though mammograms aren't a good screening tool in young women, they can still help in the evaluation of a breast lump or abnormality.

So although the message is that many women don't need a formal and vigilant breast self-exam each and every month, you should still stay in tune with your body and report anything unusual to your doctor. Take your time in the shower to give your breasts the once over. For now, that's good enough.

The Skinny on Mammograms

Mammograms are X-rays of the soft tissue of the breast, used to screen for breast cancer at an early stage before it is detectable as a lump. Mammograms are also used to evaluate a breast lump in order to determine the best treatment. At what age should you start having them? Screening mammograms are recommended for women starting at age forty. There is some controversy about the effectiveness of mammograms in the forties, but the data is clear that for women in their fifties, early detection of breast cancer by mammogram makes a difference.

I'm filling you in on mammograms here because you may be wondering why you aren't scheduled for one at your age or want to know what to expect when you do have one, and to tell you how important it is to have yours on schedule when it's your turn.

The reason mammograms are not a good screening tool in younger women is that in youth, breast tissue is dense, containing more fibrous and less fatty tissue. This dense tissue looks white on a mammogram. Breast cancer also looks white on a mammogram, appearing as little specks of white known as microcalcifications.

You'll hear your doctor talk about calcifications and microcalcifications, but it's usually microcalcifications that have the potential to be precancerous or cancer—even though most are benign. Because white on white does not show up, breast cancer is missed on the mammogram in young women much more frequently than in postmenopausal women. Calcifications are bunches of calcium in your breast. They could be caused by an injury, breastfeeding, or treatment for breast cancer, and most women have them at some point.

As women age, and especially after menopause, their breasts are more fatty and have a grayer appearance on mammography, so cancer shows up much better against this background.

Mammograms are X-rays of the soft tissue of the breast, used to screen for breast cancer at an early stage before it is detectable as a lump. Mammograms are also used to evaluate a breast lump in order to determine treatment plans. You'll hear debate about when mammograms should start and how often you should have them. Screening mammograms are recommended for women starting at about age forty, though there is some controversy about this (some authorities are recommending starting later). Always discuss your situation with your doctor to decide what is best for you. Some women need to start having mammograms earlier than others and some women can start later than age forty. Only you and your doctor know what is best for you.

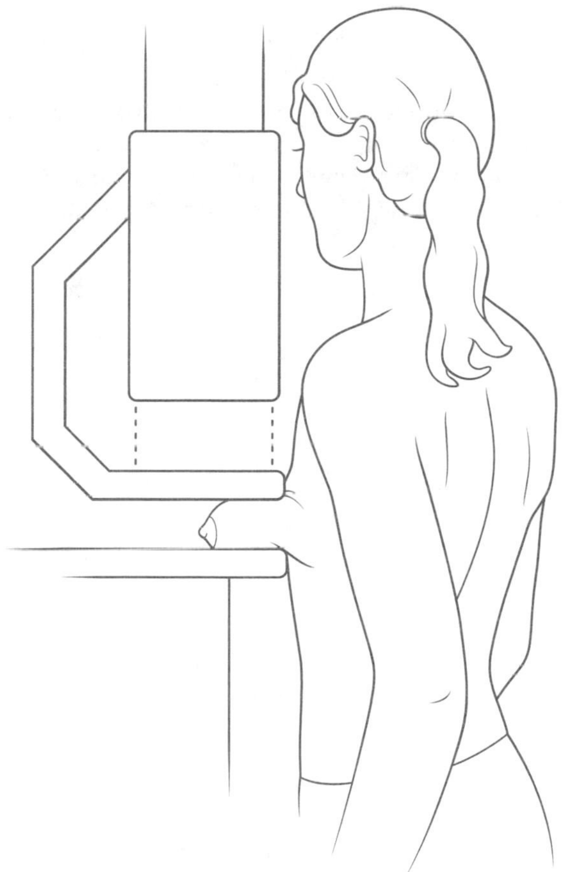

REAL LIFE QUESTION: Does a mammogram really hurt?

Yep, for about three seconds per picture (a couple of pictures will be taken of each breast). They have to squeeze your breasts in the machine to get a good image. But it hurts less than having your eyebrows waxed.

In the waiting room, women like to compare the "ouch" factor and talk about what kind of breasts hurt the most—bigger or smaller. I only know one patient who could compare the two, because she'd had breast reduction surgery. She swears that larger breasts hurt more, but also said that "it hurts a lot less than getting hit by a toy my son threw."

REAL LIFE FACT: Breast Cancer Screening Guide

Be familiar with how your breasts feel and what's normal for you. After age twenty, have a doctor check your breasts every year. At age forty, talk to your doctor about when to start annual screening mammograms. If you have a family history of breast cancer (especially in a mother or sister), or if a family member carries the BRCA1 or BRCA2 gene mutation, mammograms might be recommended earlier.

Digital Developments

Digital mammography is a technological advance that allows the radiologist to adjust the contrast, brightness, and magnification of breast images without additional exposure of the patient to X-rays. It is sort of like the difference between digital and film photography. One advantage is that you can save the image in a computer, which makes it easier to give this information to another doctor when necessary. Digital mammography may be better for young women, because the technical adjustments can help radiologists evaluate dense breasts.

MRI and Breast Cancer Diagnosis

MRI stands for magnetic resonance imaging. An MRI machine is a big magnet that reads the electromagnetic qualities of the body's cells. It does not use radiation.

In recent years, MRI has been used to help in breast cancer diagnoses. MRI works by finding body masses that contain lots of blood vessels, like cancer. Often you'll be screened twice in the same appointment. After the first set of pictures, you'll have a dye injected to give the pictures more contrast. The dye travels through your body and is picked up first by cancerous tumors that have lots of blood vessels.

But some benign conditions, like fibroadenomas, also have lots of blood vessels and so can be mistaken for tumors. MRI may also miss the more slow-growing tumors that lack blood vessels. There is hope that MRI may one day become a good screening tool, especially for high-risk young women whose dense breasts are hard to screen with mammography. Right now, though, mammography, even though it's not perfect, remains a better screening tool than MRI. MRI may be used in some cases as an additional evaluation tool when a lump is found and mammography is inconclusive, but not as a primary screening tool.

The problem is that MRI produces too many false positive results, meaning it finds an abnormality when one doesn't exist, which leads to unnecessary anxiety and medical testing. It's also expensive. And if you are claustrophobic, you will need some powerful relaxation techniques or even a tranquilizer (and a friend to drive you to the appointment and back). To learn about what an MRI test feels like, see chapter 1, Meet Your Body and Your Doctor.

The Breast Defense Is a Good Offense

Our breasts are powerful physical reminders of being women. Yes, they're sex organs, which is an important role in a fulfilling sexual relationship. At the same time, our breasts are how we feed our babies, so they feel like a very special part of us that unites mothers in a unique way. So remember that decisions you make about the cosmetic appearance of your breasts now may change your ability to breastfeed later.

The bottom line in breast health is this: understand your breasts and know what is normal. Know what health measures you can take now to make a difference in decreasing your risks later in life.

Now we're headed farther south! We'll explore your reproductive system, starting with the vagina and **cervix**, and then go through the information you need to know to have a healthy body, whether you are planning to have children or not.

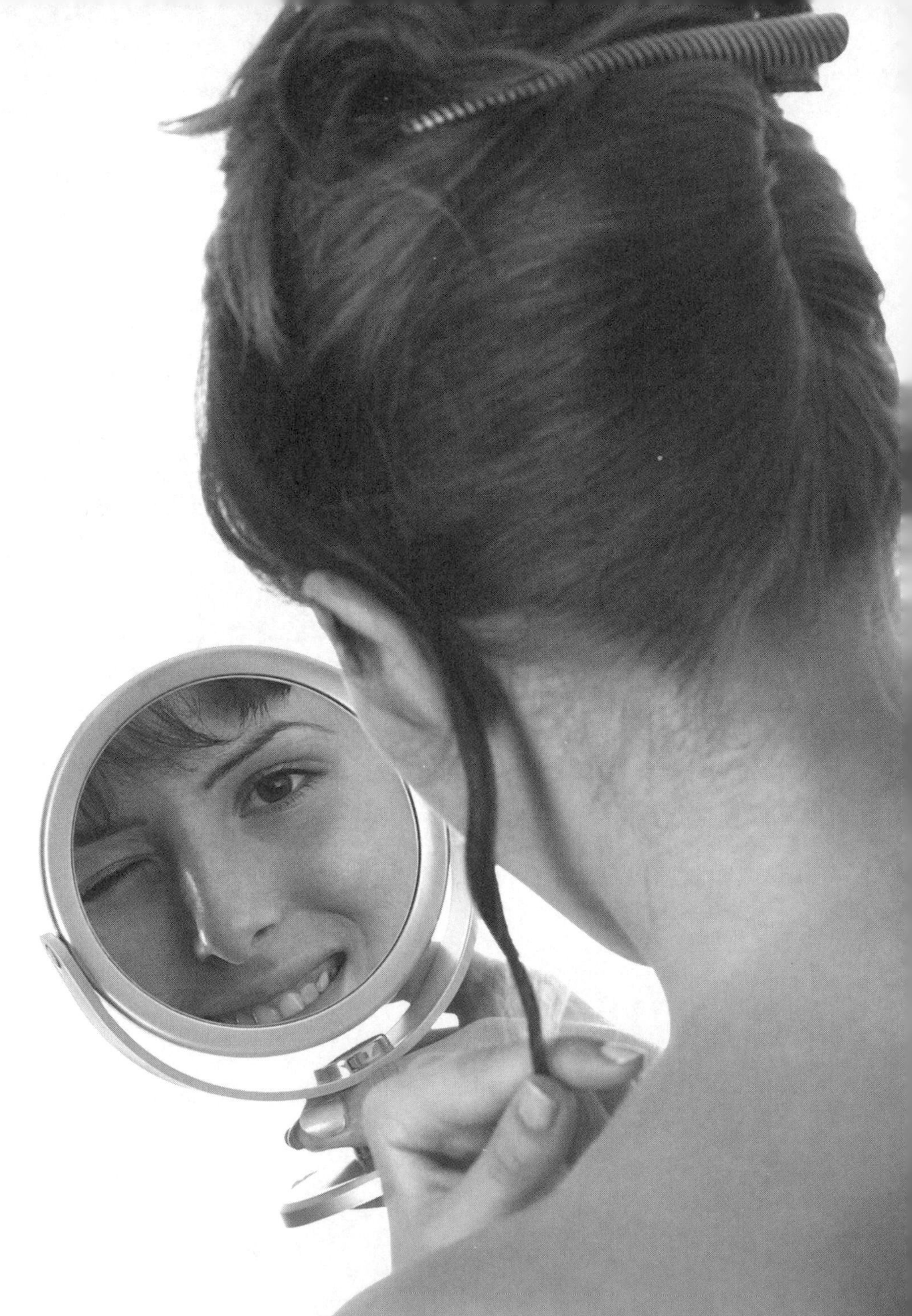

Grab your mirrors, girls.
We're going in.

your vagina and cervix

I hate to bring your mother up when we're talking about the vagina,

but it's helpful to understand our society's changing attitudes about our bodies.

If your mother is an older woman, she has never seen her "privates." She sees no reason to introduce herself to them and she leaves the acquaintance entirely up to her doctor. Her sex life most likely has never involved the kitchen table, your father's workplace, or the TV room floor.

If your mother is a baby boomer, however, there's a chance that she was part of the "get to know your vagina" movement. At her assertiveness-training class, she either made macramé plant hangers or pulled out a mirror to take a good look at the plumbing down there. For many women at that time, it felt empowering to drop their granny panties and explore the forbidden, mysterious world of the vagina—and in a group no less! For your generation, this probably sounds insane.

Which brings us to you. How much do *you* really know about your vagina—a complex, vitally important part of your anatomy? It's much more than the passage that allows babies to make their way into the world and that enables those wonderful feelings of sex. The vagina is really its own little ecosystem, and it's your job to keep it in balance. In this chapter, I'll explain how to do

NOTE TO SELF

Don't sleep with your underwear on. Ventilate!

that and I'll also cover those annoying things that can go wrong.

The Vagina Demystified

If your biology teacher were describing your vagina, s/he would say it is a muscular, stretchy tunnel lined with cells that produce lubrication and **mucus**, and that all kinds of different **bacteria** and microorganisms live naturally within it. A young teacher would stand there dying inside as s/he explained this to a classful of clowns, who would start laughing at the word "tunnel" and would be on the floor by the time s/he got to "mucus." An older teacher would make slides of bacteria and show them on the big white wall to gross you out before lunch, and then laugh about it in the faculty room.

In this mini ecosystem of yours, there is a two-way highway. Things go in—tampons, or the penis, sperm, and various other items that enter during sex. In exit mode, the lining of your **uterus**, the **endometrium**, is shed each month as your period.

Your vagina also has an incredible ability to stretch and expand to allow babies to be born. I've delivered thousands of babies, and I still can't quite believe that the **cervix** and the vagina can stretch like that. It's almost magic. Here we are, a species that can bleed for five days and not die, and then we can open a hole in our body the size of a baby's head. You couldn't sell that as a science fiction story, because it's just too unbelievable.

The Cervix

Your cervix, located at the top of your vagina, is the doorway to your uterus. It's the tollbooth. The cervix is a round structure that feels like a firm ball, and I've known many women who reached way up and felt it and thought something was wrong up there. You might expect it to be open all of the time, but it doesn't feel that way. It's firm like the tip of your nose, because it is made of similar firm connective tissue.

REAL LIFE FACT: Let It Breathe

Keep yourself as dry between your legs as possible. After a sweaty workout, change out of your damp exercise clothes or wet swimsuit as soon as you can. Wear cotton panties, wear loose pants as much as you can, and leave off the panty hose whenever possible. Everything you can do to air out keeps your vagina healthy. And yes, if your mother told you not to sleep with underwear on at night, she was right—ventilation is your friend.

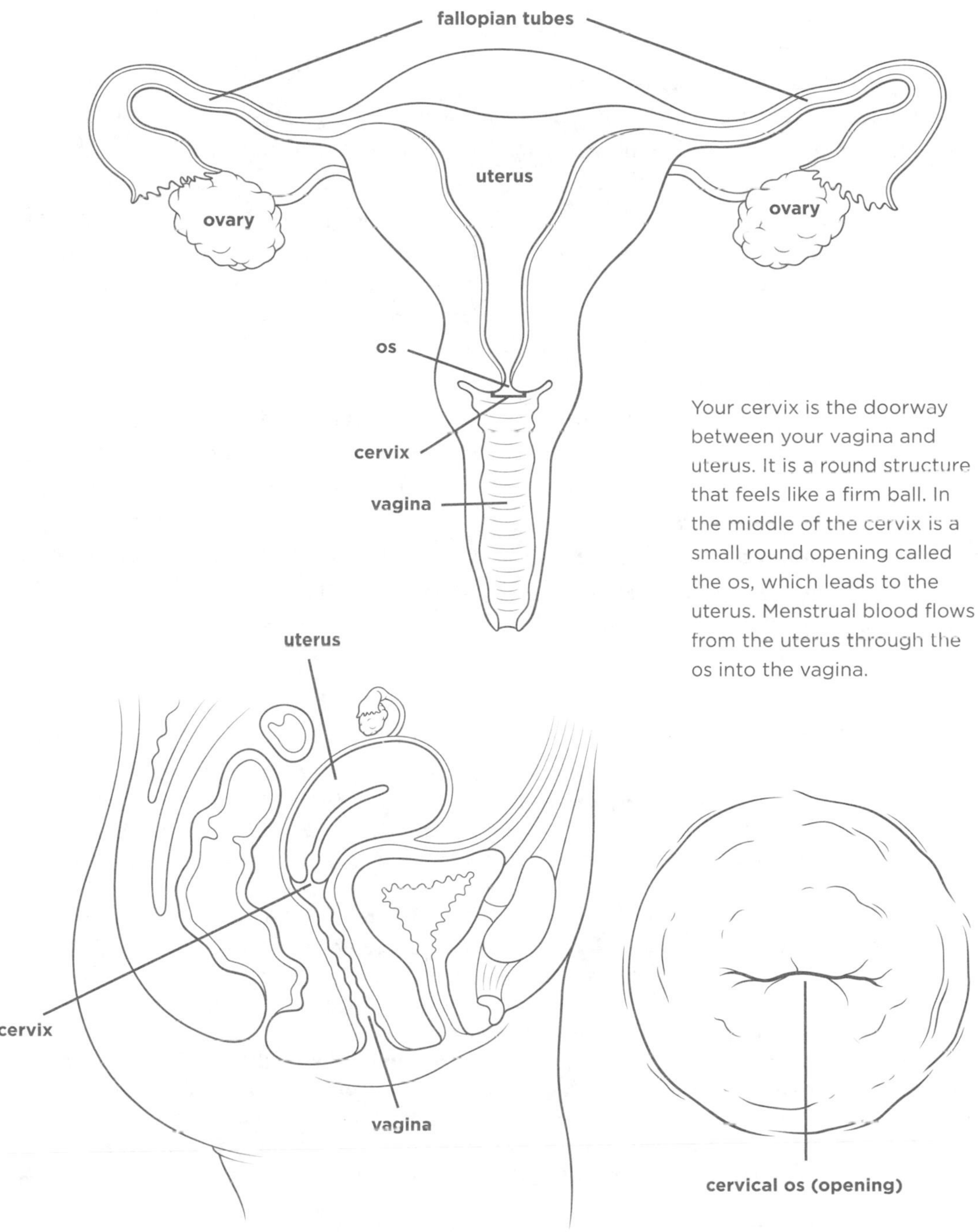

Your cervix is the doorway between your vagina and uterus. It is a round structure that feels like a firm ball. In the middle of the cervix is a small round opening called the os, which leads to the uterus. Menstrual blood flows from the uterus through the os into the vagina.

In the middle of the cervix is a small round opening called the os (pronounced OSS as in *boss*), which leads to the uterus. Menstrual blood flows from the uterus, through the os, into the vagina. During childbirth, the os dilates (expands) to let the baby pass through. The os is also where cells for a **Pap smear** are taken, because it's where most cervical **cancers** grow.

It's important to have your cervix examined during your annual physical and to keep it healthy. Be sure to have your Pap smear (see chapter 1, Meet Your Body and Your Doctor) on the schedule your doctor recommends. And remember that the Pap smear does not diagnose most **sexually transmitted diseases** other than **human papillomavirus** (HPV). You'll need to discuss other tests for them with your doctor.

Your Sexual Organs: Getting a Good Look

Okay, grab your mirror. Seriously. A hand mirror, of course, which is much easier than trying to lie on the floor in front of a wall mirror. You may need to do some gymnastic moves to see everything, but it really is worth getting to know the terrain. It can help you to improve your sex life, for one thing. So wash your hands with some mild soap, and we'll get to work.

Let's start at the front of your body. Use your fingers to spread open the outer lips (the labia majora)—the larger outer flaps that are typically covered in hair on the outside—so you can see the whole area, called the **vulva**. It's called plenty of other things too, from the soccer mom's "Volvo" to things you'll hear

REAL LIFE INFO: This Book Has Dirty Parts

Our grandmothers never called their body parts anything, not even by their proper names. Today, you'll hear a hundred different names, which change constantly. I'm including this list here not just to make you laugh—honest—but because it's useful to feel that you know what other people are talking about.

The current popular names for the female genitals include poontang, pussy, honeypot, muff, bush, beaver, twat, vadge, box, Bermuda triangle, squirrel trap, cooter, coochie, hoohah, vajayjay, crotch, pink taco, trim, kitty, goodies, bajingo, and babymaker. The C word is never, not ever, used unless you want to start a fight. The C word is *cunt*, a word so despised by older women that it is never okay to say it in front of one, especially a mother-in-law.

Men have many more names for their body parts. Nobody knows why, although many people like to guess. They have penis terms, such as dick, johnson, willy, cock, knob, prick, chicken neck, one-eyed milkman, one-eyed trouser snake, weenie, wiener, dong, schlong, pecker, tool, and joystick; and testicle terms, such as balls, nads, bollocks, happy sack, and nut sack; and terms for both, such as frank and beans, meat and two veggies, or wedding tackle.

only in rap lyrics. (In this book, we'll stick with vulva.)

Next you'll see the labia minora, the smooth inner lips of the vulva. This is one of the body's many structures that are designed to keep things from accidentally getting in there, just as your eyebrows and lashes protect your eyes. Our first stop is at the **clitoris** and the **urethra** opening, which are close together. The urethra is a tiny opening with a tiny hole, otherwise known as your pee hole. You might not be able to see it in the mirror. You can touch it, but your main job is to keep this little gal clean, because when infections brew here—and they will—it really hurts.

The clitoris is a firm, bulgy little area at the highest point of the vulva, just above the urethra, where the inner lips meet (kind of like where the pilot sits in an airplane). The hood that is formed by the meeting of the labia minora lies over the clitoris, so it is kind of under cover and not immediately apparent unless you separate your labia. It is easier to feel than to see. This hood of skin may look wrinkly. Inch for inch, the clitoris is the single most studied part of a woman's body. It is an incredibly sensitive area because it is packed with nerve endings that like sex. Stimulation of the clitoris can begin and complete an orgasm, or it can get your body in the mood

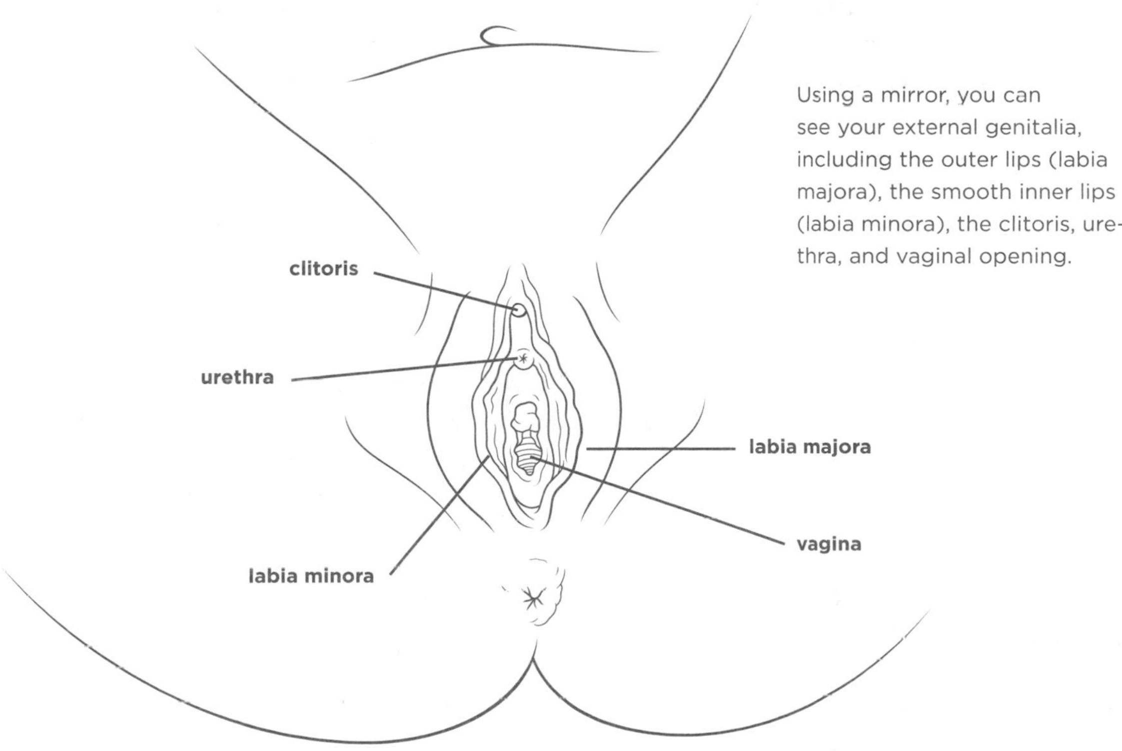

Using a mirror, you can see your external genitalia, including the outer lips (labia majora), the smooth inner lips (labia minora), the clitoris, urethra, and vaginal opening.

REAL LIFE QUESTION: It's not time for my period, so why am I bleeding?

Sometimes you bleed a little when you ovulate. It happens when the egg is released from the ovary and is perfectly normal. It's also normal to have no bleeding at all.

for vaginal sex and orgasm. It connects to the labia minora or inner lips of the vagina, with no clear line of where it begins and ends. That means it can be stimulated during sex even if nobody is touching it.

Anatomically, the clitoris is a lot like the penis—but a very tiny penis. When a woman gets sexually aroused, the clitoris becomes engorged with blood, enlarges, and hardens—much like a penis. It might even cause a tiny amount of fluid to leak when you have an orgasm. If a Ken doll were anatomically correct, he would have equipment that looks a lot like a clitoris.

People love to debate the sexual differences between the penis and the vagina, such as how many nerve endings are in each. Nerve endings are important in sex because they signal the brain that arousal is starting, and the brain can then tell the penis or vagina to get ready (sending messages to start engorgement or lubrication, for example).

What's the truth? Both organs have plenty of important nerve endings. But the nerves are more focused in the tip of the penis and in the clitoris than in the whole penis or vagina. If Dr. Helen O'Connell of the Royal Melbourne Hospital is right, nobody knows the real answer yet. Dr. O'Connell believes that the clitoris is the tip of a pyramid that is much larger and actually includes the walls of the vagina. In a *BBC News* report, Dr. O'Connell said that the total clitoris may be close to the size of a penis. On the penis side of the count, men who are against circumcision say that many nerve endings are lost with the foreskin.

Men and women are both sexual and reproductive beings. Nobody knows what is true for everybody. And the traditional method of counting the nerve endings was done by dissecting dead people, which is probably not what you and I had in mind when we signed that donor card.

The next opening below the urethra is the vaginal opening. Your vagina will be able to take in a finger, so go ahead and put one there. You will probably be able to squeeze your vaginal muscles and feel them contract around your finger. That's the same set of muscles that keeps a tampon in automatically. You'll notice that the vagina angles slightly toward your back.

Directly behind your vagina is your **anus**, the opening of your **rectum**, where your poop comes out. This isn't a great system, having all these openings right next to each other so that their contents can get mixed together, sometimes causing problems for the owner. (For more on this, see chapter 10, Your Waterworks.)

NOTE TO SELF

Limit your hot tub time. The heat, the chemicals, the other people—it's just a big germ nightmare. Please don't have sex in a hot tub either, for the same and so many other reasons, including that sex in water is only possible with an ocean full of lubricant!

What's That Stuff? Vaginal Discharge

A healthy vagina has a pH balance that is slightly acidic, with a small to moderate amount of discharge that ranges from clear to white, and from thin to thick. The color and consistency of your discharge depends upon hormone levels that vary throughout your monthly cycle.

A normal vagina has a distinct smell, caused by the many different kinds of bacteria and other microorganisms living in this small ecosystem. Your gyn may tell you that this smell is normal and therefore "not unpleasant." The human body has many such smells, none of which you would bottle and spray on your pulse points. But for your health, please leave it alone.

Special deodorants and douches are a very bad idea, because you might kill off the **lactobacillus**. Lactobacillus is the good guy bacteria found in your vagina and is very important. It's the peacekeeper among all the many microorganisms down there. These good bacteria produce acid, and this acidic environment keeps harmful bacteria and yeast from overgrowing. To keep the lactobacillus happy, don't douche, and don't use "feminine hygiene" sprays.

The vaginal walls are continually producing liquids, which we call secretions. They

REAL LIFE FACT: Bag the Douche

Remember that the vagina is like a self-cleaning oven. Its acidity keeps it clean, so douching isn't necessary, and my advice is to avoid douching altogether. It's not normal to have a vagina that smells like a field of flowers—imagine the chemicals used to create that fragrance!

Wash the external area of your vagina with gentle soap when you shower or bathe. The inside of your vagina will clean itself. Also, douching after having sex will not prevent pregnancy and should never be considered a form of birth control.

If you have a strange odor from your vagina, see your doctor.

REAL LIFE FACT: Believe It or Not

Today there are two cosmetic practices that you'll probably think I made up: anus bleaching and labia dying. Both are done with over-the-counter chemicals to keep these areas youthful looking. Apparently, some women like to have a nice, white anus, though how they know they haven't got one is another story. And I guess having pale labia is having old labia, so some women are using pink dye in their quest for youth.

I can't recommend these procedures, which use chemicals on such important and sensitive areas of skin, until there is actual research done on their safety. In the meantime, if these are big problems for you, just use a women's best beauty secret: turn out the lights.

cleanse and lubricate the vagina, like one of those indoor wall fountains, and maintain the proper acidity to prevent infection. The production of secretions changes during your menstrual cycle and increases when you are sexually aroused.

Can you ignore your vagina's discharges? Well, you don't need to be checking them all the time, but you do need to observe a few things, which you normally do by looking at the toilet paper after you pee. Discharge changes with the hormones of your menstrual cycle. You may notice clear sticky discharge that looks just like egg whites about two weeks after your period, during **ovulation**. The discharge is normal. It's caused by the **estrogen** produced from ovulation. Because it signals ovulation, it may come in handy as a way to time sex in order to get pregnant. (Having sex when you have no discharge is *not* a foolproof way to avoid pregnancy.)

Later on in your cycle, the discharge is usually thicker and whiter. This is because of the hormone **progesterone**, which is higher in the second half of the menstrual cycle. The thinner secretion helps sperm in their passage to the egg. The thicker secretion says, "We're closed."

Why Am I Dry?

Sometime after you first notice a discharge and panic, you'll have an episode of vaginal dryness and panic then, too. Most women experience vaginal dryness from time to time, usually during sex. The most common cause is a lack of **foreplay**. To get those cells pumping, take time before sex for kissing, talking out a fantasy, touching, or massage.

Common medications can also cause vaginal dryness. You use cold medications, antihistamines, and pseudoephedrine to dry out all of your **mucous membranes** so that you won't have a runny nose, but they affect all of your mucous membranes the same way, including the vagina.

Another common culprit is birth control pills, because the hormones in them can affect mucus production, although more commonly women see an increase and thickening in cervical mucus from the birth control pill. I've also noticed that antidepressants can cause dryness. Everyone is different, and it can be very hard to predict who will have side effects from medications.

The most common time in your menstrual cycle to experience vaginal dryness is, oddly, during your period; this can cause painful sex. Another common cause of vaginal dryness during sex is **condoms**, which can irritate your vagina, causing a dry, painful feeling.

Usually these issues can be fixed by using a water-based lubricant. Both partners can experiment with applying the lubricant to any number of body parts. Do not use petroleum jelly, which can damage a condom.

NOTE TO SELF

Keep chemicals out of your vagina: douches, deodorants, deodorant tampons, and spermicides. Use spermicidal jelly only if you use a diaphragm. Water-based lubricants are okay.

If this doesn't work, definitely see your doctor to rule out any vaginal infection that can also result in dryness (such as yeast or bacterial vaginosis—more on those shortly).

Does Size Matter?

When it comes to the vagina, no, size really doesn't matter. Most vaginas are about four inches long "at rest," but like your height, this can vary. I don't know many women who have measured their vaginas, and there is no myth about vagina length as there is about shoe size relating to penis size. Some teenagers have stuck a pencil up the vagina and then measured the pencil, but it's not a good idea, or sanitary, or a great use of your time. Plus, it doesn't work. By the way, the story about somebody's cousin losing the pencil and needing surgery is an urban legend, or possibly a rural one.

Most women think of their vagina as a hole or cavity inside the body, probably because it is drawn that way in illustrations. In fact, the walls of the vagina are normally touching unless something is in there. The vaginal opening is normally closed. When something enters the vagina—like a finger, a penis, or a tampon—the vagina stretches and sort of

REAL LIFE FACT: Real Life Kids

I once heard a kindergartener say that she knows the difference between boys and girls: "Boys have peanuts, and girls have pajamas."

grips it, as there are muscles in the walls of the vagina. (Please see chapter 11, Your Best Sex, for more about the vagina and sexuality.)

There are myths about exceptionally large vaginas that are the subject of comic routines. I've never seen one. As we age and experience childbirth, the muscles of the vaginal wall may slacken a bit—but they still work!

Where's My G-Spot?

I don't know. Nobody else does, either. G-spot theory dates back to 1950 and states that there is a part of the vaginal wall that will give you deeper or more frequent orgasms if it is stimulated during sex. The location is supposed to be inside the front of the vagina.

Nobody knows whether it really exists, because there's just no way to prove it scientifically. Some people who believe in the G-spot think that some women have it and some don't. If that's true, don't worry, because the clitoris is still the big powerhouse switch for sex.

My advice? If you have sex with a loving partner, show them anything that makes you love sex. That's your G-spot, and you have many of them. (For more on the G-spot, see chapter 11, Your Best Sex.)

NOTE TO SELF

Talk with your doctor about regular screening for sexually transmitted infections, and call if you develop any sores, itches, or odd odors. If you think you have a yeast infection and have never had one diagnosed or treated before, talk with your doctor before you treat it yourself.

What Can Go Wrong? Vaginitis: Ouch and Ick

Most women will have at least one episode of vaginitis during their lives. Vaginitis is not a life-and-death emergency, but the intense itching and burning south of the border can make it feel like one. Vaginitis is an **inflammation** of the vagina in which the walls are irritated and more **white blood cells** and discharge are produced as your body naturally fights off infection. Infection can result from overgrowth of normal bacteria or yeast, sexually transmitted diseases, or chemical irritants like douches.

Many different bacteria and yeast normally populate the vagina. They usually coexist peacefully and keep each other in check, but if they are knocked off balance, one may overpower the others. This leads to a decrease in the number of lactobacillus (one of the normal bacteria that lives in the vagina, keeping the peace), an increase in yeast and other bacteria, and the unpleasant symptoms of odor, discharge, and vaginal irritation. Vaginitis includes **yeast infections** and bacterial vaginosis.

Yeast Infections

Yeast vaginitis is an infection of the vagina caused by a fungus known as candida. The usual symptoms of yeast vaginitis are a white "cottage cheesy" discharge, as well as vaginal itching or burning. (I don't know why we always use food to describe vaginal discharge.) Sometimes women notice burning during urination or dryness or pain with intercourse.

Generally, women develop yeast vaginitis after a change in the vaginal environment—due to antibiotic use, bubble baths, douching, wearing wet bathing suits, using deodorant tampons, and so on—causes a decrease in the normal lactobacillus bacteria. If you are taking **antibiotics**, they'll act against all bacteria, so both the good and the bad bacteria are killed off, allowing the yeast to flourish unchecked.

I'm getting on my soapbox again about douching, but bear with me because it's important. Douching can kill off the good bacteria, leaving the bad bacteria to multiply. Douching can also upset the vagina's natural pH balance and that encourages bacterial overgrowth. Ignore those magazine ads and television commercials promoting paranoia about your natural scent. Bubble baths and soaps can cause an allergic reaction in the walls of the vagina, leading to vaginitis.

Here's another good reason not to cut off ventilation to the genital area: clothing such as nylon underwear, panty hose, or tight-fitting pants causes this area to stay moist and warm, a perfect climate for the growth of yeast infections. The same thing happens if you wear a wet bathing suit for too long. Estrogen is also a risk factor in the development of yeast infections, so women on birth control pills and pregnant women have more frequent infections.

Obesity is another risk factor for developing a yeast infection. This may be related to the association of obesity with **diabetes**, because diabetics are more prone to yeast infections. Diabetes affects the immune system, which allows yeast to overgrow. The higher sugar environment in a diabetic body allows yeast to thrive, in the vagina and elsewhere.

Vaginitis is diagnosed by your doctor or nurse obtaining a sample of your vaginal discharge and looking at it on a microscope slide. The presence of yeast without symptoms of infection does not require treatment, because yeast is a normal inhabitant of the vagina.

Treating Yeast Infections

Treatment for yeast infections is with antifungal medication. If this is your first yeast infection, go to your health care provider to be sure yeast vaginitis is the right diagnosis. Once you've had a yeast infection, you can be pretty confident you know the symptoms yourself, so it's okay to treat yourself in the future, using over-the-counter medication. If you have lots of yeast infections, it's a good idea to see your doctor, because you may have a resistant strain that requires a prescription antifungal or longer-than-usual treatment.

How do you use the treatments? You put them in your vagina. The usual form is a tablet, cream, or other form of suppository that goes into your vagina at bedtime (when you're horizontal, so it has a chance to work before oozing out) for a period of days. Antifungal creams that are available over the counter include butoconazole (Femstat 3), clotrimazole (Lotrimin), miconazole (Monistat), and terconazole (Terazol 3).

A one-tablet oral treatment for yeast vaginitis is fluconazole (Diflucan), which can be convenient in order to avoid the messy creams but is available only with a prescription since your doctor needs to be sure it is a good option for you. If symptoms do not go away with treatment, make an appointment for further evaluation.

During pregnancy, confirm your diagnosis before using any treatment. Your doctor will typically ask you to use creams instead of pills, because creams are less likely to get into your **bloodstream**—and into your baby.

We used to treat male sex partners at the same time. Now we know that yeast vaginitis is not sexually contagious, but rather an overgrowth of normal microorganisms. So your partner does not need to be treated, and you can't catch yeast from each other.

NOTE TO SELF

Your vagina is the healthiest place for a penis during sex. Anal sex increases your chances of infection because it causes tears and abrasions where germs can enter. If you do have anal sex, don't—under any circumstances—have vaginal sex afterward. You may develop a nasty infection.

If you dislike treating your yeast infections, you might feel better if you ask Mom how she treated hers. Your mother may remember when suppositories looked like giant light bulbs and you had to insert one twice a day for two weeks. Sometimes it gave you a neon yellow discharge. You're lucky! Treatment is much simpler now.

Bacterial Vaginosis

Bacterial vaginosis (BV) is caused by an overgrowth of the normal bacteria in your vagina as a result of decreased lactobacillus (good bacteria), which then decreases vaginal acidity. It is similar to a yeast infection, because it is an overgrowth of microorganisms that normally live in the vagina, but in this case the microorganism is bacteria instead of yeast.

BV is not sexually transmitted, but it usually is found in sexually active women, so it could be the sexual activity that brings it on. The infection sometimes begins after sex with a new partner, which alters the ecosystem balance in your vagina. It is usually signaled by a thin yellow, gray, or greenish, frothy vaginal discharge that is accompanied by a fishy odor (there's that food comparison again) and vaginal irritation. The odor is often noticeable after intercourse. Bacterial vaginosis is the most common vaginitis I see.

The diagnosis of bacterial vaginosis is made by your doctor by examining your vaginal discharge. One test is done by looking at the discharge on a slide under the microscope to help distinguish bacterial vaginosis from other types of vaginitis—yeast vaginitis and trichomoniasis (another STI). A sign of bacterial vaginosis under the microscope is that the vaginal cells that are normally shed become coated with bacteria. These surface cells are called clue cells. Under the microscope, they look like potato chips sprinkled with pepper. Normal lining cells look like potato chips too, but they don't have the pepper. The pepper is the bacteria sticking to the cells. (More food analogies.) Clue cells are one of the most reliable signs of bacterial vaginosis.

Besides clue cells, women with bacterial vaginosis have fewer of the normal vaginal lactobacillus bacteria. Another good test for bacterial vaginosis is called the whiff test. A drop of potassium hydroxide testing liquid is used in the whiff test, and when this solution comes into contact with a drop of the discharge from a woman with bacterial vaginosis, a fishy odor can result. Many women notice this same fishy odor after sex.

Treating Bacterial Vaginosis

Bacterial vaginosis is treated with a prescription antibiotic—in the form of either prescription vaginal cream or oral antibiotics (metronidazole vaginal cream or oral tablets, or clindamycin vaginal cream). It usually resolves completely without complications after treatment. No special follow-up is necessary if the symptoms disappear.

Just like with yeast infections, your partner does not need to be treated, because the infection is not transmitted sexually. For unknown reasons, some women get recurrent BV. Usually it can be handled by longer treatment with oral antibiotics.

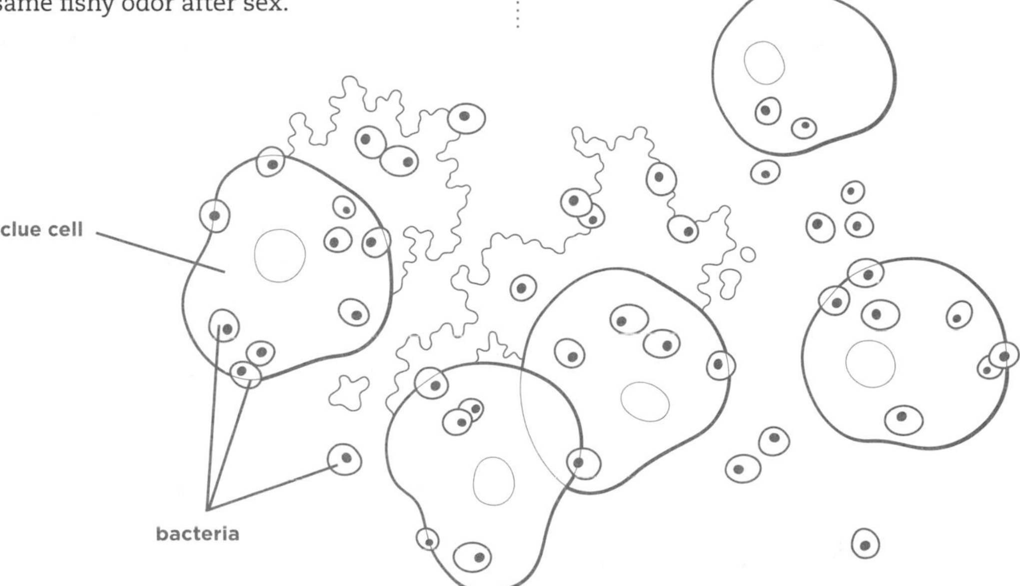

Your doctor can look at your vaginal discharge under a microscope to diagnose bacterial vaginosis. When you have BV, the vaginal cells are coated with bacteria and called clue cells.

Pregnancy and Bacterial Vaginosis

In pregnancy, bacterial vaginosis has been associated with premature delivery. Unfortunately, although treatment will get rid of the unpleasant symptoms of bacterial vaginosis, it will not lower the risk of premature labor. BV may be a red flag to health care providers to watch for signs of premature labor. Research into bacterial vaginosis and pregnancy is ongoing to help us understand how it relates to prematurity.

Vulvodynia

Vulvodynia became famous on *Sex and the City*, when Charlotte experienced pain and itching and her doctor prescribed antidepressants. The medicine was used to interfere with pain signals, but the girls laughed about Charlotte having a depressed vagina. Real women with vulvodynia experience pain, often for years, without diagnosis, and don't find it very funny. If you have pain and itching that does not sound like any of the other conditions described here, ask your doctor about vulvodynia.

Vulvodynia is a form of **chronic** pain. Besides pain and itching, you might have a burning sensation or painful sex. Although there is no cure for vulvodynia, many women can be helped with a combination of medication and self-care. Medications might include antihistamines or the use of anticonvulsants and antidepressants. This is what's called an off-label use of medication, which means that these drugs were not developed for vulvar pain but may be effective in treating it.

Self-care methods may include using lidocaine ointment before sex or holding cold compresses to the area. A cold compress can be a bag of frozen peas wrapped in a paper towel. (You don't eat or refreeze the peas once they've thawed.)

Again, don't diagnose vulvodynia by yourself. It's important to rule out other skin conditions and infections, which only your doctor can do.

The Endometriosis Mystery

Endometriosis, one of the most difficult health problems for young women, is also the one we know the least about. Let's start with what we do know. Endometriosis is a disorder named for your endometrium (the tissue that lines your uterus), and it happens when tissue that is like your endometrium grows somewhere else. This tissue may grow in your lower **pelvis**, on your ovaries, or even on your **bowels**.

Endometriosis tends to run in families, and it's a painful condition that often gets worse just before and during your period. Most of the pain is in the pelvis, but some of it may radiate. Picture rays of pain that spread down your back or legs.

Sex might also be painful, especially with deep penetration. You may have diarrhea or even pain when you poop. Endometriosis often

REAL LIFE INFO: Symptoms of Endometriosis

- **Pelvic pain that gets worse just before and during your period**
- **Painful sex, especially with deep penetration**
- **Diarrhea or painful bowel movements**

starts in your teens or early twenties, and in some cases it may cause fertility problems.

What causes endometriosis? No one really knows. It might be that cells from the lining of your uterus get loose during your period and flow through your **fallopian tubes** and out to the pelvis. Or it might be that cells in your abdomen share genetic links with your uterus lining and change into endometriosis.

It's not easy to diagnose, either. If you have some of the symptoms, you need to report them to your doctor so s/he can start to evaluate you. Evaluation often starts with an ultrasound test to rule out other things, such as ovarian cysts. With endometriosis, the ultrasound is usually normal unless you also have endometriomas—ovarian cysts made from the endometriosis cells. These are called chocolate cysts, because their fluid is thick and brown. To confirm endometriosis, surgery is usually necessary, during which the doctor is able to see the endometriotic areas or take a **biopsy** to confirm them.

Endometriosis Treatments

To treat endometriosis, we use both medicine and surgery therapy.

Because the endometrial areas behave just like the normal endometrial lining, birth control pills can decrease your symptoms. Birth control pills make the normal endometrial lining very thin, which is why women on the pill have shorter and lighter periods, and often less pain. **Progestin**-only pills, such as Implanon, the mini-pill, or Depo-Provera also work well.

REAL LIFE QUESTION: Is there a cure for endometriosis?

Menopause is the only absolute cure. However; lowering your estrogen levels will allow the endometriosis areas to shrink.

Women with difficult cases may require a type of therapy where luprolide acetate (Lupron Depot) is injected into the muscle of your upper arm or bottom, which induces a temporary **menopause**, lowering estrogen levels and causing the endometrial areas to shrink.

Surgery can also be helpful, and a minimally invasive procedure can usually be done with a laparoscope. This slender telescope is inserted through your belly button (you are asleep under general anesthesia) so the doctor can see what's going on inside your body. And then another, smaller incision (less than an inch) is made, generally just above your pubic bone, so any areas s/he finds can be cauterized (burned) away and scar tissue removed. Sometimes the effects of surgery are long lasting, and sometimes medical therapy is used to prolong the effect of surgery. Many women have both medical and surgical treatments at different times during their life.

Pregnancy often improves the symptoms of endometriosis, because the high progesterone environment that happens during pregnancy causes endometiral areas to shrink (though they can grow back later). If you have endometriosis, the treatments usually need to be continued until menopause, when it all will finally end.

Endometriosis is one of the most highly studied problems of women's health. There is a great deal of research going on—to find out how and why it happens, to find better treatments, and to find a cure for this difficult problem. Be sure to stay in touch with your doctor.

Sexually Transmitted Diseases

What the pamphlets say is true: whenever you have sex with someone, you are also having sex with everyone else they've ever had sex with. Diseases are passed from person to person, often with no symptoms. If you want a guarantee that you will never have a sexually transmitted disease or infection (STD or STI—they are the same), the only path is monogamy for you and a disease-free partner.

Most of us have more than one partner in a lifetime. How can you protect yourself? First, use a condom every single time you have sex until you are in a committed or long-term relationship. If a man refuses to use a condom, ditch him. He may complain that his pleasure is reduced, but is that worth risking your lifelong health and fertility? Kick him to the curb, right now.

Before choosing to have sex, you should already know a lot about a man. You should already know if he has any diseases and if he has a long list of sexual partners. If you don't know a man well enough to know these things, you don't know him well enough to have sex with him. You may see a culture of "bar sex," fostered on television and in movies, in which couples have sex on the first date. This is a good way to move the story line along quickly and keep the audience paying attention, but it's a very risky way to live. You probably think I sound prudish. I am, because I have seen too

REAL LIFE QUESTION: What's a microbicide and does it work?

A microbicide is a substance that can reduce the spread of sexually transmitted infections when applied in the vagina. No microbicides are available that decrease or prevent the spread of STIs, but there are several promising ones being tested. Don't believe any news about microbicides until they have been studied over the long term.

An important note if you use a diaphragm: yes, you should continue to use your spermicidal jelly with your diaphragm.

many young women whose lives were drastically altered by bar sex at twenty-one that left them unable to have children at thirty. If you are in the habit of having bar sex regularly, I, as your doctor, would want to know more about your drinking habits, and I would want your promise to use condoms.

Okay, enough with the advice. Now let's look at the common STIs and what you can do to prevent and treat them.

Herpes

We need more common words for the different kinds of **herpes** you can catch. You probably know why: At some point in sixth grade, a girl developed a cold sore on her lip. Someone in class said she had herpes. The teacher said that was true and the girl went home crying. You thought it was funny until one day that sixth-grader was your child.

What that girl had is called oral herpes or herpes simplex 1. She got it from normal contact with family and friends, such as kissing or close skin-to-skin touching. It's not genital herpes, and it's not sexually transmitted.

Genital herpes, or herpes simplex 2, is an infection caused by a sexually transmitted virus. It most commonly infects the genitals, but I've seen it on bottoms and breasts too. It is usually spread by someone who has an infectious herpes sore, but it can be spread even when it's dormant.

Herpes is a strange virus. It actually lives in the nerve endings, close to where the infection first started. Future outbreaks will always be in this same area, whenever the virus gets reactivated. There is no cure for herpes, and stress, illness, or sunlight can cause an outbreak. Some people have only a few outbreaks in their lifetime. Others have them as often as every month.

How can you tell if your cold sore is herpes simplex 1 or simplex 2? We don't normally do tests to check because we know by the location, especially if it's recurrent. While it's technically possible for a simplex 2 (genital) sore to infect the lips, it won't thrive there and recur. It thrives and recurs in the genitals. And a simplex 1 (oral) case is possible in the genitals, especially if transmitted by **oral sex**, but it won't thrive there either, so you tend to have fewer outbreaks. Simplex 1 and 2 are a lot alike at the DNA level but are still different viruses that do best in their own locations.

By the way, oral herpes is very contagious. When you have a cold sore, do everyone a favor and don't kiss anybody anywhere.

NOTE TO SELF

To avoid herpes, always use a condom, because there is *no* cure.

Hampering Herpes

Genital herpes is decreasing but is still incredibly common, with about 20 percent of Americans infected. It's more common among women than men, and the Centers for Disease Control estimates that 25 percent of women and 12 percent of men have it.

Herpes is transmitted from direct contact with someone who has a sore, which is also called a lesion.

It can also be transmitted by someone who has dormant herpes with no open sores, which is called asymptomatic shedding. For example, you know that your boyfriend has herpes, so you avoid having sex when he has a lesion. But suddenly you develop a herpes sore in your vagina after having sex with him when he did not have a herpes lesion. This is possible, because a person can be shedding virus in the absence of a lesion about 10 percent of the time. Many women know before they are about to have a herpes outbreak because they get a little tingling feeling in the area where they typically get their outbreak. Remember, too, that you don't need to have intercourse to catch herpes, because touching a lesion, such as the penis touching the outside of your vagina or labia, can transmit the virus.

Sexual transmission of herpes can be prevented by using condoms, as long as the condom covers the sore. Your best defense is to use condoms every time you have sex—that's *every time*, until you are in a committed, monogamous relationship in which you've both been cleared of STIs by tests.

There are medications that suppress the virus, but there is no cure today. The suppressive medications, which must be taken daily, can reduce and even eliminate herpes outbreaks and asymptomatic viral shedding. That can greatly reduce anxiety about having genital herpes, and most women find they have few, if any, side effects. There is also a vaccine in the works that shows promise, but it is still some years away.

NOTE TO SELF

Don't fall for the myth. Herpes cannot be caught from dry surfaces like toilet seats.

Health Issues and Herpes

Herpes sores are uncomfortable, even painful, and people feel embarrassed about having them. But in a healthy person with a normally functioning immune system, they aren't dangerous. Herpes doesn't cause fertility problems or affect your general health.

The one health issue to be aware of is this: if you have a genital herpes outbreak when you are going to deliver a baby, you should have a cesarean delivery instead of a vaginal delivery. A baby can contract a herpes infection from an infected birth canal. Because a newborn does not yet have a fully functioning immune system, infection can have serious consequences. Luckily, a cesarean delivery can prevent this from happening. Medication can also be used in pregnancy to suppress outbreaks at the time of delivery.

Human Papillomavirus

You've seen it all over TV. Human papillomavirus (HPV) is a virus that can cause cancer of the cervix, and it's a silent virus. No itching, no symptoms. Up to 80 percent of all sexually active young women have it. It is sexually contagious. Unfortunately, condoms don't give you complete protection because the virus can live on the scrotum and other places that aren't covered by the condom.

What does this mean for you? There are a hundred types of HPV, with four causing the highest risk. Three out of four young women are infected with HPV, but most clear the infection and don't even know they ever had it. Because more than 90 percent of HPV infections will disappear in healthy women who have an intact immune system and do not smoke, most women with HPV do not develop a precancer or cancer of the cervix. But sometimes the infection can cause cervical cancer decades later. Smoking greatly increases the risk, which is reason number seventy-eight not to smoke.

Your doctor may want to test for HPV when you have an abnormal **Pap test**, or as part of a screening routine. If you have an abnormal Pap, the HPV test can help clarify the Pap test results and determine the best follow-up strategy. A negative HPV test result often means that the abnormal cell changes were not precancerous. Sometimes the sample taken for your Pap test also can be used for an HPV test.

NOTE TO SELF

Having an STI once doesn't mean you can't get it again! Have regular screening for STIs at your physical, and always call your doctor if you have unusual symptoms.

Genital Warts

Genital warts are sexually transmitted warts caused by the human papillomavirus. They're **benign** and don't lead to cancer. They appear as small bumps in the genital area that look just like warts on other parts of your body. They may be single or in clusters that look like tiny cauliflowers (again with the food images).

In women, genital warts appear on the vulva (outer part of the genital area), in the vagina, on the cervix, or in the anal area. Rarely, warts may also develop in the mouth or throat of a person who has had sexual contact in those areas. Left untreated, many cases of genital warts will resolve on their own. But some will grow, spread, and get larger.

Genital warts usually are painless, but they may cause itching or irritation. They are very contagious, even with just one sexual contact. The warts can develop weeks to months later and can come back for years.

The HPV subtypes that cause genital warts (called 6 and 11) don't increase your risk of cervical cancer. But having one type of HPV doesn't mean you won't get another. By the way, an estimated 1 percent of the U.S. population has genital warts. That means there are probably three million adults who have it.

There is currently no cure for HPV infections, and treatment of genital warts only controls outbreaks of warts. Some doctors don't recommend immediate treatment of genital warts because it has been found that in 20 to 30 percent of those who have it, genital warts clear on their own within three months.

There are three kinds of genital wart treatments:

- Prescription topical chemicals designed to destroy wart tissue (applied to the wart)
- Surgical methods to remove wart tissue
- Increasing the immune response of the body against the warts

Studies do not show that any one of these treatments is better than another. The decision is best made by you and your doctor together.

HPV Vaccine—At Last!

A vaccine called Gardasil was approved by the U.S. Food and Drug Administration (FDA) in 2006. Gardasil works against two cancer-causing strains of HPV as well as the two that cause genital warts. The vaccine has benefits above and beyond cancer prevention, too. Every day thousands of women deal with repeat Pap smears, biopsies, and surgical procedures for precancerous changes, all due to HPV damage. These procedures not only create stress and pain, but can also lead to infertility and premature delivery.

The Centers for Disease Control and Prevention (CDC) recommends that all women and girls ages nine to twenty-six receive this vaccine to protect against HPV. Ideally, the vaccine should be given before you have sex for the first time, because nearly any sexual encounter carries the risk of contracting HPV. The vaccine has been shown to be nearly 100 percent effective in protecting against the four strains of HPV (quadrivalent human papillomavirus for types 6, 11, 16, 18), two of which (16 and 18) are risky strains of HPV that cause 70 percent of cervical cancers. For women from ages twenty-six to forty-five, another vaccine is available in Europe and Australia but has not yet received FDA approval in the United States.

For women up to age twenty-six who have already been diagnosed with HPV, doctors are recommending that they still should be vaccinated, because infection with one strain of the virus may not protect against other cancer-causing types of HPV.

The current treatment schedule is three injections over a six-month period. No one is sure yet how long protection will last, but it appears the vaccine remains effective for at least five years. Longer-term studies will be needed to see whether booster shots are necessary.

Cervicitis

Cervicitis is an inflammation of the cervix, usually caused by infection. Half of all women will have it over a lifetime. Cervicitis by itself is not an STI! I include it here because it can be caused by STIs, and you are at a higher risk for it if you have high-risk sexual habits: more than one partner, a high-risk partner, or not using a condom every time that you have sex.

The treatment for cervicitis will depend on what caused it in you. In some women, it's caused by douching, latex condoms, or spermicides. You won't believe what else can cause it: leaving something in there. A forgotten tampon—yes—happens to many people, a lost condom, a forgotten **diaphragm**, or a cervical cap for birth control that gets left behind. If you discover an object yourself, remove it and call your doctor to make sure that you haven't developed an infection.

Chlamydia and Gonorrhea (the Clap)

Chlamydia and **gonorrhea** are the most common STIs in the United States, and they are most common among younger people. The frightening statistics are that 75 percent of women and 50 percent of men infected with chlamydia or gonorrhea have no symptoms. They are "silent" infections.

Some women do get symptoms about three weeks after exposure, but the symptoms can mean many things, so please don't self-diagnose! You might have a smelly or yellow discharge, vaginal irritation, vaginal bleeding after sex, pelvic pain, or painful urination. Men with chlamydia can have burning urination and a painful penis. The good news is, it's easy to find out whether you have an infection, and it's easily treated and cured with antibiotics.

The very bad news: Untreated, chlamydia or gonorrhea can cause scarring and inflammation of the fallopian tubes and ovaries—called pelvic inflammatory disease (PID). PID can cause infertility and chronic pelvic pain and can increase the chance of an **ectopic pregnancy**. (An ectopic pregnancy happens when a fertilized egg cannot reach the uterus, so the pregnancy develops inside the tube or, rarely, in other locations like the **ovary** or abdomen, instead of traveling down the tube and implanting inside the uterus.) Ectopic pregnancy endangers the life of the mother and can require emergency surgery.

Women with chlamydia or gonorrhea are also three to five times more likely to get **HIV** (the virus that causes **AIDs**). We think that's because STIs inflame your tissues, which gives the HIV virus easier access to your bloodstream.

NOTE TO SELF

Penicillin does not treat chlamydia. Don't go to the medicine cabinet, and don't self-diagnose this dangerous infection.

Diagnosis and Treatment of Chlamydia and Gonorrhea

There are several tests that can be used to diagnose chlamydia and gonorrhea. Your doctor may test some cells by swabbing your cervix, or s/he may test your urine. Be aware that a Pap test is not a test for chlamydia or other STIs.

Both conditions are treated with antibiotics. Prompt antibiotic treatment can prevent damage to pelvic organs. However, antibiotic treatment does not reverse any damage to the reproductive organs.

Screening for Chlamydia and Gonorrhea

It's a good idea to be screened for chlamydia and gonorrhea at your annual exam if you are a young woman and you are sexually active, even if you have no symptoms of chlamydia or pelvic inflammatory disease. Older women with a new partner or multiple sex partners should also be screened. And all pregnant women should have a screening test for chlamydia and gonorrhea.

If infected with chlamydia or gonorrhea, women should be rescreened three to four

REAL LIFE INFO: Spermicide Does Not Protect You Against STIs (or Sperm, Either)

Spermicides are gels, creams, suppositories, foams, and sponges that work as contraceptives by destroying sperm. They are appealing because women can buy them over the counter. How well do they work? Not very. About 25 percent of women are pregnant after the first year of use.

The most recent studies have shown that the spermicide nonoxynol-9 (N-9) may actually increase the risk of STIs by irritating the tissues of the vagina and anus. Damaged tissue gives easier access to infections, just as a cut on your hand is more likely to become infected than normal skin. This is especially worrisome with HIV.

N-9 is found in some sexual lubricants, some lubricated condoms, and contraceptive products designed for vaginal use (foams, creams, jellies, films, and suppositories).

What should you do? Use a low-risk condom instead, and make sure you do not use condoms that contain N-9. How can you be sure? Bring your own!

REAL LIFE QUESTION: Am I at risk for STIs?

It all depends on your past, present, and future sex life. You're more likely to be infected if:

- **You or your partner has had sex with more than one person.**
- **You or your partner has had an STI in the past.**
- **You don't use condoms every time you have sex.**

You can lower your risk of getting an STI by:

- **Not having sex until you are in a committed relationship.**
- **Having sex with only one partner—one who has tested negative for STIs.**
- **Using a new latex condom every time you have sex.**

months after antibiotic treatment is done, because reinfection (from a partner who never took the prescribed medicine) is a key risk factor for PID, and because new, resistant bacterial strains are emerging.

Syphilis

Syphilis was a devastating and incurable disease for centuries. Unlike chlamydia and gonorrhea, it has symptoms of sores. It is impossible to diagnose these yourself, as the sores often imitate other conditions, so always head to the doctor's office with sores. Syphilis is treated with antibiotics.

Untreated syphilis leads to organ damage, insanity, and death. Literature is filled with stories of syphilis. In real life there have been millions of cases. In one of the worst chapters of the history of racism, the U.S. Public Health Service and the Tuskegee Institute of Alabama recruited African-American sharecroppers for a study. Three hundred of the men had syphilis. They were not treated—even after a cure was discovered—for the purpose of studying its progression to death. Many of our current laws and practices governing medical research ethics were established to prevent such an outrageous crime from ever recurring.

Syphilis traveled the world, carried by explorers, conquerors, and war. People often named it for its supposed origin, calling it "the French disease," for example. The CDC has another interesting fact about syphilis: among women, it is most common in the twenty to twenty-four age group, but in men it's most common among men thirty-five to thirty-nine years old.

AIDS and HIV

More than a million people in the United States are living with AIDS or HIV (the virus that causes AIDS). This disease attacks the immune system and is one of the most devastating diseases around the world today.

For a long time there were theories—and even conspiracy theories—about where the disease came from. We finally know how it started: from hunting and eating infected chimpanzees. Long ago, chimps ate monkeys that were infected with a similar virus. We don't know how the disease evolved, but when viruses cross species there is often a puzzle involved. In parts of Africa, it's a common practice to hunt and eat chimps, which transmits the HIV virus to humans. It's then transmitted to other humans through sex or contact with body fluids, including blood and semen. It then travels where people travel, up and down highways and air routes.

AIDS is believed to have reached the United States in 1977. Before anything was known about it beyond the symptoms, it was considered first a Haitian disease and then a gay men's disease. It's heartbreaking to look back at this period in American history and to recall the ignorance that surrounded AIDS victims. It's an accident of history that these groups were the first on our continent to be affected. Today 65 percent of women with HIV will get it from sex with a man. Worldwide, 90 percent of new AIDS cases are now passed along in heterosexual sex between a man and a woman. Today, the face of AIDS is all too often that of women and children. Tragically, infected women with HIV/AIDS can pass the virus on to their infants during pregnancy and breastfeeding. Thankfully, transmission is preventable with careful medical care.

Research has shown that HIV is more likely to be passed from men to women than from women to men during sex. Women have a larger area of vulnerable mucous membrane (basically the whole vagina), there is a larger quantity of body fluids (semen) transferred from men to women, and small tears can occur in the vagina and cervix from sex, which allows the virus access to the bloodstream.

NOTE TO SELF

Spermicidal birth control products do not protect you against STIs (they *increase* the chance, especially for HIV), and you have a one in four chance of becoming pregnant. Those are lousy odds. So always pack your own condoms. You can avoid spermicides, and you can be sure that the condom is new (that is, if you don't carry the same ones around for months without using them). There are many condoms in wallets and glove compartments that are older than you are. Bring your own.

A woman is more susceptible to HIV infection if her immune system is compromised as a result of other infections, including other STIs, like chlamydia, or poor nutrition. Some experts believe that young women are more vulnerable because cervical cells of adolescents are more penetrable by the HIV virus. Condoms have been shown to greatly reduce HIV transmission.

Over the last twenty years, the HIV/AIDS epidemic has evolved to become a heterosexually transmitted disease that is raging through developing countries, where health care is scarce. In the United States we're seeing it in younger people. All of humanity will benefit from strategies to prevent transmission. Research is moving rapidly, and many of us may live to see the eradication of this devastating disease, but for now you can protect yourself only by practicing safe sex.

If you already have AIDS or HIV, you will need much more information than this book contains. You will need to be treated by experts. Your doctor should be able to help you to find the best experts in your area.

How can you keep yourself safe from AIDS and HIV? The only absolute guarantee is total abstinence from sex and from anything that brings you in contact with infected blood, such as using drug needles. Like all doctors and mothers, I think abstinence was a great idea a century ago, when most of us got married shortly after puberty. Today, many people get married a decade or more after puberty, which is a very long time to wait, especially in a culture that promotes sex heavily. So have safe sex and only safe sex, whether it is vaginal, oral, or anal. And know your partner well before you have any sex at all.

There Won't Be a Test

I hope that your vagina is no longer a mysterious dark tunnel that you know nothing about. Get to know yours so you can keep it healthy, and pay the same attention to your vagina that you do to other parts of your body. Give it preventive care and have your doctor treat it when it is unhealthy. Above all, never let embarrassment, shyness, or anxiety—with sexual partners or with doctors—get in the way of your health and happiness.

Two small but powerful organs are a big part of your sexual health. Now that we've looked inside the vagina, in the next chapter we'll travel through the fallopian tubes and learn more about those important little ovaries.

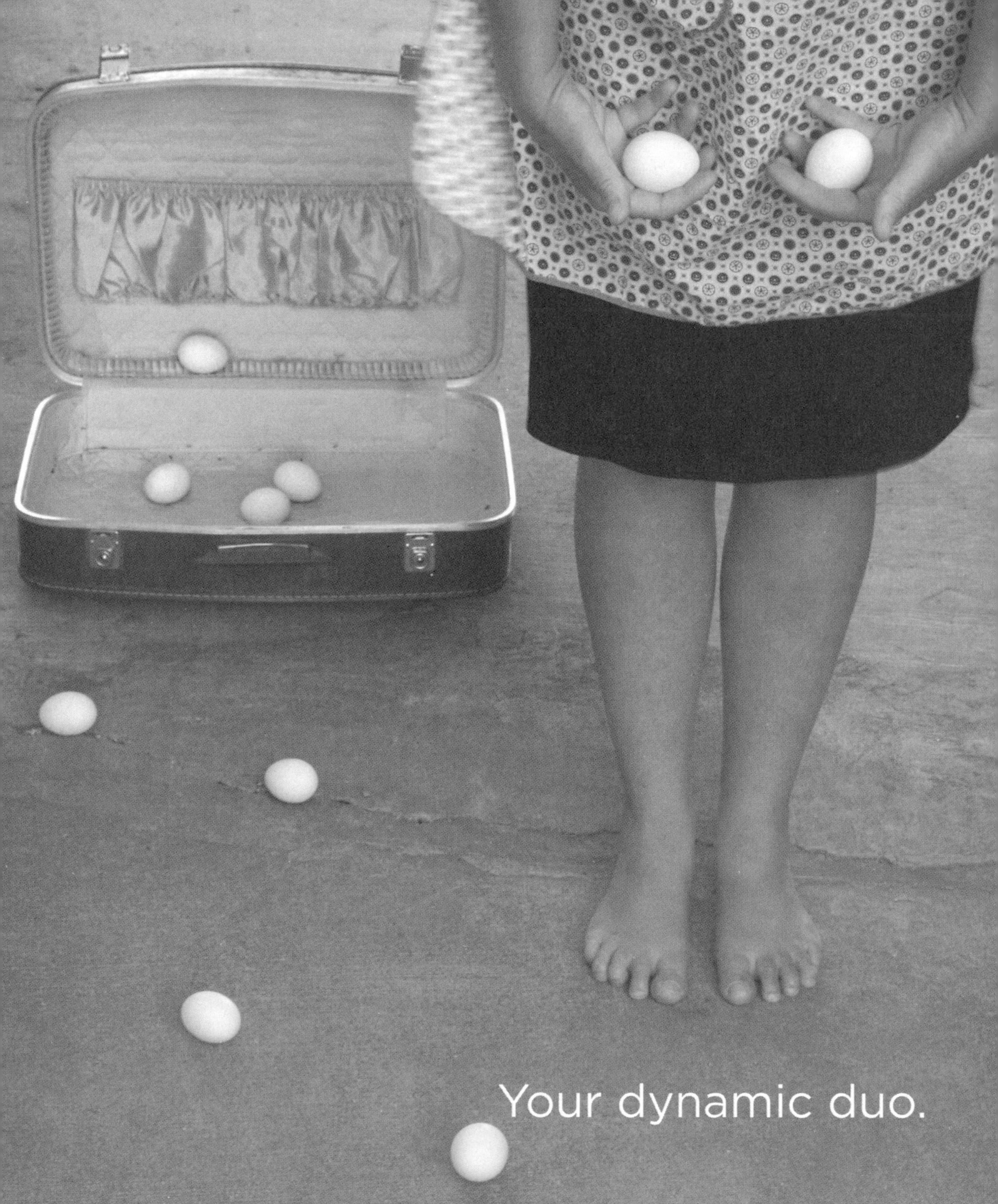
Your dynamic duo.

your ovaries

Your ovaries are small organs, the size of plums, buried deep in your **pelvis**. But don't be fooled by their size—they are powerful hormone factories and removing them can have major health effects.

Ovaries produce **estrogen** on a signal from your pituitary **gland**. You need estrogen for pregnancy, for strong and healthy bones, for blood vessels free of **plaque** buildup, and for a nicely lubricated and elastic **vagina**. Estrogen also works closely with **progesterone**—another hormonal product of your ovaries—to prepare your **uterus** every month for the implanting of a fertilized egg. But before we get too deeply into what ovaries do (**ovulation**), let's take a closer look at the fertility functions of these energetic little hormone powerhouses.

Ovaries, Hormones, and Fertility

Your ovaries lie on either side of your uterus. They hold all of your eggs, each of which could become a baby when fertilized by sperm. Women generally ovulate about once a month. We don't know for sure, but I think we have two ovaries to help us reproduce—if one fails, the other can take over. Just like the **kidneys**. Ovaries actually take turns each month, with one on duty and one off.

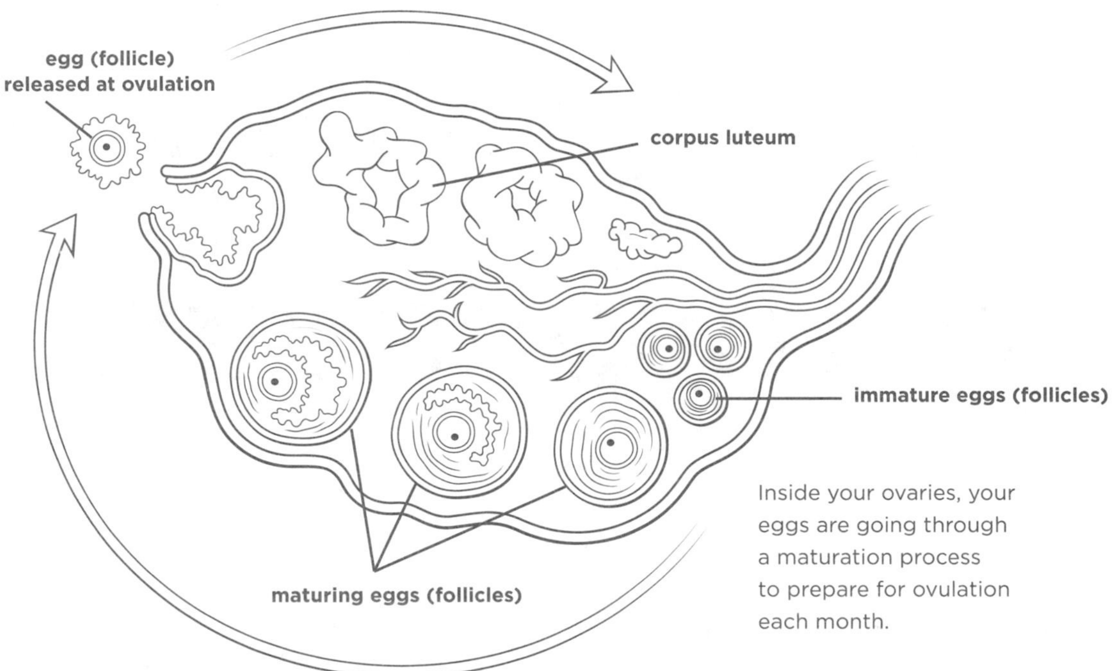

Inside your ovaries, your eggs are going through a maturation process to prepare for ovulation each month.

Every month during your menstrual cycle, a group of eggs starts to develop. Each egg is carried around inside a **follicle**, which is a tiny bag filled with liquid. Eventually one gets ahead of its neighbors in size and becomes the dominant follicle that gets to release its egg.The other, smaller eggs that never make it to ovulation dissolve. The egg travels from the **ovary** through the **fallopian tube** to the uterus. If it's not fertilized, the egg disintegrates. If it is, it will plant itself in the lining of the uterus and start to grow there.

As you go through the menstrual cycle, the ovaries produce different amounts of estrogen, progesterone, and **androgens** (male hormones) at specific times. You can't see them, hear them, or smell them, but your hormones are the managers of your reproductive system. Estrogen levels are generally higher in the first half of your menstrual cycle, and progesterone levels are higher after ovulation. Besides estrogen and progesterone, your ovaries also produce a small amount of testosterone (an androgen), throughout your cycle.

NOTE TO SELF

If you think you don't have any male hormones, think again!

REAL LIFE INFO: Do I have *all* the eggs I'm ever going to have?

That's what we've believed for years. But when researchers at Massachusetts General Hospital discovered that mice continue to make new eggs, the news stunned the research world, which has worked for so long under the assumption that eggs are created and then deteriorate. The questions researchers are asking now is whether all mammals have this capability or just mice, and does it mean that humans can make new eggs?

Why does it matter? Right now we know that as you and your eggs age, it becomes more likely that you'll be infertile or that your baby could have birth defects. If it's possible for mammals to make new eggs, could women somehow grow new eggs too? The discovery will likely have an impact on fertility treatments, but we won't know the answer for decades.

Each of these three hormones has a different function in fertility and pregnancy. Estrogen thickens the lining of your uterus, the **endometrium**, to prepare it for a fertilized egg to implant, creating a nine-month home for the growing baby. (**Menopause** means that your ovaries stop producing estrogen.)

Progesterone springs into action after ovulation. It makes sure that the uterine lining feeds the fertilized egg when it plants itself in the uterus. If fertilization doesn't happen, progesterone then becomes an antiestrogen—it cancels out the estrogen and causes your period, when your uterus sheds your endometrium. As you can imagine, without progesterone, your uterine lining could build up and become very thick, maybe even precancerous.

Testosterone is thought of as a male hormone, but women normally have it in their bodies too. Most of the testosterone gets converted by **enzymes** in your ovaries into estrogen, but a small amount of **testosterone** makes its way into your body. Testosterone in women is thought to be involved in your sex drive. In men, testosterone helps to regulate fertility, sex drive, and muscle mass.

NOTE TO SELF

Sperm can live in your body for five days! So it's important to know when you are ovulating if you are trying to get pregnant—or avoid it.

Ovulation

Most women ovulate—release an egg—about halfway through their menstrual cycle. If you have a twenty-eight-day cycle, then ovulation occurs around day fourteen. This can vary, though, from about day ten to day twenty of your cycle.

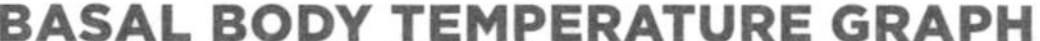

BASAL BODY TEMPERATURE GRAPH

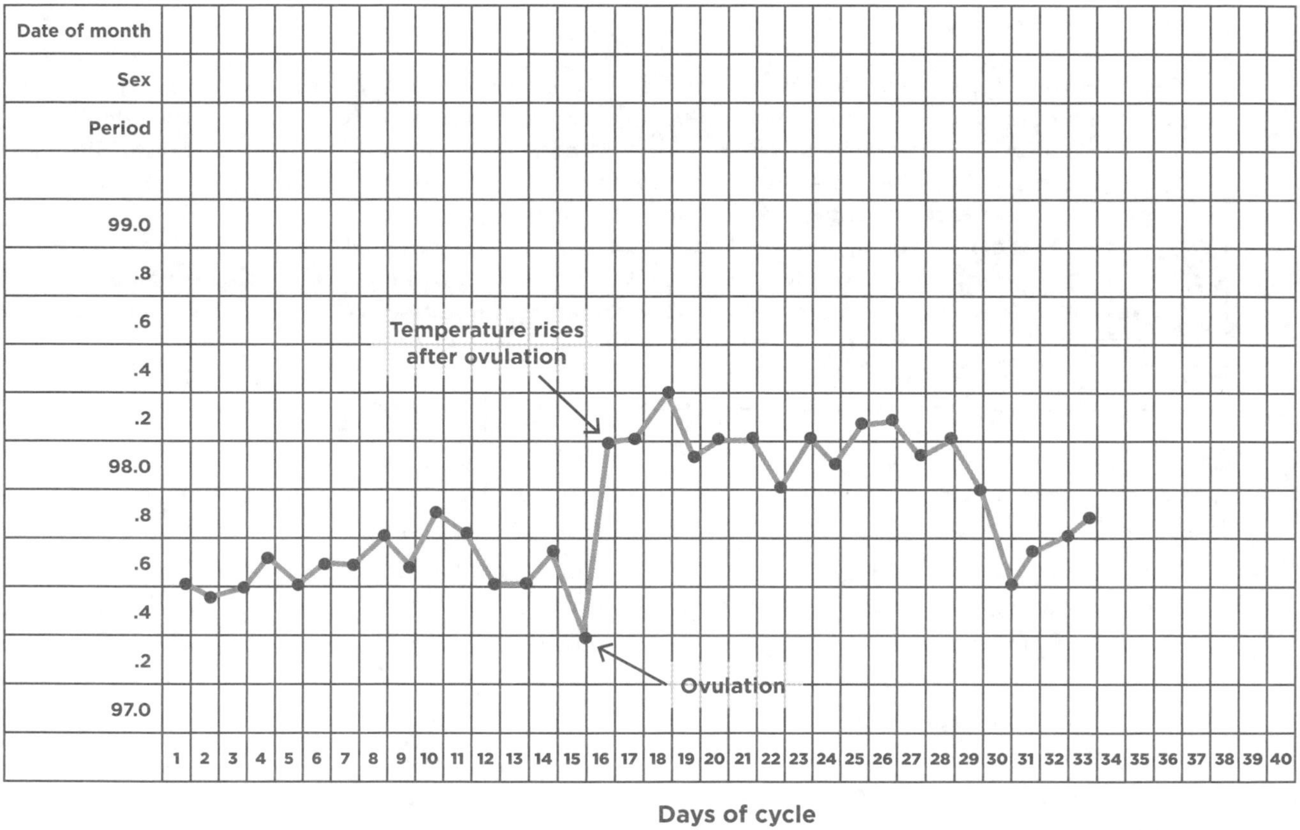

Basal body temperature: Your temperature rises just after you ovulate. Tracking this each month can give you an idea of when you are fertile, whether you are trying to become pregnant or avoid pregnancy.

When you ovulate, you are fertile for about twenty-four hours. The sperm can live in your body for about four or five days, so there is a five-day window of fertility each month. Whether you are trying to become pregnant or avoid pregnancy, it is important to know when you are ovulating. This isn't mysterious: your body sends you signals each month, so all you have to do is learn how to read them!

I go over some of these signals in detail in chapter 15, Your Reproductive System, so I'll only give you some simple reminders and new tips here. Just remember that none of these tips are meant to be used as birth control methods. Monique's father liked to say that he and Monique's mother "had the natural method completely mastered . . . right after our eighth child was born."

Basal Body Temperature

Record your temperature every day before you get out of bed or drink anything. Over time, charting your temperature will show you a pattern of temperature increases and decreases that will show you your ovulation pattern.

Cervical Mucus Monitoring

It's normal to have mucous discharge in your vagina. The color and consistency of this **mucus** changes with the hormones of your menstrual cycle, and these changes can be used to help determine where you are in your cycle.

To monitor cervical mucus, use your thumb and index finger and reach into your vagina to get some on your fingers. Yes, seriously. Then stretch it between your thumb and index finger to test for the consistency and look at the color. Before ovulation, in the first few days following menstruation, you'll have little or no discharge. As you approach ovulation, larger amounts of a white, creamy discharge appear. When you examine it, the mucus should break easily, before your finger and thumb are about a quarter of an inch apart. As your cycle goes on, there will be more mucus, and right around ovulation, the mucus turns clear and sticky and resembles egg whites. It is the thinnest, clearest, and most abundant at this point in the cycle. This egg-white mucus is very stretchy. You can usually spread your finger and thumb somewhere between half an inch and an inch apart before the mucus breaks. After ovulation, there is a big change in the mucus. It returns to the sticky white stage and doesn't stretch as much, and there is again a feeling of dryness around the **vulva**.

Most women I've talked to are not too excited about this method, but try it anyway. The mucus easily washes off.

Pain in the Ovary

About one in five women experience pain during ovulation, also known as mittelschmerz, a German word that translates as "middle pain." Typically, the pain is deep in your pelvis, just below your hipbone, and usually happens about two weeks before your period. It may feel like a cramp, twinge, sharp pain, dull ache, or uncomfortable pressure feeling. It will be off to one side in your lower pelvis, depending on which ovary is releasing an egg that month.

The expanding egg stretching the outer covering of the ovary may be what causes ovulation pain. The duration of the pain varies from a few minutes to forty-eight hours. In most cases, ovulation pain doesn't mean that anything is wrong and is a helpful fertility alarm bell.

What Can Go Wrong: Ovarian Cysts

Ovarian cysts are fluid-filled sacs (like little bags) that form on your ovaries. In some cases, ovarian cysts can be quite harmless—and actually play an important role in ovulation. In other cases, they can be painful and even dangerous.

Cyst Symptoms

The most common symptom of ovarian cysts is pain. Usually, the pain is low in the pelvis on one side. Sometimes the pain comes on rather suddenly and then stays as a constant and low, dull ache. Other times it's a crampy pain that comes and goes. Sometimes pain from cysts is felt only during sex. And sometimes a cyst causes pressure or fullness in the abdomen. Ovarian cyst pain is not brought on by eating, and pain that is made better or worse with eating is more likely to be about your digestive system than your ovaries.

Many ovarian cysts are asymptomatic (causing no symptoms) and are found during a routine pelvic exam. However, they can rupture unexpectedly, either through sex, during a pelvic exam, or just because they grow large enough and, like a balloon filled with too much air, the cyst wall gives way. When this happens, often the pain comes on suddenly and is severe. If a cyst becomes twisted, you may experience spasmodic pain that is very intense but comes and goes. Often, during the twisting, you have both pain and nausea. If it bursts, the fluid it releases can irritate the abdomen and is painful. If you have these symptoms, call your doctor immediately. Please don't try to diagnose yourself.

Cyst Diagnosis

Ultrasound is ideal for looking at ovarian cysts, and in most situations is better than a CT scan or MRI imaging. An ultrasound uses sound waves to create images of the body. It can be used to confirm a cyst's presence and may determine what type of cyst it appears to be. An ultrasound can also show the size and location of a cyst and tell us whether it appears to be **benign** or harmful.

Sometimes ultrasound is done through your abdomen, in which case you will need to have a full **bladder** during the test, as this allows the picture to be clearer. You will drink a lot of water and really need to pee, but the technician will beg you to wait. You'll be able to hold it, but will run for the bathroom when the test is over.

Or, depending on the location of your ovaries and the cyst, a vaginal probe ultrasound may be done. This is a small probe that is covered by a **condom** and inserted gently into your vagina. Because the ovaries often lie just above your vagina, it can be the better view. It's about as uncomfortable as a pelvic examination, but lasts longer. Many women prefer having the vaginal probe over having to hold a full bladder. Other women can't stand the probe!

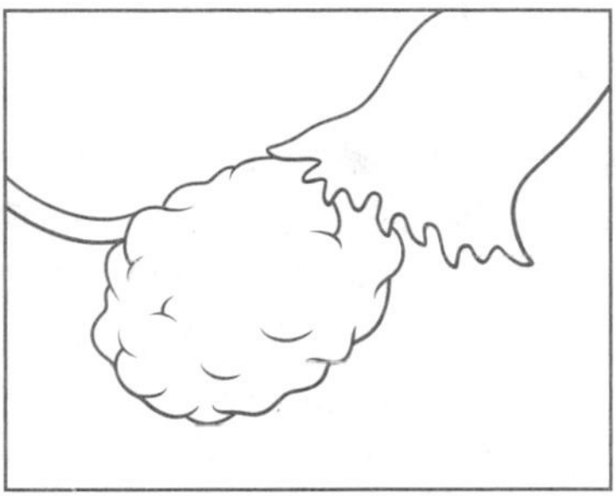

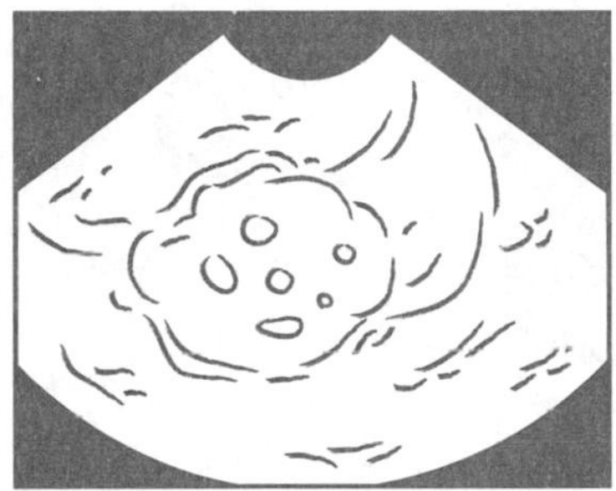

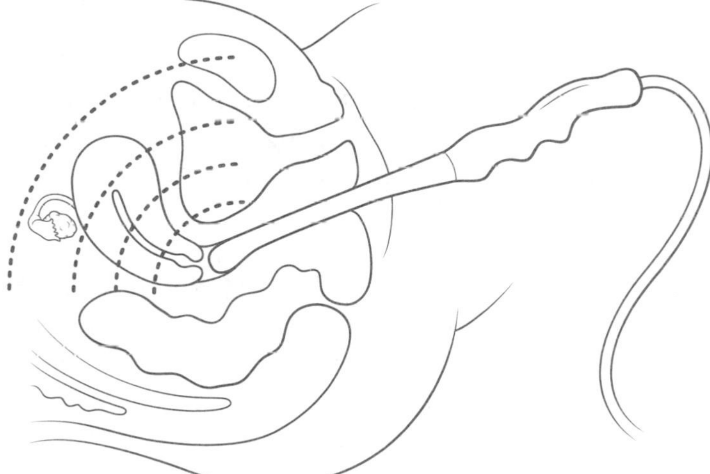

Ultrasound is ideal for looking at ovarian cysts (above right). A vaginal ultrasound (left) is a small probe covered by a condom that is inserted into the vagina to see the ovaries (above left) more clearly.

Are All Cysts the Same?

Ovarian cysts fall into two categories: cysts that are part of the normal functioning of your ovaries and cysts that may cause problems. We ought to have a different name for the functional cysts so they wouldn't cause so much worry! Let's start with these.

We all have two types of functional cysts. They each have a job, they arrive every month, and then they leave.

- **Follicular:** Your eggs are in little follicle bags. Guess what each egg looks like on an ultrasound? A cyst. If this **follicular** cyst doesn't break open to release the egg, it may continue growing and then disappear after one to three months.
- **Corpus luteum:** After ovulation, in the space where the egg used to be, a small cystic area develops and produces the hormone progesterone. It's called the

corpus luteum. It lasts about two weeks and then dissolves. This type of cyst is also normal.

On to the second category. These three types of cysts can cause problems.

- **Endometriomas**: These cysts develop in women who have **endometriosis**, a condition in which tissue identical to the lining of the uterus grows outside of the uterus (where it doesn't belong), such as on the ovary. The tissue may attach to the ovary and form a cyst filled with blood. The old blood turns dark brown and looks exactly like chocolate sauce. That is why these cysts are also known as chocolate cysts. They can be painful during sex and during your period, and sometimes they can even cause pain every day.

- **Cystadenomas:** These benign cysts develop from cells on the outer surface of the ovary. There are two types of cystadenomas—serous and mucinous. Serous cystadenomas are filled with a thin watery fluid and can grow to be from two to six inches in diameter. Mucinous cystadenomas are filled with a sticky, thick gelatinous material and grow to be, typically, anywhere from six to twelve inches in diameter. There have been rare cases of neglected cysts measuring forty inches across and weighing over one hundred pounds.

- **Dermoid cysts:** These strange cysts develop from the ovary's germ cells—the cells that become the egg and the beginnings of all human tissues. They are therefore able to make many body tissues. The cysts are filled with sebaceous, oily material, and may contain hair, teeth, and other tissues. They can grow to be very large and cause pain.

Treatment of Cysts

Treatment of ovarian cysts depends on many things, including the type of cyst, its size and location, the type of material it contains, whether you have pain, and your age. For functional cysts, we might wait and watch. Functional cysts tend to dissolve over time as the menstrual cycle progresses, and treatment is usually not needed. Most women are asked to return after about two menstrual cycles for a follow-up ultrasound, to make sure the functional cysts have resolved. If the cyst is still present, your doctor may recommend that it be removed surgically. Occasionally, functional cysts (follicular or corpus luteum) can bleed or cause the ovary to twist, and in these cases sometimes surgical removal is necessary.

Women who frequently develop ovarian cysts can consider going on birth control pills. The Pill can reduce the number of functional cysts your ovaries make because it prevents ovulation and the subsequent formation of follicular or corpus luteum cysts. The Pill won't help a cyst you already have to go away more quickly, but it will prevent future cysts.

For endometrial cysts, cystadenomas, and dermoid cysts, the treatment is usually to remove the cyst surgically, unless it is very small and you and your doctor decide to follow it closely with ultrasound. These cysts are all benign. Most of these cysts can be removed laparoscopically (see sidebar), so that the incisions are tiny and your recovery is shorter.

In most cases a cystectomy is done, which removes just the cyst and leaves the ovary behind. Sometimes a piece of your ovary must be removed, and in rare cases the whole ovary is taken out. If this happens, as long as you still have your other ovary, you will still be fertile. The other ovary somehow knows that it is now alone, and it will ovulate every month instead of every other month.

If cysts are large, if they appear cancerous, if they rupture and you need emergency surgery, or if you live in a place where laparoscopy is not readily available, you may need a laparotomy. Laparotomy is the more traditional approach to surgery, in which an incision is made in your lower abdomen—usually a horizontal "bikini" incision just where your pubic hair begins—and the cyst is removed.

Polycystic Ovary Syndrome

Polycystic ovary syndrome (PCOS) is a complex syndrome of irregular periods and hormonal imbalances. Women with PCOS have ovaries that produce higher than normal amounts of androgens, which can interfere with ovulation. This causes irregular periods.

In each cycle several eggs begin to develop in women with PCOS, just as in normal women. However, with PCOS, often a dominant follicle does not emerge, and ovulation doesn't always happen. So instead of being released during ovulation, the eggs build up as small cysts that don't quite make it to ovulation, remaining in the ovary in a state of arrested development. Eventually, after several cycles

REAL LIFE QUESTION: What is laparoscopy?

Laparoscopy is a minimally invasive surgery done under general anesthesia. For ovarian cysts, a very small cut is made below or inside your belly button, and a small instrument that looks like a tiny telescope is inserted through the cut into your abdomen. The telescope has a camera attached, and the surgeons watch the operation on a video monitor to guide them while they work. A second or third tiny incision may be made above your pubic bone and on your lower abdomen on the side opposite the cyst. Through these ports, your doctor will insert long slender instruments to operate on the cyst—scissors, dissecting instruments, and electrocautery instruments (which use heat to remove tissue and stop bleeding). Today, more and more operations are being performed this way, because it causes less scarring and takes less recovery time.

that don't end in ovulation, the ovaries may become enlarged with these undeveloped eggs. Because ovulation doesn't happen regularly, women with PCOS have irregular periods. In severe cases, there are no periods at all.

Although PCOS has been known since the 1930s, we still don't know exactly what causes it. PCOS can run in families, so there appears to be a genetic component. Recent research has found that altered **insulin** production and insulin sensitivity in the body is part of the syndrome. Women with PCOS may produce too much insulin, which signals their ovaries to release extra male hormones.

Despite the large amounts of insulin in their system, women with PCOS are resistant to the effects of insulin, which can often result in **diabetes** during pregnancy or later in life, especially in women who are overweight.

Being overweight seems to worsen the symptoms of PCOS. Untreated, PCOS can lead to infertility, excessive hair growth, acne, diabetes, **heart disease**, abnormal bleeding from the uterus, and endometrial **cancer**. The good news is that, although there's no cure for PCOS, it can be treated. The most important step is diagnosing the condition, because when you get treatment for PCOS, your chances of having serious side effects are reduced.

NOTE TO SELF

PCOS is the mystery disease that can explain period difficulties, extra weight, acne, and unwanted hair.

Symptoms of PCOS

Women with irregular or no periods should be evaluated for PCOS. Signs and symptoms may include:

- Irregular periods (or no periods)
- Abdominal discomfort
- Very heavy periods
- Weight gain, obesity, or difficulty maintaining a normal weight
- Increased hair growth on your face, chest, abdomen, nipple area, or back (a little hair in these places is normal)
- Thinning hair on the head (alopecia)
- Acne and clogged pores
- Darkened, thickened skin around the neck, armpits, or breasts

How Is Polycystic Ovary Syndrome Diagnosed?

Your doctor will ask you some questions about your menstrual cycle and perform a physical examination to look for signs of PCOS. Blood tests will then be done, which may include **thyroid**, insulin, and other hormone tests. An ultrasound may be done to look at your ovaries and to determine if you have cysts or other abnormalities. Because cysts are not always visible, though, this test is not always helpful.

Treatments for PCOS

Although there's no cure for PCOS, the condition can be treated and managed.

If you are overweight, it's important to try to regain a healthy weight. Weight loss can be very effective in lessening many of the health conditions associated with PCOS, such as diabetes. Sometimes weight loss alone can restore hormone levels to normal, causing many of the symptoms to disappear or become less severe. Exercise is a great way to help fight the weight gain that often accompanies PCOS.

The Pill is another excellent treatment for PCOS. The estrogen in the Pill helps to reduce the male hormone levels in your body to a normal range and to regulate your menstrual cycle. Birth control pills may also help control acne and excessive hair growth.

Other medications used to treat PCOS include antiandrogens, which reduce the effects of excess androgen and can help clear up skin and hair growth problems. Another medication, metformin, which is commonly used to treat diabetes, can lower insulin levels. It's especially helpful for women with diabetes or women who are trying to get pregnant.

Although the medications used to treat PCOS will slow down or stop excessive hair growth for many women, they won't get rid of hair that has already developed. There are lots of different types of products available to help get rid of hair where you don't want it. Depilatory creams can remove facial hair on the upper lip or chin. Tweezing, waxing, threading, and pumice treatments are other methods you can use at home or have done professionally to manage hair growth. Electrolysis and laser surgery can remove unwanted hair permanently, although they are more expensive. Current laser treatments are unlikely to remove fair hair.

If you have severe acne as a symptom of PCOS, it may improve with the medications that help PCOS. If it doesn't, a dermatologist may also be able to recommend medications to help. (Also see chapter 4, Your Skin.)

Ovarian Cancer: The Silent Killer

Ovarian cancer is the eighth most common cancer in women and the fifth leading cause of death from cancer. It occurs when cells in the ovary grow in an uncontrolled, abnormal way and produce tumors in one or both ovaries. It usually occurs in women in their sixties, and is rare—but not unknown—in young women. President Obama's mother, S. Ann Soetoro, died of ovarian cancer at age fifty-two, and Gilda Radner, a comedienne who was a member of the original *Saturday Night Live* cast, died at age forty-two.

Ovarian cancer has a fatality rate higher than 70 percent, mainly because the disease is usually not diagnosed until it is in an advanced stage. Your chances of surviving ovarian cancer are better if the cancer is found early. But the disease is difficult to detect in its early stage, and only about 29 percent of ovarian cancers are found before tumor growth has spread into tissues and organs beyond the ovaries. In most cases the disease has already advanced before it's diagnosed.

REAL LIFE FACT: The Pill Reduces Ovarian Cancer Risk

Despite the rumors, taking the Pill may actually help prevent ovarian cancer. The number of times you ovulate in your lifetime is a major risk factor for ovarian cancer—the lower the number, the better. Because the Pill stops ovulation, it lowers the number and decreases ovarian cancer risk. Protection can last for up to thirty years after stopping the Pill, and protection increases with each year of use. Ten years of using the Pill reduces the risk of ovarian cancer by up to 80 percent.

There are several types of ovarian cancer. The most common type, epithelial carcinoma, begins on the surface of the ovaries. Germ cell tumors, another type, begin in the egg-producing cells of the ovary. And stromal tumors, a third type, are found in the supportive tissue surrounding the ovary.

Ovarian Cancer Risks

Usually, the more times a woman ovulates in her lifetime, the higher her risk of developing ovarian cancer. Women who have never had children are more likely to develop ovarian cancer than women who have had children. In fact, the more children a woman has had, the less likely she is to develop ovarian cancer.

A woman's chance of having ovarian cancer also increases if she has one or more close relatives (mother, daughter, or sister) with the disease. Rarely, women may inherit genes that increase the risk for ovarian cancer substantially. And women with a history of breast, endometrial, or **colon** cancer also have a greater chance of developing ovarian cancer than women who have not had these cancers.

Other factors decrease a woman's risk of getting ovarian cancer, including childbearing, the use of oral contraceptives, and having a **tubal ligation** or **hysterectomy**.

Symptoms of Ovarian Cancer

Until recently, doctors thought that early-stage ovarian cancer rarely produced any symptoms. But new evidence has shown that many women do have signs and symptoms before the disease has spread. Being aware of them may lead to earlier detection. Symptoms tend to be nonspecific, and include **gastrointestinal** discomfort, pressure in the pelvic area, frequent urination, lack of energy, and swelling or bloating of the abdomen. These symptoms, particularly when they're new, happen almost daily. If you feel them and they are severe, call to see your doctor and ask for an appointment very soon. If you have a mass, or lump, the doctor will give you a pelvic exam and a rectal exam, because they work best together. An ultrasound can also help with the diagnosis.

The symptoms of ovarian cancer tend to act like other conditions, including digestive problems. It's not unusual for a woman with ovarian cancer to be diagnosed with another condition before finally learning she has cancer. Look at the list of symptoms in the sidebar. A woman might be pregnant or have painful gas and have the same symptoms!

The difference seems to be persistent or worsening signs and symptoms. With a digestive disorder, symptoms tend to come and go, or they occur in certain situations or after eating certain foods. With ovarian cancer, there's typically little change—signs and symptoms are constant and will gradually worsen.

Remember that the sooner ovarian cancer is found and treated, the better the chance for recovery. Don't use your time diagnosing yourself, but call the doctor instead. If the doctor is not available, ask to see a nurse, who will speed things up for you if s/he suspects cancer.

Screening for Ovarian Cancer

Aren't there any early screening tests? Unfortunately, no. First, ovarian cancer doesn't seem to have a long precancerous stage (as in cervical cancer, for instance) that would give us a chance to diagnose the cancer early. With ovarian cancer, you can have an ultrasound showing perfectly normal ovaries one month and an ultrasound showing ovarian cancer the next month.

You may have heard some excitement about using a CA125 tumor marker to detect ovarian cancer. A tumor marker is a substance made by a tumor that can be used in tumor detection through blood testing. If a particular substance increases in your blood, your doctor knows something is brewing. Serum CA125 has been the tumor marker most extensively studied in ovarian cancer.

At first, studies of CA125 seemed promising when it was found that more than 80 percent of ovarian cancer patients had elevated levels of CA125. The problem is that other benign conditions, including fibroids,

REAL LIFE FACT: The Subtle Early Symptoms of Ovarian Cancer

- **Bloating**
- **Pain in your abdomen or pelvis**
- **Stomachache, meaning that you don't feel like eating or just can't eat**
- **Having to pee more often or more urgently**
- **Lower energy level**

REAL LIFE INFO: Can I really sell my eggs?

Yes. Take a quick look on the Internet and you'll see this topic everywhere. Fertility clinics recruit women, typically between the ages of twenty and thirty, and pay them for egg donations. And researchers are doing the same thing in some labs, but the practice has been banned in many places after a 2005 scandal in South Korea in which employees were used for egg donation in a project that was plagued with ethical and scientific flaws.

This issue has actually united pro-choice and pro-life activists because both groups want more regulation, especially rules that prohibit the abuse of low-income women who haven't been given thorough education about the issue.

Should you donate your eggs? It's your decision, but before you make it, insist on being given a thorough training about the risks. They are real. The process involves hormone shots and surgery—and neither one should be taken lightly.

endometriosis, pregnancy, and just having your period can also elevate CA125. As a result of this research, ovarian cancer began to be overdiagnosed and many women had unnecessary surgery.

Unfortunately, overall death rates did not differ much between screened and unscreened women, because levels of CA125 often do not increase until women have advanced-stage disease. And the diagnosis was missed in 50 percent of patients with stage I ovarian cancer because they turned out to have normal CA125 levels.

CA125 does not appear to be the answer. The one piece of good news is that CA125 has turned out to be useful for women already diagnosed with ovarian cancer and even breast cancer. Over time, it can show a pattern that the disease is decreasing or increasing. It can help to make decisions about chemotherapy. For example, if the tumor marker remains the same for months of one type of chemo then suddenly rises, it might be time to switch to another treatment.

Today, the only way to reliably diagnose ovarian cancer is with surgery to examine the ovary, **biopsy** any suspicious lumps, and remove the cancer. Women at high risk for ovarian cancer may also be offered prophylactic oophorectomy (removal of both ovaries to prevent cancer) if they don't plan to have children. It's the only method that we know of to reduce the rate of death.

Transvaginal sonography (ultrasound done with a vaginal probe) plus regular CA125 testing is another way for women who decline oophorectomy to be screened, but this combination is still unreliable. Women at high risk for ovarian cancer due to family history (those with two or more first-degree relatives with ovarian cancer or premenopausal breast cancer) and women of certain hereditary backgrounds (such as Ashkenazi Jews) with only one affected family member should also be offered genetic testing and ovarian cancer screening.

In some preliminary studies, a new technology called **DNA microarray** is being tried as a method of screening. How does it work? Imagine that you have to study each individual runner in a marathon race in which thousands and thousands of people are running over a long distance. How difficult would it be to stand at the finish line and interview each one of thousands of people? Today, that's how biology studies your genes: one at a time.

With the microarray technology, we could watch the whole marathon and study all of the runners at the same time. We could see every complex action and interaction that takes place. Let's say it starts to rain, which makes the road slippery and causes the first runner to fall. That makes others trip and fall, too. Everything has an impact on everything else and we would see all of it at once. If we could study your genes all at once, someday we might be able to see a tiny change in one gene that is found in most women with early stage ovarian cancer. That would give us a method of early detection. And then maybe we would discover that the first gene was changed by a second gene having been exposed to an environmental factor. That would give us a hint at prevention. We're a long way from answers, but microarray technology does give us hope.

Even though good routine screening tools are not currently available, if we can work with patients to recognize the pattern of symptoms, we can help to diagnose it early.

Your Ovaries: The Source of Life

The ovaries are vitally important organs that hold the genetic material for future generations. Take comfort in knowing that ovarian cancer is a relatively rare disease, especially in young women.

Ovaries are your source of fertility. You may be at the age when you're about to use your ovaries to start a family, or you may be trying to avoid pregnancy. Either way, it's helpful to learn as much as possible about birth control and family planning—a complex, exciting, and sometimes exasperating subject, and the focus of the next chapter.

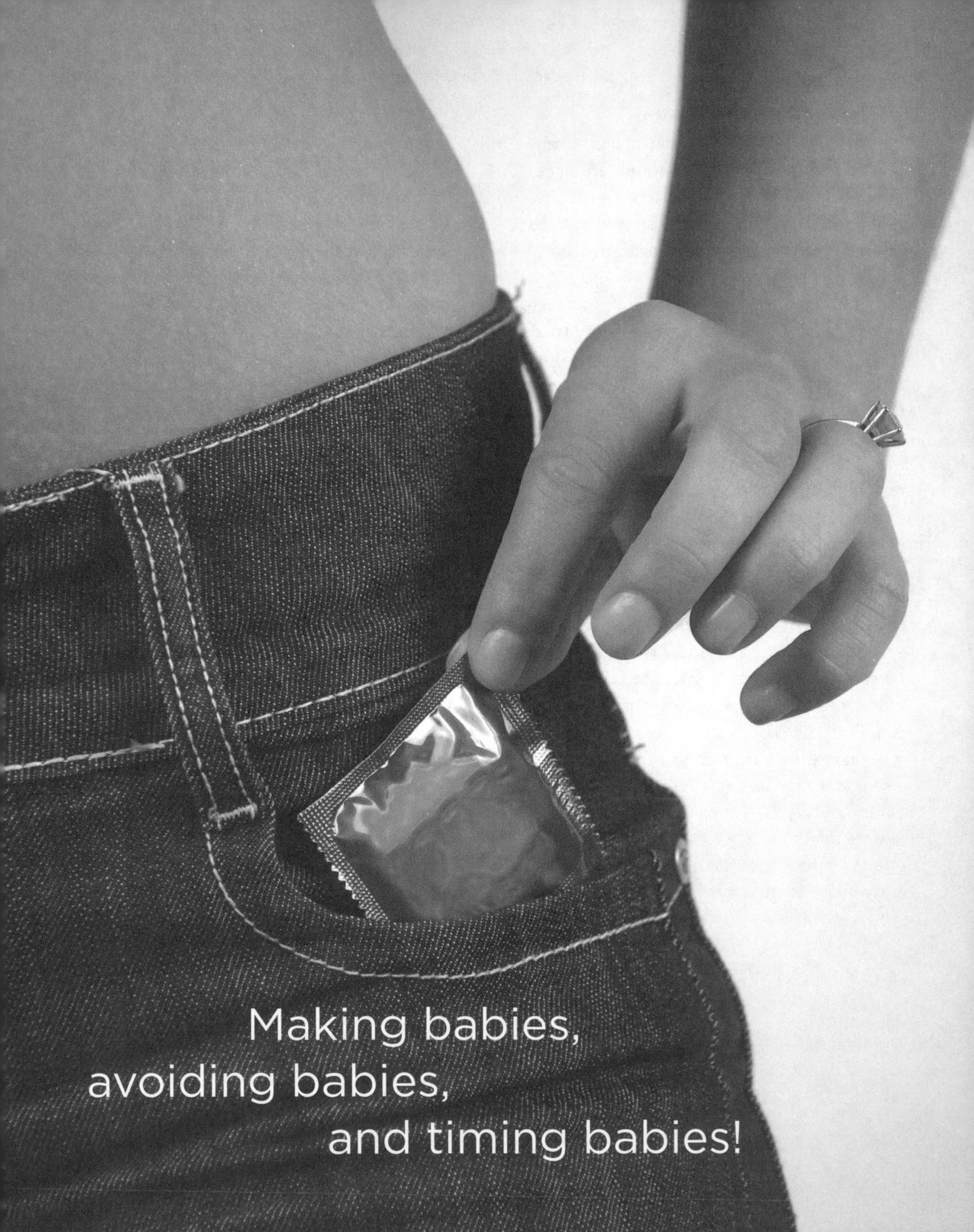
Making babies,
avoiding babies,
and timing babies!

your reproductive system

What do all of these things have in common: sex on a first date, the Pill,

legal abortion, and fertility treatments? They're all things that didn't happen or weren't available when your grandma, and maybe even your mom, was your age.

Having sex on the first date was a teenager's secret fantasy and a parent's nightmare, because the Pill wasn't released until the 1960s and abortion wasn't legal in most states until 1973. Nobody even imagined that we'd need fertility treatments, probably because nobody could imagine wanting more children. When your grandparents were young, children came like clockwork after you got married and had no method of birth control except the rhythm method, **diaphragms**, and **condoms** as thick as your arm. Having a large family is wonderful if you choose it and are prepared for it, but when nature forces it on you, it's a different happy ending.

So the women who lived in those times say you have nothing to complain about because compared to their lives, yours is so easy. To them, we live in a magical world of medicine in which everything about pregnancy is a choice.

But . . . it isn't. Unplanned pregnancies still happen. And couples still struggle with infertility. For all of our miracle treatments and tests, your fertility system still depends on you. You've heard it a few times in this book: healthy life, healthy body. Your reproductive system is like a big theme park—a fun place, but it needs tons of maintenance.

What Is Your Reproductive System?

Okay, okay, I can already hear many of you objecting to the term *reproductive system*. If you are getting older, you might refer to it as your nonreproductive system. If you are still young, you might call it your Dear-God-please-don't-let-me-reproduce-right-now system. And if you don't even think about reproduction, you might just call it your toy box!

Simply put, this is an incredibly complex system that has only a few visible signs other than pregnancies and, eventually, **menopause**. You may have PMS or PMDD (see page 48) and you have your period. Some women feel their egg burst from the **follicle** during **ovulation**, which is called mittelschmerz. (One of my patients calls that moment the Ethel Mertz.) And that's about it for noticeable signs. But there's a whole lot of stuff going on down there! So let's get to it.

Menstruation: My Friend, Aunt Flo, *la Regla*

Let's start with an illustration of your reproductive system (see page 319). Are you surprised to see a brain in this picture? Without your brain, none of this works, so let's talk about the connection between the brain and your reproductive system.

Your period is one part of your monthly menstrual cycle. On day one in the brain, the pituitary **gland** makes follicle-stimulating hormone (FSH). Remember that follicles are little bags containing an egg. Each of your two ovaries has zillions of follicles, each containing immature eggs. FSH makes these grow into mature eggs. Normally, just one egg becomes the dominant one each month. We don't know how "she" is selected but I like to think she runs for office. Of the eggs volunteering for the job, she is the dominant candidate.

The eggs release **estrogen**. Among the many other jobs estrogen performs, which you discover only when you start making less and less of it in a few decades, is to cause the lining of the uterus to grow. It's making it ready for a fertilized egg to be planted and nourished.

Back to the pituitary. It gets the message that the egg is ready to be released. It sends out luteinizing hormone (LH), which tells the eggs their winning candidate can go free. The egg bursts from the follicle and heads down the **fallopian tube** to the uterus (ovulation).

Although you may be looking for a good time, the egg is looking for a mate. If the egg meets sperm, it is fertilized and will plant itself in the lining of the uterus (also called the **endometrium**). The egg lives for twenty-four hours, and sperm live for four to five days, so there's a period of up to five days in which you could become pregnant. Now you can see why "counting days" or other rhythm methods don't work too well to pinpoint the window of fertility.

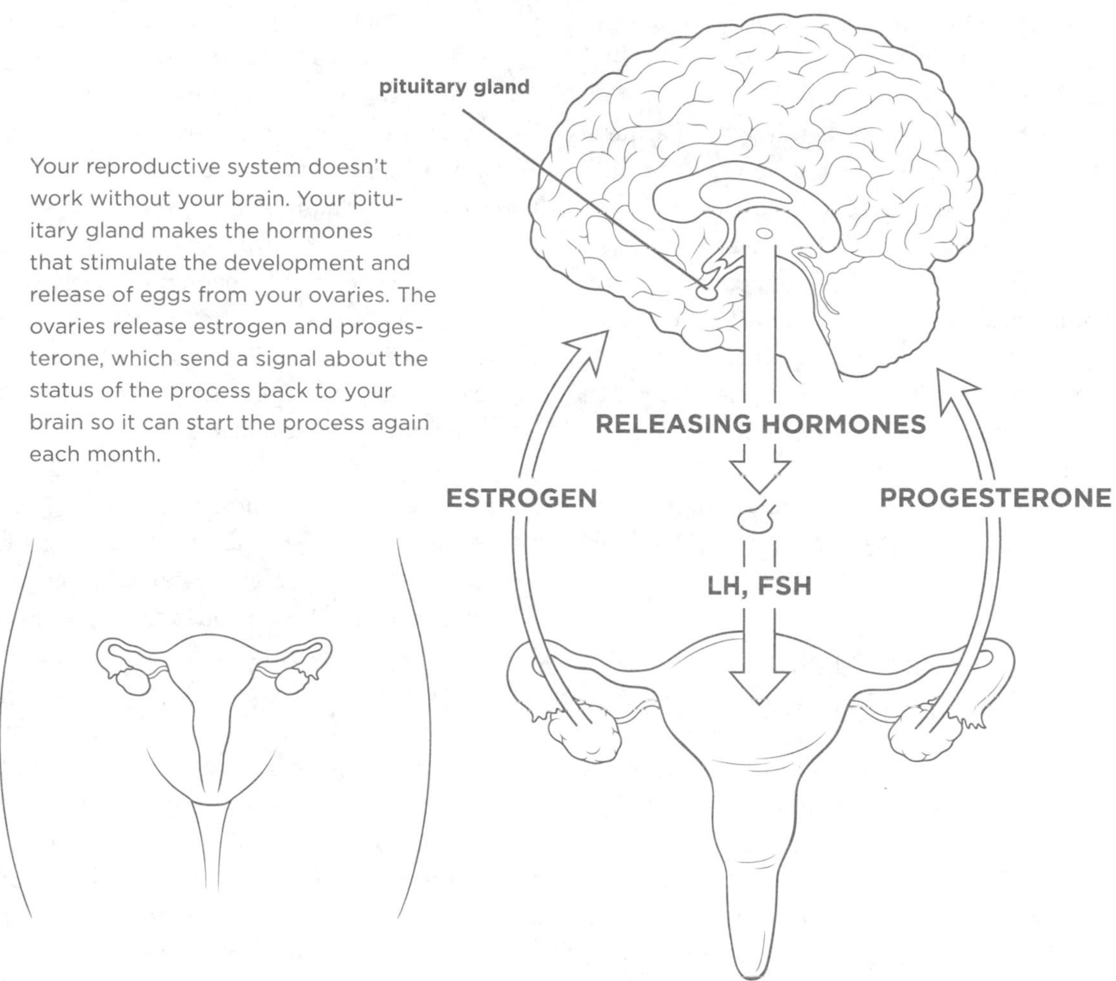

The follicle, having released an egg, is transformed into a cluster of cells. It starts producing **progesterone**, which gets the lining of the **uterus** ready to nurture the egg. It also causes your basal body temperature to go up, which is why we encourage women who are trying to have a baby to take their temperature every morning. That does not make this a reliable birth control method, either. Just ask Grandma, but not in front of Mom. ("Oh, no, dear, we weren't planning another baby, she was a complete shock!"—better left unsaid.)

The follicles wait to see if a fertilized egg is implanted. It usually isn't. So the level of hormones drops and the lining of the uterus starts to break up and flow out through the **vagina**. That's what we call your menstrual period.

Although the average length of a menstrual cycle is twenty-eight days, that's only an average. I see a wide range of normal cycles that are shorter and longer. Anything from twenty-one to thirty-five days is normal. You should ask your doctor if you are concerned.

After a few days or a week or so, your period is over and the new cycle begins. We count the cycle from the first day of your period to the first day of your next period. If your period begins on March 1, then starts again on March 28, you have a twenty-eight-day cycle.

The Best Feminine Hygiene Products

I don't know who invented the term *feminine hygiene*, but I wish it would go away. It makes it sound like women are dirty and we need all those products in the drugstore aisle to keep us clean. Doctors would actually prefer if you avoided all of those products. In our fantasy world, we'd like you to keep your privates covered the old-fashioned way: with a big cotton diaper. Your vagina would breathe a lot better than it can in a tight little pair of satin undies plus panty hose, which both suffocate you. But, because we realize that the cotton diaper won't happen, for you or for me, please just follow a few simple tips.

Always (now there's a little pun) choose a product without deodorant, especially tampons. I know the manufacturers make the products look safe, but deodorants will disrupt the climate of your vagina. It's like inviting a **yeast infection** to come and stay.

If you use tampons, use the smallest one you need for your flow and change it often, sometimes many times a day. Leaving a tampon in for too long can cause a dangerous infection, and leaving one in when you're dry will make it painful to remove. It could give you abrasions along the vaginal wall, which, again, will allow infection to come right in.

It used to be that everyone who could figure them out used tampons. Now that pads are so much improved in length, width, absorbency, and wings (not to mention the adhesive strip, which freed women from sanitary belts—ask Grandma about those!), they are a real option. Try them out when your period is at its lightest and see what you think.

REAL LIFE FACT: A Man's Worst Nightmare

One patient asked her husband to go to the drugstore and buy her some pads. He came back, looking pale, and asked, "Why does your period make you need . . . wings?"

REAL LIFE QUESTION: What's a basal body temperature?

As you chart your daily temperature, we want it to be *basal*, or "the base." This means you take it as soon as you wake up, before you get out of bed, before you drink anything, with no interruptions. If you are a morning sex couple, you'll have to wait a minute.

Many women use a tampon and a pad at night. There's nothing wrong with that, as long as you change them both first thing in the morning.

And by the way, not only can you still buy those cotton diapers for your period—you can also buy reusable cotton tampons, too. A major laundry decision. For other health tips, see chapter 13, Your Vagina and Cervix.

"Family Planning"— Birth Control

Now that you know more about your cycle, you can begin to understand what we call family planning. The term refers to all types of birth control, including temperature taking.

Before the 1960s, before the Pill, women had ingenious ways to prevent unwanted pregnancy. The problem? None of them worked reliably. Women would count the days from when their period began and then guess when ovulation might start—not knowing that sperm can live for four or five days, and an egg lives for a day, so that there are truly five days when you can become pregnant.

Some women used temperature taking to figure out when they were ovulating. We use this method to aid fertility today, but it's not foolproof for contraception. In ancient times, women relied on the moon, or rituals, or herbs. Eventually, as medicine became science based, it failed to include this folk medicine among its tools. Now we know that some of the seeds and herbs used by ancient women gave them some control over fertility. They probably had more control than a sophisticated woman of the eighteenth century. The ancient methods don't work as well as modern methods, but they are still interesting to know about. And by the way, the Pill, ironically, was the result of modern fertility research!

Let's look at the various methods we can use today for family planning, along with the pros and cons.

The IUD

The intrauterine device (IUD) is the most common reversible method of birth control used in the world today. The IUD is roaring back into favor after a disaster in the 1970s when it first became widespread. A faulty version called the Dalkon Shield caused serious health problems and raised questions about IUD safety. There seemed to be more pelvic infections associated with this particular IUD, and in 1974 the Dalkon Shield was removed from the market.

Media attention caused women to worry about other IUD models, even though they proved safe and effective. Fearing litigation, manufacturers withdrew IUDs from the market. But now they're back, and for the right user, today's IUDs are safe and effective. If you're looking for a long-term, yet reversible method of birth control, the IUD may be a great option.

The IUD is a small plastic device that your doctor puts inside your uterus through your **cervix** in a quick office procedure. The IUD contains copper or hormones (**progestin**) that keep sperm from joining an egg, like a little chaperone. Both the copper and the progestin IUD prevent fertilization by making it harder for the sperm to get to the fallopian tubes or by reducing the ability of sperm to fertilize an ovum. (We don't know exactly how they do that.) IUDs also alter the lining of the uterus, which, in theory, may prevent implantation of a fertilized egg.

The IUD is highly effective at preventing pregnancy (a failure rate of less than 1 percent), as good as getting your tubes tied, yet it is immediately reversible. It's a good method for women who want more long-term birth control. Its popularity is increasing as we learn more about its safety and convenience. It's a good choice for monogamous couples who want to space their children apart or do not want children right now.

Your ability to become pregnant returns quickly when the IUD is removed. In the past, most doctors used IUDs only in women who were done having kids. Today IUDs are being used much more often in younger women who think it may be several years before they want children. It is slightly more difficult to place an IUD in a woman who has not been pregnant, so you'll need to go to a doctor experienced in IUD placements, and be prepared for some cramps with the insertion.

With the IUD, there is nothing to think about or do before having sex. The ParaGard (copper IUD) may be left in place for up to twelve years, the Mirena (hormone IUD) for five years. The Mirena may reduce menstrual cramps and result in lighter and shorter periods, whereas copper IUDs may increase cramps and result in heavier and longer periods. Some women use the Mirena IUD to control heavy or painful periods. It's important to be cleared of any sexually transmitted infections and to be monogamous (have sex with only one partner who has sex only with you) when you use an IUD because of an increased chance of tubal infection if you have a sexually transmitted infection when the IUD is placed. Rare complications of the IUD are perforation of the uterus during insertion, infection during insertion, and **ectopic pregnancy**.

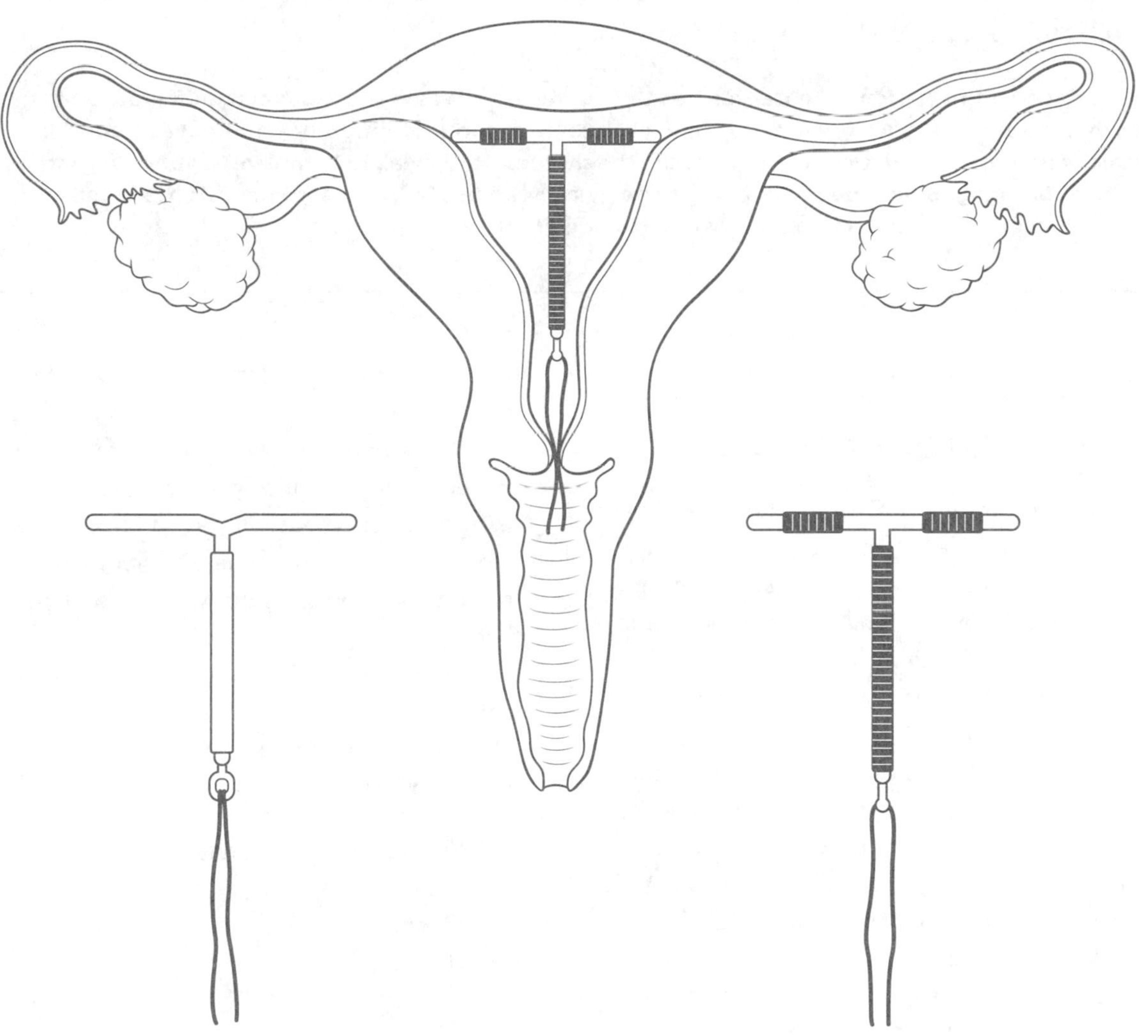

The interuterine device (IUD) is a small plastic device that is inserted into your uterus to prevent pregnancy. Both the progestin hormone IUD (Mirena; above left) and the copper IUD (ParaGard; above right) work by preventing an egg from joining sperm.

REAL LIFE FACT: The Most Common Methods of Birth Control in America

According to the National Center for Health Statistics, the Pill is the most common method of birth control used in America. On a state level, there are lots of different preferences from the male condom, tubal ligation, vasectomy, and the shot to withdrawal, IUD, implant, diaphragm, and natural planning. Since the most recent survey was done in 2002, I'm sure the IUD has climbed much higher on the list. Its popularity has exploded in the last few years.

Combined Hormonal Contraception

Combined hormonal contraception methods, which include the Pill, the patch, and the vaginal ring, all work through the basic concept of preventing ovulation. They use synthetic hormones similar to the estrogen and progesterone made by your ovaries to stop ovulation and prevent pregnancy.

They also work (in case your pill-taking skills aren't perfect and an egg slips out) by thickening the cervical **mucus** to keep sperm from joining the egg. They change the lining of the uterus, which may prevent a fertilized egg from planting itself.

None of these hormonal contraceptive methods protect against sexually transmitted infections—you'll need to use condoms to reduce that risk. And in case you're wondering, the most recent scientific research suggests that the use of combined hormone methods probably does not increase the risk of developing breast **cancer**, even with long-term use.

Remember that your ability to become pregnant returns quickly as soon as you stop using these methods. So you will need to use another method immediately if you stop, or if you're planning a family, you won't need to wait.

There may be side effects for some women using combined hormonal contraceptive methods, but these usually clear up after two or three months of use:

- Bleeding between periods
- Breast tenderness
- Moodiness or depression
- Headache
- Nausea
- Weight gain or loss
- Changes in sex drive

You'll notice that I mention weight gain or loss. This is another of those science and medicine versus experience problems. First, remember that the Pill today does not cause weight gain like earlier versions did. Even though there is no scientific connection between the Pill and weight change, some women still have that experience and we can't be sure why.

Keep in mind another problem of combined hormonal contraception. Whenever you change a hormone drug, including the Pill, your hormone levels will change with it. As you try different methods—the patch, low-dose, regular dose—you may notice that you feel different. Some women go through hormone changes with little trouble. Many women feel a big difference that is very hard to manage. It can feel like menopause or like changing antidepressants. Be sure to talk with your doctors about your symptoms. You may be able to adjust to the change over a few weeks, or you may feel like you've been dropped in hell and want to go back to your prior method immediately. We have no way of predicting who will have which reaction. Pay attention to your symptoms and don't keep them to yourself. Your doctor needs to know.

Rare but Serious Side Effects of Combined Hormonal Contraception

There are some women who should not use combined hormonal contraceptive methods at all. The risk of serious side effects increases

REAL LIFE FACT: Body Benefits of Hormonal Birth Control

Besides their contraceptive benefits, combined hormonal birth control methods have other health benefits. The birth control pill reduces the risk of ovarian and endometrial cancer, pelvic inflammatory disease, fibrocystic breast changes, ovarian cysts, and osteoporosis (loss of bone mass). And all combined hormonal birth control methods can provide you with some protection against:

- **Irregular or painful menstrual cycles**
- **Infection of the fallopian tubes (pelvic inflammatory disease), which often leads to infertility**
- **Ectopic pregnancy (in the fallopian tubes)**
- **Noncancerous breast lumps**
- **Ovarian cysts**
- **Cancer of the ovaries**
- **Cancer of the lining of the uterus**
- **Menstrual cramps**
- **Iron deficiency anemia that results from heavy periods**
- **Acne**
- **Excess body hair**
- **Osteoporosis**

after age thirty-five and with smoking, and also if a woman has conditions that put her at risk for heart attack, such as **diabetes**, high blood pressure, or high **cholesterol**, and certain inherited conditions that increase the risk of blood clotting. If you are in one of these groups, combined hormonal contraception should not be the first-line choice for you. If you smoke, remember that the risk of complications for you is always higher than for nonsmokers—and the risks outweigh the benefits over age thirty-five if you smoke.

Serious problems don't happen often, but I want you to know what to look for. Some women develop high blood pressure. The most serious complication of combined hormone use is getting a blood clot in the legs, lungs, heart, or brain. Women who are bedridden by surgery have an increased chance of having blood clots. The immobilization plus the estrogen increases the risk.

If you need a major operation or have a medical problem, such as a broken leg, that keeps you in bed for a long time, it's important to tell your doctor that you're using hormonal contraceptives so that precautions can be taken to minimize your risks.

Serious problems usually have warning signs. Report any of these signs to your doctor as soon as possible:

- Changes in your vision such as blurred or double vision
- Pain or swelling in a leg or arm
- Chest pain
- Severe headaches
- Sudden onset of shortness of breath or spitting up blood
- Developing a yellow color in the whites of your eyes or your skin
- Breast lump
- Heavy or prolonged vaginal bleeding
- No period after having a period regularly every month (sometimes this can be normal)

When you choose a birth control method, consider all of these risks and side effects. Read the sections below for more information, and talk with your **gynecologist** to help you to make the important decisions about what to take or whether you should take anything. I'll give you my opinion, too.

The Pill

If you use the birth control pill, you *must* take one pill per day every day. If you are a skipper, you'll soon be a mother. The closer to the same time that you can take your pill each day, the more effective it will be as a method of birth control. Although this is a simple and easy method, some women find that remembering to take a pill every day can be a problem for them. If that's you, pick another method!

Compared to the 1960s version of the Pill, today's pills are all low-dose (30 to 35 micrograms of estrogen). If you are troubled by nausea or persistent breast tenderness, you can try one of the ultra-low-dose pills (20 to 25 micrograms of estrogen). Sometimes you can get more breakthrough bleeding on these very-low-dose pills, but this doesn't make the pill less effective for birth control. It's more of a nuisance.

Most pill packs contain seven days of placebo pills (sugar pills) in addition to the hormone pills. It's while taking these placebo pills that you get your period. Some of the newer brands of pills have fewer placebos, some with only four placebo pills, and others with placebos only four times a year. One new pill has no placebos at all, which means you never get your period.

If your pack contains placebos and you want to move the date of your period (away from a vacation or a special event, for example), you can simply skip the placebos one month and shift your period to a different time for the next cycle.

Vaginal Ring

The latest popular option in hormonal contraception is the vaginal ring. It's simple: you insert a small, flexible ring deep into your vagina for three weeks and take it out for the fourth week, during which time you get your period. It releases hormones that protect against pregnancy for one month, and it's up to 99.7 percent effective in preventing pregnancy. It can be a good choice for pill skippers.

The advantage of the ring is that there is no pill to remember to take daily, so the ring may be more effective than the Pill for some women. It doesn't require a fitting by a clinician (the diaphragm does) and does not require the use of spermicide. There is nothing to put in place before sex, as it stays in place for three weeks. Most surveyed women report being very happy with the ring.

Some possible downsides to the ring include increased vaginal discharge or irrita-

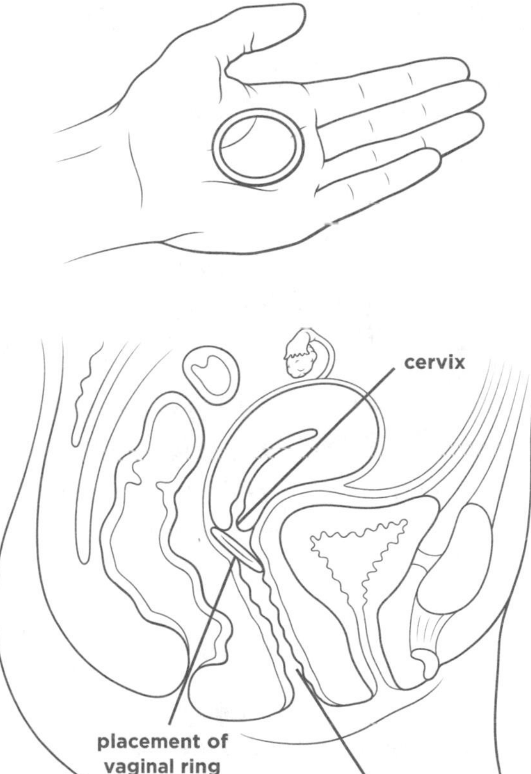

The vaginal ring is a form of hormonal contraception that you insert deep into your vagina. You leave the small, flexible ring there for three weeks, and then take it out during the fourth week to get your period.

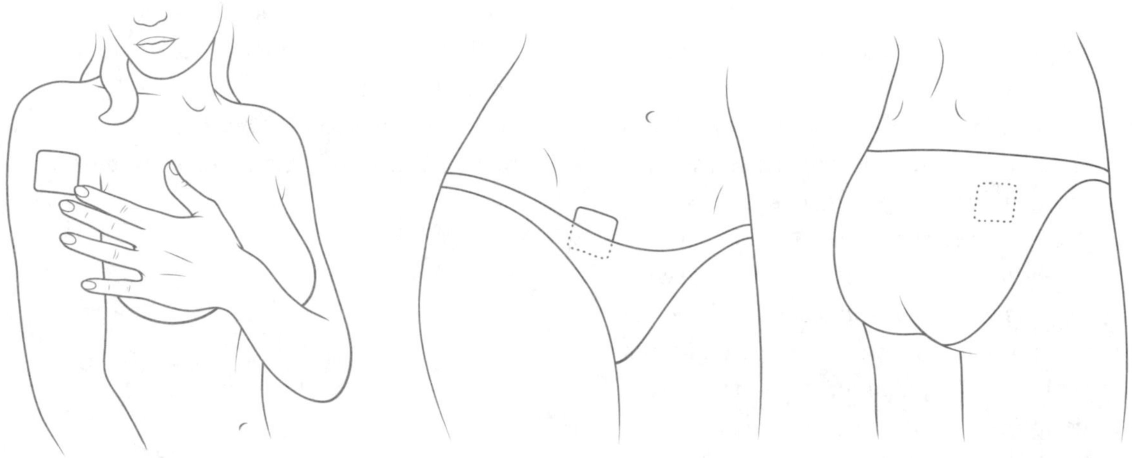

The patch is a form of hormonal contraception that you stick on your arm, waist, or buttocks. You replace the patch once per week for three weeks in a row, and then you remove the patch for the fourth week to get your period.

tion. And some women have said they don't like the idea of having something in their vagina. Surprisingly, most women can't feel it in there, and most partners won't notice it during sex.

The Patch

The patch is a thin plastic patch that you stick onto your skin—recommended locations are the buttocks, abdomen, upper outer arm, or upper torso. It is replaced once a week, and stays on constantly for that week. Each week you take it off and replace it with a fresh one, for three weeks in a row. No patch is used in the fourth week, during which time you get your period. It works best when it is changed on the same day of the week for three weeks in a row.

The patch is a very effective method of birth control. Fewer than one out of every one hundred women who use the patch will become pregnant with perfect use. That's compared to eight out of every one hundred Pill users who become pregnant with typical use. Most women find the patch a good alternative to the Pill if they have trouble remembering to take the Pill. However, the patch may be less effective for women who weigh more than 198 pounds.

Some women are more comfortable with a patch on their skin than placing a ring in their vagina. But the one disadvantage compared to the ring is that although you can place the patch in places covered by clothing, it can be noticed if you don't have much on. And some women find that the patch doesn't stick well, especially if they've used lotions on

REAL LIFE FACT: The Dung Method and Other Ancient Birth Control Methods

Several ancient cultures created a very early version of the sponge for birth control. Women would stuff their vaginas with crocodile dung or other dungs of choice to cover the area around the cervix. It's awful to imagine how many infections women and men got from "the dung sponge."

Alternatively, women in ancient times also used preparations of herbs and leaves mixed with oils or juices as birth control. In ancient Greece, the juice of one local plant became such a popular birth control method that it quickly became extinct.

And some cultures used a method similar to the rhythm method, but they believed that the fertile time happened during the period.

their body. So remember that you have to use the patch perfectly for it to work.

Progestin-Only Contraceptive Choices

Progestin-only contraception contains only progesterone analogues (synthetic versions of the hormone), unlike combined hormonal contraception, which contains both estrogen and progesterone analogues.

Like combined contraception, progestin-only contraception works by keeping your ovaries from releasing an egg. It's not as consistent in stopping ovulation, though, and relies heavily on thickening your cervical mucus so that sperm have a harder time getting through to reach the egg. (Imagine them trying to swim through mud.) Progestin-only contraceptives also change the endometrial lining in your uterus to make the environment less receptive to a fertilized egg.

Who should use progestin-only contraception? Most women prefer combined hormonal contraception because it is slightly more reliable in preventing pregnancy and has fewer side effects. However, progestin-only contraception may be safer for women who smoke, have high blood pressure, are overweight, or have a history of blood clots. It appears that it's the estrogen component of hormonal contraception that increases the medical risks with these conditions.

A small number of women have side effects such as nausea or headaches from the estrogen in the Pill, so progestin-only contraceptives may be a better choice. Progestin-only contraception is also a good choice if you are breastfeeding, because the estrogen found in combined hormonal contraception can decrease your milk supply. There are several types of progestin-only contraception: the mini-pill, the shot, and implants.

The Mini-Pill

The mini-pill contains only the hormone progestin. There is no estrogen in it and there are no placebo pills. You take one pill every day of the month.

The most common side effects of the mini-pill are irregular periods, spotting, and having no periods. Daily progesterone causes thinning of the lining of the uterus, so it's normal if your periods are light, as there is little or no lining to shed at the time of your period. Headaches are less common than with the combination pill. Other possible side effects include breast tenderness, nausea, weight gain or loss, appetite changes, swelling due to fluid retention, and an increase or decrease in sex drive.

Users of the mini-pill need to take one pill every single day. If you forget to take a pill, the mini-pill is less forgiving than the combination pill at preventing pregnancy. Like all birth control pills, the progestin-only pill does not protect you from getting a sexually transmitted disease.

Progestin Implant

The progestin implant (Implanon) is a device that's placed just under the skin of your upper arm, where it constantly releases small amounts of the synthetic hormone progestin. It must be placed and removed by a clinician in a minor office procedure using local anesthetic. It is about the size of a wooden matchstick and is not noticeable under your skin. It lasts for three years. Then it must be removed and a new implant placed. It was approved for use in the United States in 2006.

The advantages of this method are that you don't have to think about it at all for three years. It works in the same way as other forms of progestin-only contraception. Its advantage lies in giving continuous long-lasting birth control, with no pills to take daily. It can be removed if you decide you want to get pregnant, and you'll be fertile again very quickly. With the implant in place, your periods become lighter over time, and in about a third of women, they stop altogether. This is considered a "good" side effect.

Some women still worry that missing a period means they're pregnant. However, because this is a highly effective method of birth control, most doctors and women who use it feel comfortable with that. The downside is that it is common to have irregular spotting for several months, and in some cases even longer, after the implant is first placed. It's impossible to predict who will have the side effect of irregular bleeding, and it doesn't always go away with time.

The Shot

Medroxyprogesterone acetate, or the shot (Depo-Provera), is a slow-release progestin injection given in your bottom or your upper

The progestin implant is a form of hormonal contraception that is placed just under the skin of your upper arm in a minor office procedure. It is highly effective at preventing pregnancy because women with the implant don't have to remember to do anything like take a pill or change a patch.

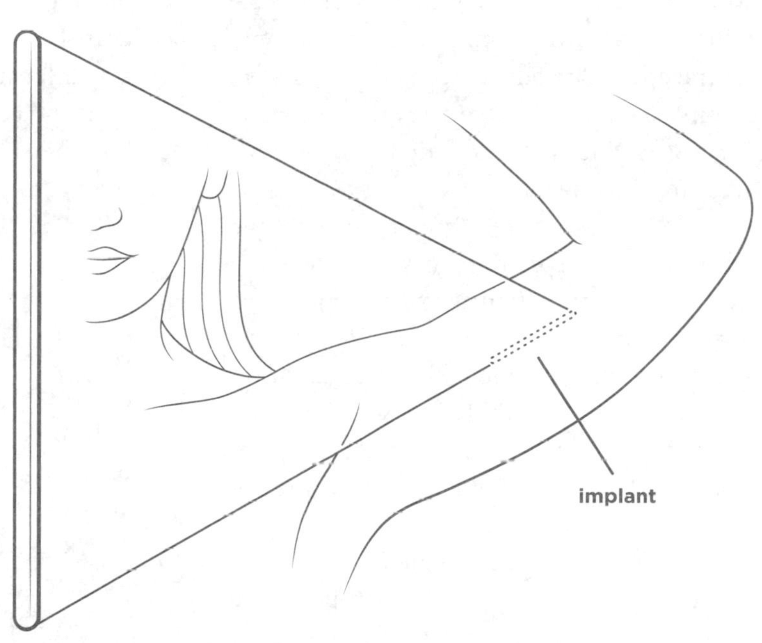

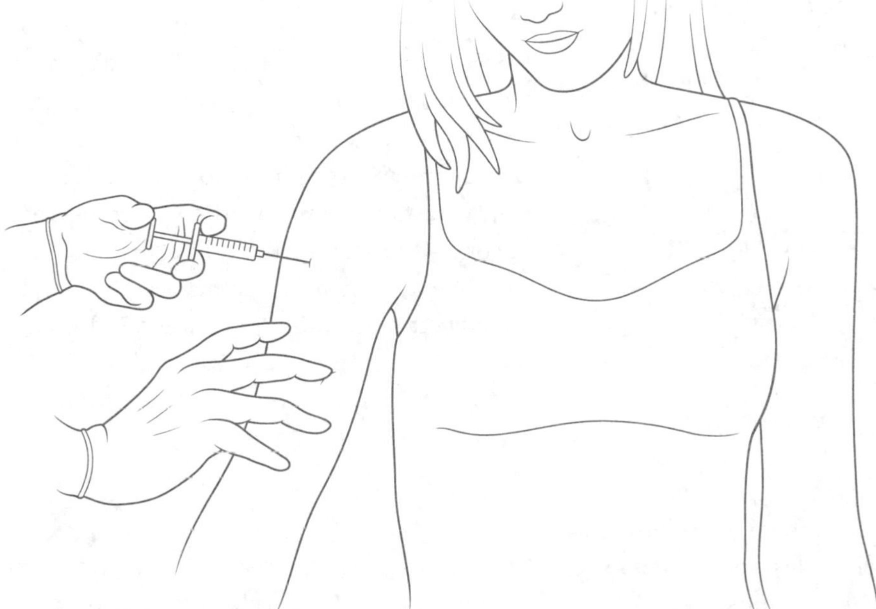

The shot is a form of hormone contraception that is injected into your arm or bottom once every three months.

arm once every three months. It works in the same way as other forms of progestin-only contraception. Its advantage is that you have to think about it only once every three months, although it does require a trip to the doctor's office for the injection.

At the beginning, it's common to have some irregular bleeding, and most women stop having their period after a few injections. Having no periods is considered a "good" side effect, and many women choose the shot for this reason. But as with the progestin implant, it can take time to get used to that, as we are so used to the period signaling that we are not pregnant.

There may be some delay in your ability to get pregnant after shots are stopped (nine to ten months), as it can take some time for the hormone to completely clear out of your system. Some women notice weight gain with the shot, and long-term use has been associated with bone loss and **osteoporosis**, though most of this reverses when the shot is stopped.

Barrier Methods—Diaphragm, Cap, Shield, Condom

Female barrier methods are devices that a woman places in her vagina or over her cervix to form a physical barrier to prevent sperm from reaching the egg. Most of them work with a spermicide, which overpowers sperm. The two must be used together for most barrier methods to work effectively. With the exception of condoms, barrier methods are fitted by a health care provider and require a prescription. Their major advantages are their lack of hormones and the fact that women control their use.

Diaphragm

The diaphragm is a barrier method in which you place a shallow cup over your cervix just before sex. You add spermicide, and sperm are prevented from joining the egg, both by the physical barrier and by the spermicidal agent. You need to add more spermicide for every act of sex. It's important that you leave the diaphragm in place and, if you have sex again, use an applicator to add some more spermicidal cream or jelly. It must stay in place for at least six to eight hours after sex.

Its disadvantages are that it can be a bit messy, it creates a small risk of **bladder** infection in some women, and it can be left in place for only twenty-four hours. Some men and women find that the insertion time can cause a drop in sexual arousal, others do it together, or some women insert it in advance.

The diaphragm is about 71 to 86 percent effective in preventing pregnancy. It does not protect against sexually transmitted infections. It is nonhormonal and has no major health risks.

Cap

The cap is a barrier method in which you place a small cup over the cervix just before sex. You

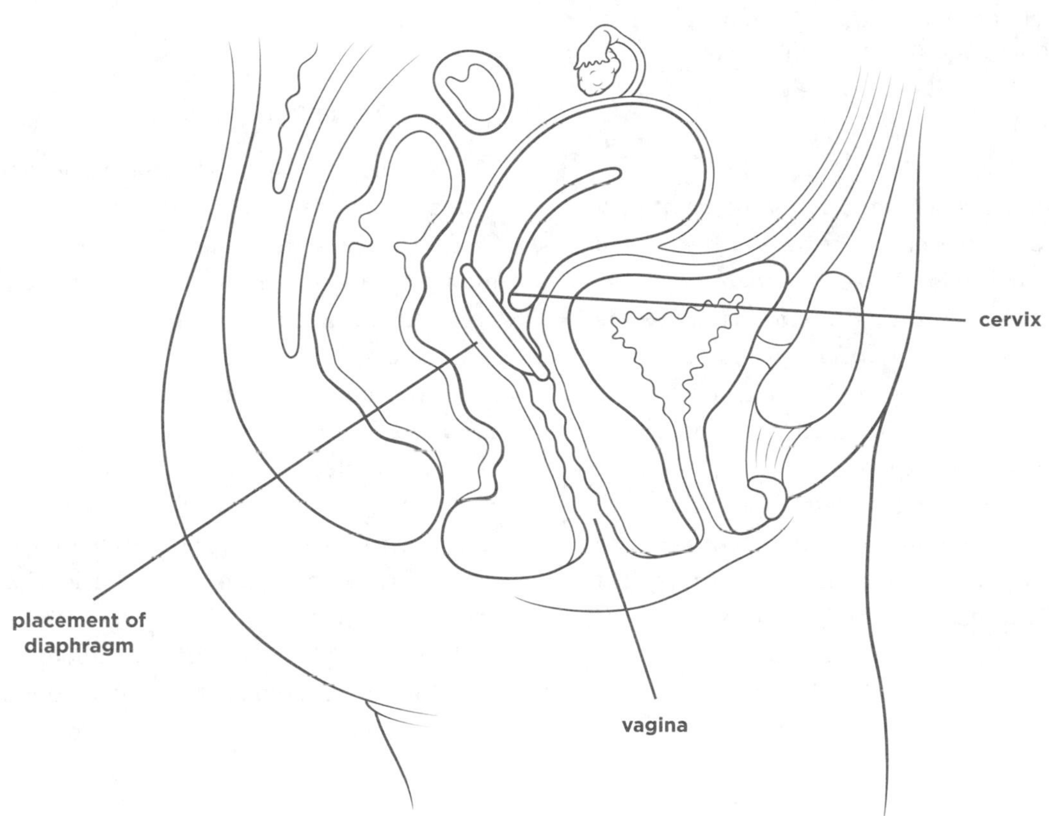

The diaphragm is a form of barrier contraception that is inserted into the vagina and placed over the cervix just before sex. You leave the diaphragm in place for six to eight hours after sex to prevent pregnancy.

put spermicide into it, and it works exactly like the diaphragm. The disadvantage is that not all women can be fitted for a cap, because it comes in only a few sizes and not all female anatomy matches it.

The cap can be left in place for up to forty-eight hours, and more spermicide must be applied for more sex. Because the cap is smaller than the diaphragm, it seems to cause fewer bladder infections, and some women find it more comfortable than a diaphragm. It's nonhormonal and has no major health risks. It does not protect against sexually transmitted infections.

If you have never had children, the cap is about 86 percent effective as birth control, but after you have children and your vaginal shape changes a bit, the cap drops to 71 percent effectiveness.

Shield

The shield is also a barrier method, but it does not fit over the cervix like the diaphragm and cap. Instead, it is pushed up into the top of the vagina, where it naturally expands so that the vaginal walls hold it in place. It's one-size-fits-all and does not need to be fitted individually. Some women find it difficult to use, and rarely, some partners can feel it.

The shield can be left in place for up to forty-eight hours. It's nonhormonal and has no major health risks. It does not protect against sexually transmitted infections.

If you have never had children, the shield is about 85 percent effective as birth control, but after you have children and your vaginal shape changes a bit, the effectiveness of the shield may decline.

Female Condom

The female condom is a sleevelike device that a woman inserts into her vagina, where it is held in place with a ring similar to the one on a diaphragm. Another ring stays outside the vagina, where it lies against the labia. The female condom is 79 to 95 percent effective in preventing pregnancy. It is made of polyurethane, a type of plastic, and is the only female-initiated contraceptive that prevents both pregnancy and sexually transmitted infections. It's available over the counter.

Many women don't like the idea of a female condom even if they haven't tried it. There are plenty of theories about why. They're not as reliable as a male condom, they cost more, and they look weird. Educa-

REAL LIFE FACT: Latex Allergy Caution

Most male condoms and the diaphragm contain latex. Latex allergies are becoming increasingly common. If you notice vaginal or rectal itching or swelling after using these birth control methods, you may have latex sensitivity and should ask your doctor. It's another good reason to pack your own condoms!

Several types of condoms are suitable for people allergic to latex. Lambskin condoms (made from the intestinal lining of lambs) have no latex. Unfortunately, although lambskin condoms can protect against pregnancy, they do not provide a barrier against sexually transmitted infections. Try condoms made of polyurethane instead. The major brands are making them, and you can expect more in the future.

> ## REAL LIFE FACT: Goodyear . . . Condoms?
>
> **Charles Goodyear, the maker of tires, invented vulcanized rubber, which was a new process of making rubber that changed manufacturing, including the production of condoms! In the 1800s, condoms were easy to get, although they were a little different from the flavored, colored, and ribbed versions we have today. Get this: condoms were meant to be *reused.* Men were supposed to wash them before and after sex and then store them in a little box.**
>
> **Incidentally, condoms are *not* mentioned in Goodyear's online corporate history.**

tion about the female condom is more widespread in developing countries where women do not feel they can demand that a partner wear a condom. And I think that some women just plain feel that a man should step up and handle this job.

Male Condom

Condoms have been around for a long time. They were used by the ancient Egyptians to protect themselves from disease and infection. And today condoms come in every size, color, and even flavor. You've probably seen packaged condoms in purses and medicine cabinets, and old ones scattered in litter. There are no age restrictions on buying condoms, and they are available without prescription in drugstores, supermarkets, and even vending machines. They're vitally important both for birth control and for preventing sexually transmitted infections.

The condom is a barrier method that covers the penis before sex with a sheath made of thin latex, plastic, or the original material, lamb intestines. It's very effective when used right. Success at preventing pregnancy ranges from 85 to 98 percent.

The major advantage of using condoms is that they protect against sexually transmitted infections (as long as they cover the affected area). They are easy to get, simple to use, and have no health risks. Condoms can deteriorate if they are exposed to too much heat or sunlight, so it's best not to use a condom that has been stored in your back pocket, your wallet, or the glove compartment of your car.

For information on how to use a condom, see chapter 11, Your Best Sex. And remember: the best way to protect yourself is to use your own condoms. Pack your own!

Spermicides

Over-the-counter spermicides work by killing sperm. They come in various forms: foam, cream, jelly, film, or suppository. Spermicides are inserted deep into your vagina shortly before sex to immobilize sperm and keep them from joining the egg. Spermicides are

71 to 82 percent effective in preventing pregnancy. They *do not* protect against sexually transmitted disease. Failure rates for spermicides alone are worse than for most other methods of birth control.

Caution: Using the spermicide nonoxynol-9 many times a day, or for anal sex, may irritate tissue and increase the risk of **HIV** and other sexually transmitted infections.

The Sponge

Oh, the sponge, immortalized on *Seinfeld*. You can't get it in the United States anymore, so I'm not going to go into detail here. Yes, they were easy and comfortable, but they didn't work very well. They were a one-size-fits-all sponge, soaked in spermicide. But again, they didn't work!

Sterilization

Sterilization is a harsh word. We like to say, "having your tubes tied," because it sounds so routine, but I use the word sterilization because it's very important for you to know that these methods are permanent.

Sterilization is a permanent method of birth control. It can be done for either men or women. It should be used only if you are certain that you are done having children. Although technically reversible, the rates of successful pregnancy after sterilization reversal are not high, and the procedure is very expensive.

NOTE TO SELF

Many of my patients opt for female or male "tube tying." If you are still fertile but do not want more children, these are effective tools. Remember that the procedure is easier for men. Only you can decide if it's right for you and your partner.

Tying the Tubes for Women

Tubal ligation is a surgical procedure in which the fallopian tubes are blocked off to provide permanent protection against pregnancy. They are not actually *tied*. There are several different

REAL LIFE FACT: Ranking Contraceptive Effectiveness

When contraceptive methods are ranked by effectiveness based on general use, the IUD, implant, patch, and injectables have the lowest failure rates (1 to 3 percent), followed by the Pill (8 percent), the diaphragm and the cervical cap (12 percent), the male condom (14 percent), periodic abstinence (21 percent), withdrawal (24 percent), and spermicides (26 percent).

Source: 1995 National Survey of Family Growth

methods—they can be cut, burned, clipped, or plugged from the inside. The advantage of this procedure is that there are no lasting side effects and no effect on sexual pleasure, and it is highly effective. Despite the common myth that it affects your hormones or your menstrual cycle, tubal ligation simply interrupts the tunnel in which the egg and the sperm meet, keeping them permanently apart. Your hormones remain unchanged.

The disadvantage is that it is a surgical procedure and requires anesthesia, which means it has some medical risks. Because it is permanent, some women later regret it, and it is not easily reversed. It has a small failure rate, and if pregnancy does occur, then there is an increased risk of a dangerous ectopic (tubal) pregnancy.

Laparoscopic Tubal Ligation

In laparoscopic tubal ligation, a telescope with a camera attached is placed through a small incision under your belly button, and a second small instrument is place through an even smaller incision just above your pubic bone. Through this, the surgeon burns through or clips the tubes. The procedure requires general anesthesia, which although safe for most people, has some risks. The advantage is that it works immediately.

Postpartum Tubal Ligation

In the hours to days after you have a baby, your uterus is still fairly large, with the top just under your belly button. Doctors can access your tubes with a small incision under your belly button. Your tubes can be reached, cut, and "tied." The procedure requires either a spinal or general anesthesia, and it adds a bit to the recovery time of having a baby.

If you are having a C-section, a postpartum tubal ligation can be done after the birth. It only adds a few minutes and does not increase the recovery time. The advantage of doing a tubal ligation postpartum is that you are in the hospital anyway, so it's an efficient way to get things taken care of if you know for certain that you are done having children.

Be careful about making that decision while you still remember the pain of labor. Consider this option long before delivery to give it the careful thought it deserves.

No-Incision Method: Hysteroscopic Tubal Sterilization

A no-incision method for tubal sterilization is now available. It's usually done under local anesthesia with an option of some intravenous sedation. A doctor inserts two small, soft metallic coils (called microinserts) through the vagina, cervix, and uterus into the fallopian tubes. A small, telescope-like instrument called a hysteroscope is inserted into the vagina and through the cervix. Fluid moving through the scope helps the doctor to see the opening of the tubes from inside your uterus. The microinserts are positioned in the opening of the tubes. Once in place, the coils cause scar tissue to grow, blocking the tubes.

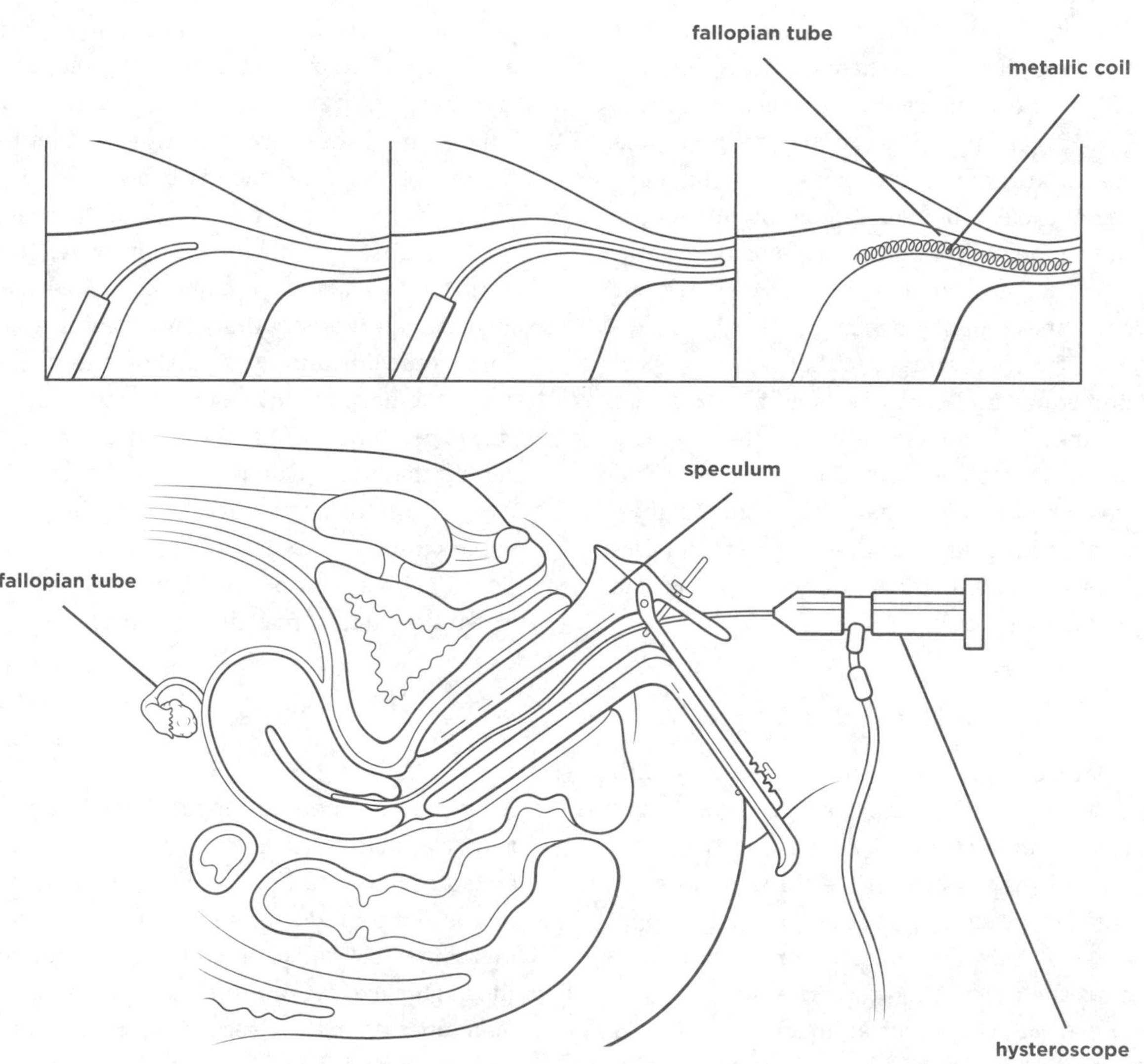

Hysteroscopic tubal sterilization is a no-incision method in which two small metallic coils are inserted through the cervix and uterus into the fallopian tubes. After being positioned at the opening of each tube, the coils cause scar tissue to grow and permanently block the tubes.

It is 99.8 percent effective at preventing pregnancy. Three months after insertion, a test called a hysterosalpingogram (HSG) is performed to make sure the tubes are permanently blocked. HSG is an **X-ray** test that takes pictures of the uterus and fallopian tubes after a dye has been inserted through the cervix. Until the HSG shows that the inserts are in the correct position and the tubes are blocked, another method of birth control must be used. The advantage of this method over traditional tubal ligation is that there are no incisions on the abdomen, healing is quicker, and there's no visible scarring. It's a safer method for obese women. The disadvantage is the three-month wait before it is known to be effective.

Male Sterilization—Vasectomy

Vasectomy is a permanent method of male birth control in which the **vas deferens**—the tubes through which sperm are carried to the penis—are blocked off. An incision is made on each side of the scrotum (sometimes a single incision is made in the center, and sometimes an incisionless puncture method is used), and the vas deferens are located. A small section of each tube is removed, tied, burned, or blocked with surgical clips. It is an office procedure that takes about fifteen to twenty minutes and is safe and effective.

Side effects include temporary bruises, swelling, or tenderness of the scrotum. It does not affect sex drive, erections, orgasms, ejaculations, or a man's voice. This is not castration! The fluid that comes out of the penis will simply have no sperm in it. It takes about three months for the sperm to completely wash out, and a semen analysis must be done to be sure there are no sperm left before you rely on the method for birth control.

You'll notice that this procedure really is simpler than the options available for women. While many men are very anxious about anything happening around their genitals, your doctor will advise you to go the male route. Again, only you and your partner can decide.

It's Not Too Late: Emergency Contraception

You forgot to take your pill. He didn't pull out in time. The condom broke. You were sexually assaulted. Whatever the circumstance, you had unprotected sex. Now is the time for emergency contraception.

Emergency contraception is a method of preventing pregnancy after having unprotected sex. It is often called the morning-after pill, but emergency contraception can be used before the morning after or up to five days after. Emergency contraception is an important way to prevent unintended pregnancy.

Do not rely on emergency contraceptives as your only protection against pregnancy if you are sexually active or planning to be, because they are not as effective as ongoing contraceptive methods.

In the United States and some other countries, emergency contraceptive pills are available over the counter. Your doctor can also provide you with emergency contraception by prescription (if you have insurance, it may be cheaper to obtain it that way) and help you to decide which method is right for you. It's also a good idea for women who use barrier methods to have a supply of emergency contraception on hand, in case of condom breakage or misuse of other barrier methods.

Emergency Contraceptive Pills

Morning-after pills can reduce the risk of pregnancy if started within 120 hours (five days) after unprotected vaginal intercourse. The sooner they're taken, the better. If started within seventy-two hours, they can reduce the risk of pregnancy by 75 to 89 percent.

Plan B is the brand name for the progestin-only emergency contraceptive pill, which is the most effective oral method for preventing pregnancy in an emergency. It's also the preferred method, since it has fewer side effects. These pills are available to women over age seventeen at pharmacies without a prescription. Girls under age seventeen need a prescription.

When combined hormones—estrogen and progestin—are used (combined oral contraceptive pills in higher doses), nausea, vomiting, and cramping can be common side effects. It's best to make the effort to obtain the progestin-only version whenever possible.

Copper-T Intrauterine Device

Emergency IUD insertion within five days of unprotected intercourse is 99.9 percent effective for preventing pregnancy in emergencies. This is a good method in an emergency if you plan to keep the IUD in place long term, or if you have medical reasons why you can't take emergency contraceptive pills.

NOTE TO SELF

Emergency contraception is not an abortion pill. It prevents pregnancy from ever happening in the first place.

Birth Control Methods That Often Don't Work

There are many reasons women use the following methods, which don't work very well. People living in the developing world often have no access to modern methods. And some people in the United States can't afford health insurance or a lot of medicine and think these are cheaper options. (I always remind them that a $1 condom is a lot cheaper than an unplanned pregnancy.) Young people often believe that these methods work because an older partner has told them so to manipulate them into having sex. Remember, these methods are not going to protect you like the contraceptive options described above will.

Withdrawal

In the withdrawal method, the man pulls his penis out of the vagina before he ejaculates sperm. This method is 73 to 96 percent effective, depending upon whether he gets out in time. Pregnancy is always possible, because the pre-ejaculate can contain sperm. He may ejaculate before pulling out, and sperm may be spilled on the **vulva**. And remember that withdrawal doesn't protect you against sexually transmitted infection.

"Outercourse"

Outercourse is sexual play without the penis entering the vagina. If carefully controlled, this will keep sperm from joining the egg. It is not a perfect method, as sperm can spill on the outside of the vulva and, in rare cases, can make their way up your genital tract to the fallopian tubes, so pregnancy is technically possible. Outercourse does reduce, but does not eliminate, the risk of many sexually transmitted infections. Its advantage is that it can be used when no other contraceptive methods are available. The obvious major disadvantage is that many people find it difficult to stop short of vaginal intercourse.

However, if you do it right, it's fun.

Breastfeeding (Lactational Amenorrhea Method)

Breastfeeding inhibits ovulation. For most women, breastfeeding frequently every day will prevent the ovaries from releasing an egg. It's up to 99.5 percent effective for up to six months if you have not had a period since delivery and you are breastfeeding at least six times a day and giving nighttime feedings to the baby. Breastfeeding women can consider progestin-only contraception, an IUD, or barrier methods as good options.

Natural Methods

Methods such as discharge testing and temperature taking (see page 358) can be helpful for women who have absolutely regular cycles and who are prepared to spend a lot of time thinking about and planning birth control. The advantage of natural methods is the low risk of side effects. But unless you are willing to devote a great deal of energy to this, it just won't work. It will never be completely reliable, and it gives you no protection against sexually transmitted infections.

If Contraception Fails: The Most Difficult Decisions

Nearly every sexually active woman has, at least once, stood in the bathroom with her heart pounding. She has peed on the stick; now she waits. And waits.

For some, in the end it says pregnant. The problem: She is single. She is not in good health. She has no health insurance. She's in college. She's not yet self-sufficient.

If you are one of these women, here's the first step: call the doctor's office or a family planning center. You need to confirm the over-the-counter test results and, if you are pregnant, get some advice. If your doctor is a good person to talk to, tell him or her that you'd like to know what your options are.

Your choices range from keeping the baby to adoption to abortion. The rare single mom can successfully raise a child herself. Family support makes this much more likely. If poverty and college are part of your story, life will be extremely tough.

I know you are probably at your wit's end trying to deal with this surprise pregnancy, but it's really important for you to do some careful research, whether you are considering keeping the baby, having an abortion, or giving the baby up for adoption. Why? Because this is a big decision with many possible outcomes, and you might regret your actions later if you didn't fully understand all of the issues when you made your decision.

For instance, many of the adoption sites you'll find online are actually fronts for other organizations. They pretend to be helpful adoption websites, but they are really law firms looking for babies for private adoptions, or other extremely biased groups that don't have your—or the baby's—best interests at heart. No matter what your circumstances are, this is your own decision to make, so don't let anyone else push you into doing something that isn't right for you. There are some organizations that are against single moms and will tell you how horrible it will be for you and your baby if you decide to keep it. These "adoption websites" will push you hard to give up your baby, even if you live in a houseful of loving family members who could offer you support. Other adoption websites are fronts for anti-abortion organizations.

Knowing that young women need *help* at this time, I'm shocked that there are so many questionable people "working" in this area. Right now, the last thing you need in your life is help from a biased group of people who don't know you. Even your family could be pushing you in one direction or another. It's hard to keep remembering that only *you* can make this decision. So to help you do that, I recommend that you please find a counselor or social worker who can guide you through the process. If you are pregnant due to a difficult situation such as rape, you have even more thoughts and feelings to work through, and I'd like you to have a guide. A good counselor can help you make a well-informed decision by explaining what your options are for keeping the child, having an abortion, or having an open, semi-open, or closed adoption.

Adoption

If you decide to go the adoption route, a counselor or social worker can help you figure out the legal issues and costs and give you resources to find the best family for you and your baby. While open adoption (where you

REAL LIFE FACT: The Catholic Church and Abortion

The Catholic church is a staunch pro-life advocate, meaning that it is antiabortion *and* against the death penalty. Little-known fact: In the 1960s, the church allowed contraception and morning-after pills for nuns under attack in the Belgian Congo. More recently, in 1993, the church provided the same standard for everyone, not only nuns, in Bosnia.

Contraception, including the morning-after pill, is considered by the church to be a form of self-defense in these cases. Contrary to what many people believe, the church does not expect rape survivors to carry a pregnancy that is there against God's will. Don't bet on your local pastor knowing that, but it's true. If he's telling women anything else, set him straight. Or at least tell the women.

continue to see your baby, usually on a schedule) may sound like a shocking idea, it is turning out to be an excellent option if everyone involved is comfortable and trusting.

How do you find an adoption counselor or social worker? Look for counselors who have completed Infant Adoption Awareness Training. This is a federal program to train counselors in helping women make their own decisions. If your faith is extremely important to you and you want your baby to be raised in your religion, try asking your minister, rabbi, priest, imam, pandit, or other leader for help. And this may surprise you, given their image in the media, but Planned Parenthood can often recommend a very good adoption counselor. Not every Planned Parenthood office does this, so you'll have to do some research on the options in your area.

If you are pretty sure that adoption is your choice, take a look at the reading list and links on the website of the Center for Family Connections at www.kinnect.org. A book called *Adoption Nation*, by Adam Pertman, executive director of the Evan B. Donaldson Adoption Institute, offers an interesting view of the adoption process that's worth reading. And when you are definitely sure that adoption is your choice, go to the National Council for Adoption at www.adoptioncouncil.org for next steps.

Abortion

To antiabortion activists, nothing justifies abortion, not even your life, not even if you are have been sexually assaulted. To pro-choice activists, abortion is a matter of a woman's right, which she may use as she and only she sees fit, in the event of mistakes, contraceptive failures, or birth defects, and for physical and mental health reasons. Both sides agree that preventing unintended pregnancy should be a major goal.

In the United States, abortion is legal through the second trimester, though access to second-trimester procedures is more limited in some areas of the country. Some states require parental consent for young women under eighteen, though exceptions can be made.

Almost half of all pregnancies in the United States are unintended, and almost half of these end in abortion. Most abortions, nearly 90 percent, are provided in the first trimester—the first three months of pregnancy.

Safe, uncomplicated abortion should not affect fertility. Abortion does not make ectopic pregnancy more common unless a serious infection occurs, which is rare. And it does not cause breast cancer or premature birth or birth defects in future pregnancies.

What if abortion is the best option for you? There are options, medical or surgical.

NOTE TO SELF

Abortions performed in the first trimester pose no long-term risk of future infertility, ectopic pregnancy, breast cancer, miscarriage, or birth defects.

Surgical Abortion

The two surgical methods used for an abortion are vacuum aspiration, and dilation with evacuation (D&E). Vacuum aspiration is more common than D&E and is done up to fourteen weeks after a woman's last period. D&E is usually performed later than fourteen weeks after a woman's last period. Fewer than 10 percent of abortions in the United States happen during that later period, as most women seek to end an unwanted pregnancy as early as possible.

Vacuum aspiration empties the uterus with gentle suction from a manual syringe or with machine-operated suction. D&E is a two-part procedure. The cervix is slowly opened (dilated), and the procedure is completed by emptying the uterus using a combination of suction and medical instruments.

Medical Abortion

Medical abortion is the use of medication to end an early pregnancy. Studies show that medical abortion works through the eighth week of pregnancy. There are two steps.

First, a clinician gives either an injection of methotrexate or a dose of mifepristone in tablet form. Methotrexate works to stop the pregnancy in the uterus or in the fallopian tube (ectopic pregnancy). Mifepristone (also known as RU486) blocks the hormone progesterone, which causes the lining of the uterus to break down, ending the pregnancy.

Mifepristone is used more often than methotrexate because it is more effective and more predictable. Medical abortion with methotrexate is about 92 to 96 percent effective. With mifepristone, it is from 96 to 97 percent effective.

In the second step, another medication, misoprostol, is taken in tablet form, which causes the uterus to contract and empty, similar to a miscarriage.

The process of medical abortion begins immediately after taking mifepristone or methotrexate. Some women may begin spotting before taking the misoprostol. For most, the bleeding and cramping associated with medical abortion begin after taking the misoprostol. More than 50 percent of women who use mifepristone abort within four to five hours after taking misoprostol. Heavy bleeding may continue for about thirteen days and spotting can last for a few weeks.

About 92 percent of mifepristone abortions are completed within a week. Only 75 percent of methotrexate abortions are completed in that time—it may take up to four weeks. If a medical abortion does not work, a vacuum aspiration abortion must be done. Vacuum aspiration ends a pregnancy by suctioning away the remaining contents of the uterus.

Making the Abortion Decision

Few women will admit that they've had an abortion. Some do, without regret. Some do, with remorse in different degrees.

You'll hear a lot of talk about your rights. Everybody else seems to think they own them. But only you do. The people outside the abortion clinic who yell crazy things and show terrible photographs don't. The people who act like an abortion is an everyday activity or a form of contraception—they don't own your rights either. This is a decision for you alone.

I encourage you to look at all of your choices before making a decision, unless there is a medical reason for having an abortion done, which makes the moral content of the decision much simpler. Please do not believe the extremists who think that a mother should die for a pregnancy. It's not true, not in the eyes of anybody's God.

You also have the right to be upset. No matter what decision you make, there will be times in your life when you think about it. Seek comfort from friends and loved ones, or find a support group, but remember that nobody goes through an unintended pregnancy without tears, no matter what they decide.

All doctors will encourage you to use the best contraception methods, not abortion, for family planning. That's much better for your body. Think of contraception as a form of prevention.

Stay Informed

There are many decisions that all sexually active women have to make about their bodies and only you (and your partner) should make them. Be as informed as you can be about your body, your cycle, and the options you have to keep yourself healthy. Keep this book close by as a reference so you can refer back to these chapters from time to time.

Whether you are planning to start a family now or years from now, it's never too early to learn about fertility. Now that you've learned about keeping yourself healthy and planning your family, it's time to look at how to keep your fertility going strong.

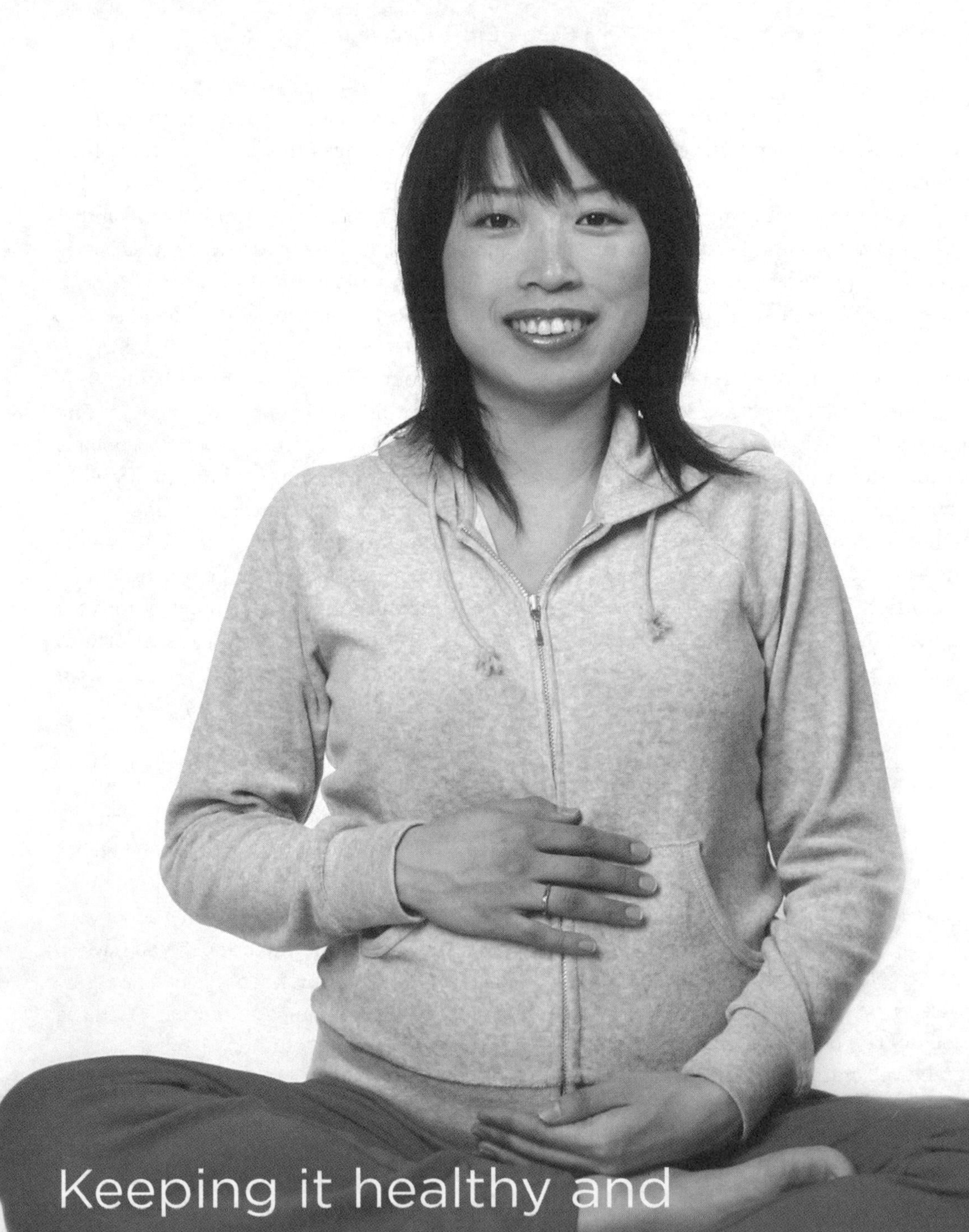
Keeping it healthy and
getting your body ready
to start a family.

your fertility

Did you know that you're born with all of the eggs you'll ever have?

Although nobody knows exactly how many, it's estimated that you have about a million eggs in your ovaries at birth and maybe three hundred thousand by the time you hit puberty. Why do we have so many eggs when we release only one every month? We don't know, and it's a big puzzle.

What we do know is that your overall health when you're young plays a big part in your future fertility. This is just one more reason to keep your body in good shape, even if kids are the last thing on your mind. Someday you may want to have children, and it's never too early to start thinking about your fertility.

Fertility: How to Protect Yours

You can protect your future fertility while you are young in the same ways that you use healthy behaviors to prevent **heart disease** and other health problems later in life. About 10 percent of the reproductive-age population in the United States is infertile. As doctors, we don't spend enough time educating people about the links between health and fertility. You can help prevent infertility in the future by educating yourself now and making lifestyle adjustments.

What's the big picture? Understand that your lifestyle does affect your health, and your health directly affects fertility. Protect your future fertility by practicing safe sex, eating nutritious food, avoiding harmful foods, not smoking, and maintaining a healthy weight. It's a short list, but it has so many challenges on it!

In this chapter, we'll talk about the best ways to protect your fertility and to get your body ready for pregnancy when the time comes.

Protect Yourself from STIs

You know that if you don't practice safe sex, you might get pregnant. And you also realize that if you aren't using **condoms** now and you become infected with a sexually transmitted infection (STI), you may have trouble getting pregnant in the future. But it never hurts to tell you again!

STIs are transmitted from person to person through intimate sexual contact, and one in three sexually active people is infected by age twenty-four. STIs are a leading cause of infertility because they often have few, if any, visible symptoms. Because people often don't know that they have an STI, they don't get treatment, and that threatens their fertility. This is another good reason to keep your annual physical appointment.

Prevention is your best approach. Use condoms until you are in a committed relationship in which both partners are tested and determined to be free of STIs, or practice abstinence until you are ready to be sexually active.

NOTE TO SELF

Abstinence is hard, I know. One patient said, "I know why they say 'practice' abstinence, I practice every weekend, but I still can't get it right."

Quit (or Never Start) Smoking

You already know a lot about smoking, but here's another huge reason to quit: Smoking is harmful to your ovaries! How much damage it can do depends on the amount and length of time that you smoke. Nicotine and other chemicals in cigarettes interfere with your body's ability to make **estrogen**, and they cause your eggs to be more prone to genetic abnormalities.

Although some damage is irreversible, stopping smoking now can prevent further damage. I don't say this lightly—I know that nicotine is an intensely addictive drug. But at some point you have to quit, and now is a good time. Don't become a grandma with an oxygen tank and a nose tube. However much you love her and tell her it doesn't bother anybody, she really, really wishes she were free of it.

Maintain a Healthy Weight

Twelve percent of all infertility is a result of a woman weighing either too little or too much. The main link between body weight and fertility is **estrogen**. One form of estrogen in your body, estrone, is produced in fat cells. If a woman has too much body fat, the body produces too much estrogen and begins to react as if it is on birth control, limiting your odds of getting pregnant. A woman with too little body fat can't produce enough estrogen, and her reproductive cycle begins to shut down. Both under- and overweight women have irregular menstrual cycles in which **ovulation** does not happen or is irregular.

Get Your Body Ready for a Healthy Pregnancy

Whether you are already pregnant or just really want to be, I want to help you have a healthy pregnancy. From foods to eat, foods to avoid, vitamins to take, activities to avoid, and more, read on for some tips on how to get your body ready. (And also read chapter 17, Your Diet, for more information on healthy eating—but remember that you'll be eating a little more once you're pregnant!)

Fabulous Folic Acid

There is a lot of evidence that getting enough of the B vitamin folic acid (or naturally occurring folate, which is found in foods) may actually decrease your future baby's chances of having a neural tube defect. (The brain and spine develop from the neural tube, and defects can cause paralysis and mental retardation.) Because neural tube development is complete in the four weeks following conception—before you even know if you're pregnant—you should start supplementing your diet with folic acid beginning at least one month before you get serious about becoming pregnant.

This simple measure can reduce your future baby's risk of birth defects such as spina bifida by up to 70 percent. There may even be other benefits too. Some studies have shown that not getting enough enough folic acid may increase a woman's risk of miscarriage and the baby's risk of cleft lip and palate, limb defects, and certain types of heart defects. In fact, because half of pregnancies are unplanned, the U.S. Public Health Service recommends that all women of childbearing age get 400 mcg of folic acid each day.

NOTE TO SELF

Folic acid—taken before you get pregnant—can help to prevent serious birth defects in your baby!

So how do you get folic acid into your diet? In the United States, Canada, and many other countries, flour and grain products are fortified with folic acid as a public health measure to prevent neural tube defects. I'm glad measures like these—adding iodine to salt, fluoride to water, and folic acid to flour—were done years ago, because I'm not sure we could get the public to accept them today. Despite this fortification, approximately 70 percent of

REAL LIFE QUESTION: Can I overdose on folic acid?

Any folic acid that you don't need is quickly discarded when you pee. Still, it's important for your doctor to know your dosage, because a high dose can make it hard to detect other vitamin problems.

women of childbearing age still don't get the recommended amount, so it is a good idea to either take a folic acid supplement or ensure you get adequate amounts in your diet.

Again, it is recommended that you get 400 mcg of folic acid per day to lower the incidence of neural tube defects. Prenatal vitamins usually contain 1,000 mcg, and regular multivitamins usually contain 400 mcg, so either of these methods of supplementing is fine before you get pregnant. Folic acid alone is available as an over-the-counter supplement, usually in amounts of 800 mcg, and one a day of these is fine as well. If you prefer to get folate from your diet, instead of the synthetic folic acid, the 400 mcg level can be reached without fortification or supplementation simply by following a good diet. Good sources of folic acid are green leafy vegetables (spinach, collard greens, Swiss chard, kale, mustard greens, turnip greens), legumes, nuts, citrus fruits, and whole-grain breads and cereals. (See the list that follows for the amount of folate in certain foods.)

Food manufacturers are required by the U.S. Food and Drug Administration (FDA) to

REAL LIFE QUESTION: Should I get my folate in food or supplements?

If you're like most people in the United States, you don't get the amount of folate you need from your diet, and research shows that the body actually absorbs the synthetic version of this vitamin (found in supplements and enriched foods) much better than the version that occurs naturally in certain foods. On the days in early pregnancy when you can't stomach your prenatal vitamin, at least take a separate folic acid supplement. (These pills are small and easy to get down.) But eating plenty of folate-rich foods won't hurt either, as the recommended daily amount you're supposed to get from your supplement is designed to add to the amount you're likely to get from food sources.

REAL LIFE FACT: What to Avoid When You're Trying to Get Pregnant

Alcohol, recreational drugs, hot tubs, too much caffeine (more than about 1½ cups per day), and fish high in mercury (shark, swordfish, king mackerel, tilefish, golden or white snapper, fresh or frozen tuna steak, orange roughy, Spanish mackerel, marlin, and grouper). And, yes, you've put it off forever, but now you have to do it: quit smoking! Talk to your doctor immediately to see if you can take any of the helpful smoking cessation medications during pregnancy, or join a program and quit now.

add synthetic folic acid when they enrich grain products such as breakfast cereals, bread, pasta, and rice so that each serving contains at least 20 percent of the daily requirement, and some breakfast cereals contain 100 percent (400 mcg) or more. Other nonfortified sources include:

- ½ cup cooked lentils: 179 mcg
- 1 cup boiled collard greens: 177 mcg
- ½ cup canned chickpeas: 141 mcg
- 1 cup cooked frozen peas: 94 mcg
- 4 spears steamed or boiled asparagus: 88 mcg
- ½ cup steamed broccoli: 52 mcg
- 1 cup strawberries: 40 mcg
- 1 medium orange: 39 mcg

Something's Fishy

You need to be a little careful about your seafood intake before and during pregnancy. Nearly all fish and shellfish contain traces of methylmercury—a compound known to be harmful in high doses to an unborn baby's or young child's developing nervous system. Unborn babies and children are more susceptible to the toxic effects of mercury than adults are, because their brains and nervous systems are rapidly developing.

Fish absorb methylmercury from the water they swim in and the food they eat. Larger predator fish accumulate the highest levels of methylmercury from their prey because they eat more fish that are higher up the food chain, and they tend to live longer. Methylmercury binds tightly to the **proteins** in fish muscle and remains there even after the fish is cooked. Mercury can hang around in your body for several weeks after you eat it, and in your **bloodstream** it can harm the neurological development of a fetus, so it is a good idea to ensure that your diet contains as little mercury as possible in the months before conception.

The FDA and the Environmental Protection Agency have guidelines for limiting exposure to mercury in fish. These guidelines are primarily for women who are trying to conceive, pregnant women, nursing mothers, and young children. They now advise eating no more than six ounces (about one serving) of canned albacore or "white" tuna a week and twelve ounces (about two servings) of canned "light" tuna and other cooked fish per week. Albacore tuna contains more mercury than the canned "light" variety, which can be relatively low in mercury. And you should completely avoid shark, swordfish, king mackerel, and tilefish (also called golden or white snapper), tuna steak (fresh or frozen), orange roughy, Spanish mackerel, marlin, and grouper because these fish are at the top of the food chain and contain the highest levels of mercury.

All this talk of mercury may give you the idea that you should avoid fish altogether while you're trying to get pregnant. Remember that fish is an excellent source of protein, vitamins, and omega-3 fatty acids—all of which are essential for your future baby's development. There's no reason to put the kibosh on all fish. There are plenty of other tasty varieties—salmon, rainbow trout, and canned mackerel, for instance—that contain low levels of mercury and are high in healthy fats. The FDA considers these fish safe for pregnant women to eat twice a week.

Brain Booster

The baby's brain continues to develop and grow rapidly throughout pregnancy. Some recent studies suggest that this growth and development can be boosted by a diet rich in omega-3 fatty acids. The richest sources of omega-3 fatty acids are fatty fish. Fish are the only source of all three omega-3 fatty acids.

There are three principal omega-3 fatty acids: alpha-linolenic acid (ALA), eicosapentaenoic acid (EPA), and docosahexaenoic acid (DHA; not to be confused with the other DHA, dihydroxyacetone, a self-tanning product ingredient mentioned earlier in the book). However, many of the fish that are rich in these fatty acids are also high in mercury, which can be harmful to the baby's developing nervous system. Pregnant women need to focus on the fish that are low in mercury yet rich in omega-3 fatty acids.

REAL LIFE QUESTION: Can I eat sushi if I'm pregnant?

Avoid sushi during pregnancy to avoid any potential bacteria. Women in Japan continue to eat sushi, but that doesn't mean you should have it here. There can also be mercury in the sashimi (the raw fish itself). So if you go out for sushi a lot socially, try all of the cooked pieces like California rolls. It's still the real thing and you can still enjoy an evening out. In really modern sushi places, where they are making combination sushi rolls that you love, just ask them to use shrimp or other cooked fish instead of sashimi.

Two good choices are salmon and anchovies. Wild salmon is particularly rich, but farm-raised salmon is also a good source. Other sources of omega-3 fatty acids include omega-3-enriched eggs, flaxseed, flaxseed oil, walnuts, and canola oil. These foods are all good sources of one omega-3: ALA.

Omega-3 supplements are another way to get all three essential fatty acids without the worry of mercury contamination. Some experts are now recommending that women who are trying to get pregnant, are pregnant, or are breastfeeding take an omega-3 supplement containing 200 milligrams of DHA. Some prenatal vitamins also contain some omega-3 fatty acids.

Iodine— Pass the Salt Please!

Shouldn't we all have plenty of iodine in our diet, seeing as iodine is in table salt? Not necessarily. Researchers have noted a trend of iodine deficiencies in the United States. Internationally, iodine deficiencies are more common in mountainous regions such as the Himalayas, the European Alps, and the Andes, where iodine has been washed away by glaciers and flooding.

In the United States, we started adding iodine to salt in the 1920s to help avoid certain widespread **thyroid** problems, including goiter, which is a swelling of the thyroid. Iodine deficiency was a serious health problem at that time, and since salt was on every dinner table, adding iodine to it was a perfect marriage. Since then, dietary iodine levels generally have been fine.

However, a large nutrition study in the United States found that iodine levels dropped in the early 1990s and that some people may now be at risk for deficiencies. This reduction in U.S. dietary iodine intake likely has two causes: new recommendations to cut salt intake for blood pressure control, and the use of designer salts, including sea salts. Many cooks prefer sea salt because of the taste and texture, but it has no iodine in it. Also, restaurants are not required to use iodized salt, and many of them don't.

To make matters worse, a recent study found that prenatal vitamins are inconsistent in their iodine content. The investigators found that the actual content of iodine in the prenatal vitamins studied was lower than the label indicated, especially when the iodine came from kelp. The researchers recommended that iodine in prenatal vitamins should come from potassium iodine, and that women trying to conceive and pregnant women should have at least 200 mcg and ideally 220 mcg in their diet. If you are taking a multivitamin, check the label and be sure yours has iodine in it from potassium iodine.

Iodine is essential in pregnancy because it's necessary for thyroid function, and the fetus depends on the mother for thyroid hormones early in pregnancy before its own thyroid has formed. Low thyroid levels in pregnant women—even very borderline deficiencies—have been linked with lower IQs and some neurocognitive disorders in their children. So check the label, and make sure your vitamins contain at least 200 mcg of iodine from potassium iodine. And pass the salt—please!

Hot Tubs— Don't Get Hot and Bothered

You should keep from getting overheated around the time of conception and during pregnancy. An increase in your core body temperature above 102.5 degrees Fahrenheit has been associated with increases in congenital anomalies (birth defects) in babies. Yes, your temperature goes up in a hot tub. Avoid hot tubs from ovulation onward.

Caffeine— Just a Bit Is Fine

It is a good idea to lower your caffeine intake before you get pregnant, but you don't need to entirely eliminate caffeine from your diet. Keep your intake at or below 150 mg of caffeine per day. There is approximately 100 mg of caffeine in a cup of coffee, 50 mg in tea, and 30 mg in a can of soda or a chocolate bar.

Large amounts of caffeine have been shown to increase the risk of miscarriage. There have been some associations between caffeine intake and difficulties conceiving for women. This has not, however, been a consistent finding in all studies. A small amount is fine, just don't overdo it.

Smoking— Now Is the Time to Stop

Any benefit you gain from following a healthy diet and lifestyle will be canceled if you smoke. Smoking is associated with low-birth-weight babies, increased risk of miscarriage, increased risk of death in the **uterus**, and, after the baby is born, increased incidence of sudden infant death syndrome (SIDS), as well as respiratory problems in children who breathe secondary smoke.

Smokers have higher rates of many **cancers** and cardiovascular diseases. If you smoke, now is the time to quit. It is the best thing you can do for your health and your future baby's health. It's your baby's first gift to you. Again, I know it's hard. Please be honest with your doctor about your smoking so that you can get some help quitting.

NOTE TO SELF

As soon as you have some baby names picked out, write them on a piece of paper and keep it in your pocket every day. Having this reminder of why you are quitting smoking will help when the urges are powerful. The names you list can be your baby's fantasy names, not necessarily the real one. You know what I mean—Little Princess Golda Meir or Little Prince Barack Obama—the names that nobody else knows. One patient's fantasy name belonged to a horse she loved. Yours can be anything you want, as long as it helps you stop smoking.

Alcohol

During the time before conception, when you are trying to conceive, alcohol can decrease fertility. Avoid alcohol from ovulation onward, until you know whether or not you have become pregnant in a given menstrual cycle.

An occasional drink during pregnancy carries no known risk, but because no level of drinking is known to be safe, it is probably best to avoid alcohol entirely. If you would like to cook with alcohol, simmering for approximately ten minutes will remove most of the alcohol content, which should make it safe to consume.

Don't be shocked if the world scorns you if you drink or smoke during pregnancy. Sure, Jackie Kennedy did it. So did your grandmother. Knowing what we know now, we shouldn't.

Drugs

This is easy for me to say and may be hard for you to do, but it's urgent. Do not use recreational drugs if you are trying to get pregnant! Speak with your doctor frankly if you need help. If you are addicted to drugs, it is nearly impossible—and dangerous, too—to quit on your own. Also check with your doctor if you are taking any over-the-counter drugs, including cold and headache medications, or prescription drugs.

Vaccinations

Before you get pregnant, take a minute to review your vaccinations with your doctor. Many vaccine boosters can't be given during pregnancy, so the time before conception is the ideal time to be sure you are up-to-date.

- **T-dap:** T-dap is a combination of three vaccines that protects against tetanus, diphtheria, and pertussis (whooping cough). Pertussis was once common among teens and young adults in the United States. This vaccine serves as a booster so you don't get it, and especially so newborn babies don't get it. It's especially important that new mothers are immune, so they don't pass a case on to their newborns.
- **Chicken pox (varicella):** If you had chicken pox as a child, you most likely have lifelong immunity and don't need this vaccine. However, if you had the vaccine as a child, and not the disease, then you might need a booster. Either way, have your doctor check with a blood test to be sure you are immune to chicken pox. Getting chicken pox in pregnancy can be serious, and it can also cause birth defects in the baby.
- **Human papillomavirus:** Ideally you've already had your series of three anti-HPV shots by now, but if not, get them before you get pregnant (it takes six months to get all three of the HPV vaccination shots in the series to become fully immunized), because you can't get the vaccine during pregnancy, and you need to get it before you turn

twenty-seven or your insurance won't pay for it—and it's expensive! If you happen to get pregnant before you are finished with the series of three, you can get the remainder after you have the baby.

- **Measles, mumps, rubella (MMR):** You probably had this vaccine as a child, but in some women the rubella immunity fades with time, so have your doctor check with a blood test to be sure yours is still good. If not, you need a booster, because rubella (German measles) can cause birth defects if you get it during pregnancy.

Fertile Ground: Increasing Your Chances of Getting Pregnant

You are finally ready to start a family. Planning ahead for pregnancy can have a big impact on the health of your future baby. A few simple diet and lifestyle adjustments can increase your chances for having a healthy pregnancy and a healthy baby.

Until now, you've probably spent a lot of years trying to not get pregnant. Now you need to reverse course and have sex when you have an active egg. Now that you are trying to get pregnant, learn to recognize the clues that your body provides and have sex on those days that are likeliest for conception. After ovulation, the egg lasts only about twenty-four hours. Sperm can live up to four or five days in your body, so having sex as much as five days before ovulation can result in pregnancy. Be sure to read chapter 14, Your Ovaries, for more detail.

Menstrual cycle lengths—the number of days from the first day of one period until the day before the next period—can vary from woman to woman. The average cycle is twenty-eight days, with ovulation on day fourteen, but cycles from twenty-one days to thirty-five days are normal. The range of days to ovulation is from twelve to sixteen days. So you need to estimate when your next menstrual period is due to start, then count backward from that day twelve to sixteen days. (The second half of the menstrual cycle tends to be more constant, which is why we recommend counting backward instead of forward.) Those are the days during which you are most likely to ovulate. This process can be a little unpredictable, but there are other signs and body changes to look for (as we discussed in chapter 15, Your Reproductive System), in addition to the calendar, that will help you recognize ovulation.

NOTE TO SELF

Learn the secret language of your body to find out when you are most fertile.

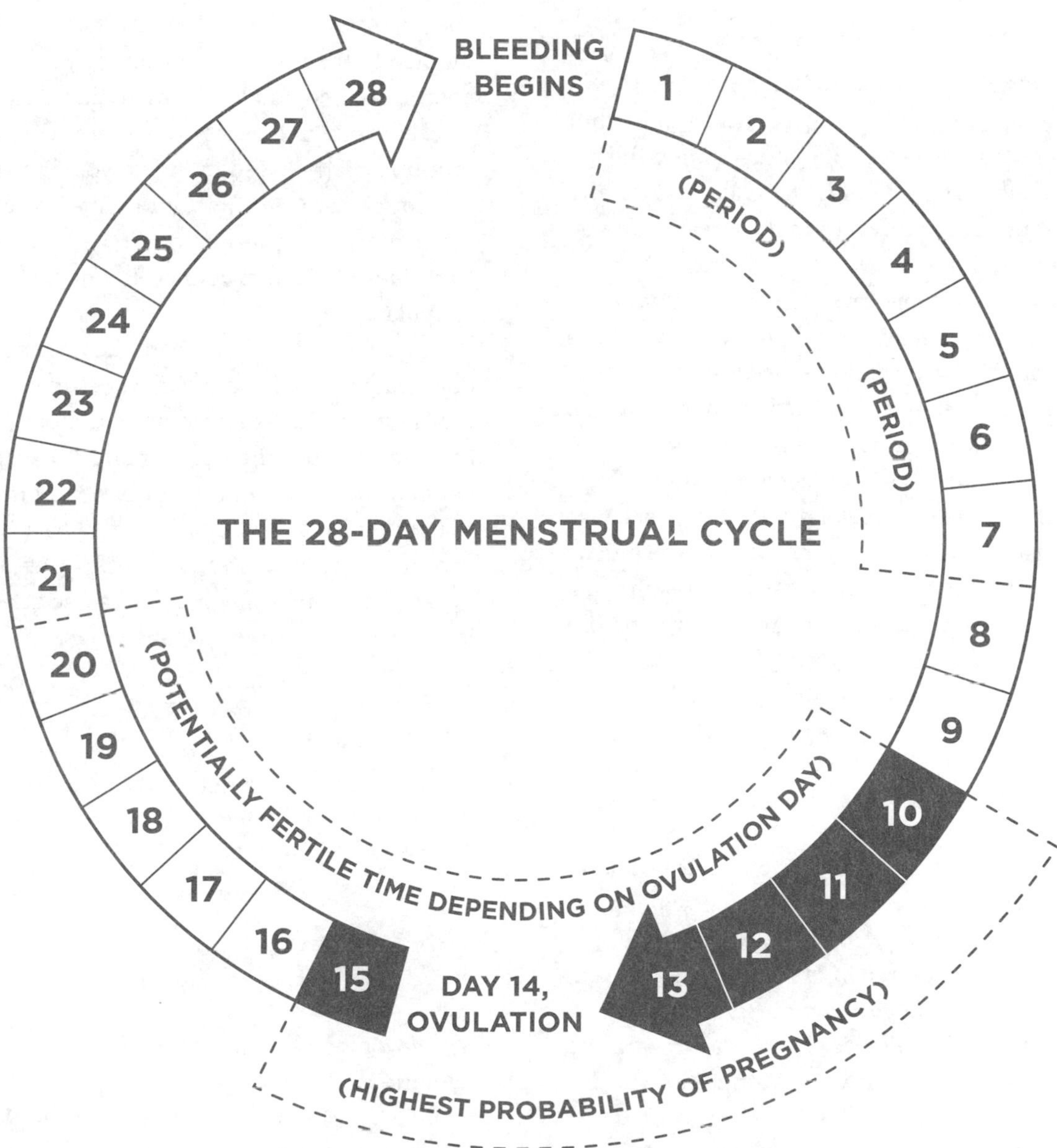

Timing it right: The average menstrual cycle is twenty-eight days, with ovulation happening on day fourteen (although ovulation can vary from day twelve to day sixteen). The egg lives for twenty-four hours and sperm can live for four to five days, so there's a period of up to five days during which you could become pregnant.

Meaningful Mucus

Cervical **mucus** is produced by your **cervix** (the opening to the uterus at the top of your **vagina**) and leaves your body through the vagina. It changes in amount, color, and texture throughout your cycle, and this can give you clues about when you're ovulating.

The first few days after menstruation this mucus is usually absent, followed by mucus that is sticky; it then changes to a creamy texture. As you approach ovulation, the mucus increases in amount, becomes thinner and clearer, and looks just like raw egg whites. Now is the time to get cooking, so to speak, because you are now fertile! After ovulation, the mucus dries up for about two weeks and results in a reduced amount of vaginal discharge before menstruation.

When You're Hot

Another fairly accurate way to track ovulation is to record your basal body temperature. Basal body temperature is your body temperature measured immediately after waking up, before you do any physical activity. Ovulation causes an increase of 0.5 to 1 degree Fahrenheit in your body temperature, so monitoring it with a very sensitive basal body temperature thermometer is one way of estimating the day before ovulation.

Just after ovulation your basal body temperature goes up and stays up for approximately the next twelve to sixteen days, until you menstruate. Because your temperature goes up after ovulation, you cannot use this method to time sex. If you wait for your temperature to rise, you'll miss ovulation. But you can keep track and use it to estimate ovulation in future cycles based on when you ovulated in prior cycles. Charting your temperature on a calendar over several months will give you some idea of when in your cycle you are likely to ovulate.

Start taking your temperature on the first day of a period at about the same time each morning. Keep the thermometer right at your bedside to reduce the need for any movement before taking your temperature. Record these temperatures on a graph to chart a line so you can more easily see temperature shifts. The lower temperature just before the rise at ovulation is the best time for conception.

NOTE TO SELF

During your highest fertility days, have sex every thirty-six hours. It increases your chances of conceiving.

Oh! My Aching Ovaries

Some women get a mild ache or pain during ovulation. About 20 percent of women can actually feel the release of an egg from their **ovary**. It's called mittelschmerz. But don't count on it alone to tell you when you're fertile, as so many things can cause little twinges of pain.

REAL LIFE FACT: On Trying to Get Pregnant

One patient said, "It took us six months to conceive, and we went about it enthusiastically—in the beginning. The freedom of unprotected sex every thirty-six hours was fabulous. But by the end, you don't feel that way so much, whether male or female. I went from telling my husband, "Come to bed, my darling love," to just sighing, "Oh, hurry up."

Stay Tuned

Tuning in to your body's clues and changes over three or four months will give you an idea of when ovulation probably will occur, so you can time sex to increase your chances of becoming pregnant. Don't get discouraged if it doesn't happen on the first few tries, even if your timing is right.

On average, couples have about a 30 percent chance of conceiving with unprotected sex per cycle, and it takes an average of four to six months for the average couple to conceive. If after a year of trying, or after six months if you are over thirty-five, no pregnancy occurs, it's a good idea to see your doctor to begin some preliminary investigation with both of you.

Pregnant Moment: Timing It Right

You should have sex daily, every other day, or, best of all, every thirty-six hours on days ten through twenty of your menstrual cycle to maximize your chances of timing it right to hit ovulation.

If you want to time things more exactly, you can use an over-the-counter ovulation predictor kit. Available without a prescription, ovulation predictor kits detect the surge in luteinizing hormone (LH), which signals the release of an egg, just before ovulation. They're easier to use and often more accurate than the basal body temperature method, and they can predict ovulation twenty-four to thirty-six hours in advance and help you time sex to maximize your chances of conception. Using an ovulation predictor kit, you should have sex on the day the kit shows the LH surge and again the next day.

When you are trying to get pregnant, sometimes all the pressure can take the fun out of sexuality. Using the ovulation kit can make it so there are only two days per month that you have to have sex. The others are up to you. But the kits are not foolproof. Sometimes false LH surges can take place before the real one, especially if your urine has become concentrated, such as from dehydration.

Age: How Old Is Too Old?

It's a fact that fertility decreases with age. We are born with a set number of eggs. Because no new ones are formed during your life, the number of eggs steadily declines over time. As you age, the quality of your eggs also goes down, resulting in a slow decline in pregnancy rates in the early thirties. The decline speeds up in the late thirties and early forties. Few women over forty-five are still fertile. Unfair as it may seem, the age of the male partner doesn't appear to matter nearly as much. Sperm from older men often have the same fertilizing potential as sperm from younger men.

This doesn't mean that you should run out and get pregnant right now if you are twenty-nine. But you should understand the facts. Every woman's body ages at its own rate, and there is no way of knowing for sure what your fertility will be like, say, ten years from now. You want to wait until you are ready to make such a big choice, but you can't wait forever. Despite all the choices that have opened up to women in the last few decades, there remains one enduring fact. The biological clock never quits ticking. The difficult truth is that as women age, fertility declines.

Where I live, many women have their babies in their thirties and even early forties. School meetings look like grandmother conventions. These women are more exhausted by raising children than a thirty-year-old would be, true. But their choices work for them and their lives, and they seem very happy. The child's teenage years seem to be the toughest, because by then Mom is going through **menopause** and will not be easy-breezy while giving driving lessons.

Egg Freezing and Other High-Tech Options for Fertility

It's the ultimate career woman's dream: work now; conceive later. Can this be possible? There are advanced technologies that can help you have a baby when nature doesn't work out. In vitro fertilization (IVF) is a method of assisted reproductive technology that combines an egg with sperm in a laboratory dish. If the egg is fertilized and begins cell division, the resulting **embryo** is transferred to the woman's uterus where it will, if all goes well, implant in the uterine lining and develop into a baby. IVF may be performed in conjunction with medications that stimulate the ovaries to produce multiple eggs, to increase the chances of successful fertilization and implantation. If more embryos are produced than are needed, the extra ones can be frozen for future use.

Assisted reproductive technologies such as IVF have given older women some hope of pregnancy when nature has quit and gone home, but even this runs up against the physiological limitation of aging eggs. No one understands exactly what happens to eggs after several decades of waiting in the body. When you are twenty, 90 percent of your eggs are normal. By the time you are forty, 90 percent of your eggs are abnormal, meaning they won't be able to grow into a pregnancy.

Is it possible to prevent eggs from aging, to keep them frozen in time until you are ready to use them? By freezing eggs instead of embryos, you eliminate the need for a partner before taking action. Has technology advanced enough to allow eggs that last forever? Promising research is going on now, but we are not yet ready to offer this option routinely to all women.

The trouble is that eggs are more difficult to freeze than sperm or embryos. Because they are comparatively large single cells filled with water, eggs are particularly vulnerable to the formation of ice crystals. Researchers have tinkered with the formula for decades, with some successes, but none have been consistently successful.

Very recently, though, Italian scientists have perfected a slow-freezing method that takes the temperature of the egg down a couple of degrees per second. And they've developed a new recipe for a cryoprotectant solution (liquid to protect eggs during freezing) that includes just the right amount of **nutrients**. With their techniques, they've averaged a 17 percent pregnancy rate from frozen eggs. This is actually close to the success rate with frozen embryos, which is a much more mainstream practice.

Egg freezing is an expensive bet—and far from a guarantee. It's usually better, if possible, to have the "baby conversation" with your partner sooner than later and find a way to balance work and family together.

Passing the Pregnancy Test: How to Find Out

Your period is late. Are you pregnant? Today, you can find out in the privacy of home with highly sensitive and accurate urine pregnancy tests.

Home pregnancy tests measure the presence of a telltale hormone in your urine called **human chorionic gonadotropin (HCG)**. This hormone, produced by cells from the placenta, first gets into your bloodstream when the fertilized egg implants in your uterus, about six days after fertilization. The amount of HCG in your body then increases rapidly over the next few weeks, doubling about every two days. By fourteen days after fertilization, around the time you would expect your period, some home pregnancy tests may be able to detect the hormone in your urine and give you a positive result. Some can even detect it a few days before then. Home pregnancy tests have improved over time and are very sensitive, even to low levels of pregnancy hormones.

Be sure to check the expiration date on the urine pregnancy test and make sure it's still valid, especially if you've had it around for a while. If you've been storing the test anywhere that gets moist or warm (like the bathroom), it may have deteriorated, so it's best to throw it away and get a new one. When you're ready to test, read the directions carefully because they'll vary with different brands. Some require you to urinate in a cup and then, using a supplied dropper, place a small sample in a testing well. Others let you pee directly onto a stick.

The tests also vary in how they display results. Some show pink or blue lines on the test strip. Others show a red plus or minus sign in a window. Most have a control indicator (often a second line or symbol) that's supposed to indicate whether the test is valid. If the control indicator doesn't show up properly, the test may be faulty. If the test shows a negative result, wait another few days or a week and try again if you still haven't gotten your period. If you ovulated later in your cycle than you thought, you may have taken the test too early to get a positive result. For best results, try taking the test first thing in the morning, when your urine is most concentrated.

NOTE TO SELF

If you are pregnant, don't ignore abdominal pain or abnormal bleeding. You might have an ectopic pregnancy.

Pregnancy Tests Are Not Always Perfect

Whatever you do, don't assume that one negative result means you're not pregnant. If you don't get your period as expected, remember that you still might be pregnant. Using first morning urine is a good way to make sure the HCG in your urine is concentrated, making it easier for the pregnancy test to return a positive result if you are pregnant. If you want to test in the middle of the day, you will want to limit fluid intake for several hours to make sure your urine is not diluted.

If you have been at this for a while, and get a negative result, talk with your doctor about it. Generally, doctors advise doing some fertility testing after a year of trying if you are under thirty-five, or after six months if you are older than thirty-five.

False Positives

If the test says you're pregnant but you're not, this is called a false positive. Sometimes the test is just wrong. Sometimes, though, you get an early positive result and then get your period soon after. In this case, you may have had what's called a chemical pregnancy. That means a fertilized egg implanted in your uterus and developed just enough to start producing HCG but then stopped developing for some reason. This happens with about 30 to 50 percent of all fertilized eggs; for some reason they're incapable of developing into and surviving as an embryo.

If you have a false positive result, you'll go on to get your period (though it may be a little heavier and a few days later than usual). Your chances of having a false positive are lower if you wait to take the test until a week after your period is due.

Take Charge of Your Future Fertility Today

Although age is a vital factor in your ability to conceive, it's not the only one. There are proactive, effective measures that you can start using now to help preserve your fertility later on and help to ensure the health of your babies.

By planning ahead, you can start taking charge of your future fertility today, and you can maximize both your own health and your future baby's with these simple steps for living healthy. It's easy to forget that in the past there were many potential problems during pregnancy. Today we assume that any risks are taken care of by vaccines and vitamins. These help, but you have to do your part by living healthy—for yourself and for your future babies. Start today.

In the next chapter, we'll look at diet and talk about what you should eat and drink in order to keep all of your body's systems healthy and humming along.

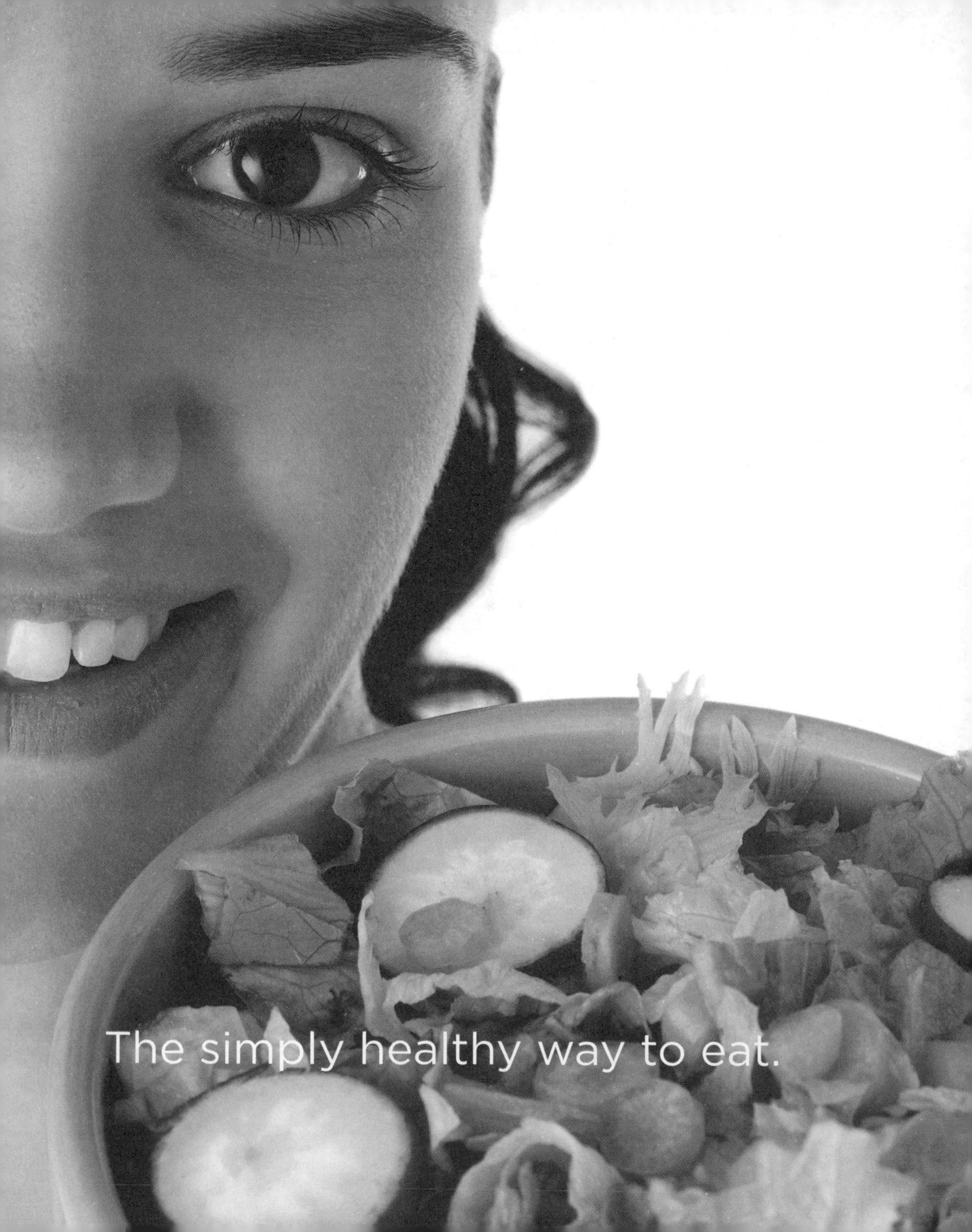
The simply healthy way to eat.

your diet

Where do you get your information about healthy diets? Maybe you start

with the U.S. Food and Drug Administration (FDA) food pyramid—and then read a hundred articles by nutritionists who say they don't like it. Maybe you follow the advice given in health magazines—and then realize that those same magazines are filled with two-thousand-calorie cake recipes that you can't resist making. Maybe you follow the tips mentioned on a TV show or by a celebrity who had a team of five people helping her to lose five pounds. Or maybe you follow any program that has good before-and-after photos. I'll let you in on a secret: those "afters" also had a team to help them get to their goal weight and, once they did, that team dropped them like a hot, twice-baked, butter, sour cream, and bacon potato.

Why does it seem so complicated to have a good way of eating? Because every day you see a new report on what you *should* be eating. One day it's butter and bacon, and the next it's cabbage soup. There are celebrity diets, celebrity mom diets, French diets, Mediterranean diets, all-grapefruit diets—you name it, it's got a diet, from high protein/low carbohydrate to low fat/high carbohydrate, and everything in between. Google the

NOTE TO SELF

Don't know what to eat? This chapter gives you a personal recipe for good health.

phrase "diet plans" and you'll get millions of results.

It can be difficult and confusing to know what's best for you. So in this chapter, I'll sift through the media noise to help you understand what the latest research has shown to be the healthiest style of eating.

NOTE TO SELF

The days of the low-fat diet are over!

Back to Basics: Simply Healthy Eating

When you eat for health, other issues, such as weight, tend to take care of themselves. It's true—forget about the scale and focus on the food. Let's talk about how to do it.

If you've tried a few diets, that not what you'll find here. This is a plan for life. Any diet that causes you to obsess on certain foods or forbids others creates a stressful anxiety about food—and you know by now what I think of stress. No more diets that make you feel obsessed about food and every morsel you eat.

I also want you to eat enough. I don't want you starving yourself at 1,000 calories a day, or even 1,200. You should know by now that your body goes into "famine" mode when you do that, and you will only gain more weight when you go back to normal eating. For anyone who is concerned about health or weight, the plan I'll describe is simple and inclusive, and it works.

So what am I recommending? That you adopt a new way of normal eating. Forget the low-calorie craziness and focus on *learning*. It works, it lasts a lifetime, and it has room for chocolate. A healthy diet consists of a wide range of whole grains, healthy fats, lean proteins, and fresh fruits and vegetables. On a healthy diet you greatly reduce your unhealthy saturated and **trans fats**, **cholesterol**, sugar, and alcohol. Recent research has shown that the recipe for health consists of a moderate amount of unrefined **carbohydrate**, a moderate amount of protein, and a moderate amount of unsaturated fat. The days of the low-fat diet are over. Scientific evidence has suggested that a low-fat diet is not necessary for health, as long as the fats you eat are from healthy sources.

NOTE TO SELF

Eating disorders are a serious, complicated problem. But they are *not* about food. See chapter 2, Your Head, for more information.

How to Create Your Simply Healthy Eating Style

Eat fruit two or three times per day. Eat mountains of vegetables, just limit the starchy ones like potatoes. Choose healthier sources of proteins, like beans, nuts, fish, poultry, and eggs. Eat legumes (a fancy word for beans, peanuts, and peas). Legumes are plants that make edible seeds or seed pods, aboveground or under. Have legumes one to three times per day. Fish, poultry, and eggs are healthy proteins that you should try to incorporate into your diet up to twice a day. (Choose low-mercury fish like salmon or anchovies.) Limit red meat to once a week. Emphasize healthy fats, such as olive oil.

Create your own "use sparingly" category. This list will include your hot-button foods, as well as my list. I'll start with red meat, butter, white rice, white bread, potatoes, pasta, and sweets. Now add your own items. For many people, that's some kind of chips. "Use sparingly" means that you buy the little bag, not the big one. See? You're not banning them for life, you're just reserving them for the occasional meal or side dish.

What happens when you ban a food for life ("I will *never* eat chocolate *again*!")? You will think about nothing but chocolate. You'll dream about it. Life will be one long day of fasting that never ends. The stress on you and your body will eventually weigh on you and you will end up eating bags of chocolate chips for breakfast, lunch, and dinner, and nothing else, for days.

NOTE TO SELF

Mom was right about vegetables (and fruit, too)!

Eat Your Fruits and Veggies

Over the past thirty years, research has backed up what generations of mothers knew. Eating plenty of fruits and vegetables can help to prevent **heart disease**, **stroke**, high blood pressure, high cholesterol, and **cancer**.

Most of us don't eat enough of these. Americans eat, on average, a total of just three servings of fruits and vegetables a day. We should aim for about nine servings a day. If this seems impossible, keep in mind that increasing your fruit and vegetable intake by as little as one serving per day can have a real impact on your heart disease risk. So do the best you can, because studies show that for every extra serving of fruits and vegetables added to your diet, the risk of heart disease drops by 4 percent.

A diet rich in fruits and vegetables can lower blood pressure. The Dietary Approaches to Stop Hypertension (DASH) trial looked at the effect on blood pressure of a diet that emphasized fruits, vegetables, and low-fat dairy products and restricted the amount of saturated and total fat. The researchers found that people with high blood pressure who followed this diet reduced their systolic blood pressure (the upper number of a blood pressure reading) by about 11 and their diastolic blood pressure (the lower number) by almost 6—that's as much as medications can achieve, and the DASH eaters did it without any medicine or side effects.

People with the highest daily consumption of fruits and vegetables (more than four servings a day) have significantly lower levels of **LDL** (bad cholesterol) than those with lower consumption. How fruits and vegetables lower cholesterol is still something of a mystery. It's possible that eating more fruits and vegetables means eating less meat and dairy products, and therefore less cholesterol-boosting **saturated fat**. Soluble fiber in fruits and vegetables may also block the absorption of cholesterol from food.

Studies also reveal a link between eating fruits and vegetables and protection against cancer. Fruits and vegetables are clearly an important part of a good diet. Almost everyone can benefit from eating more of them, but variety is as important as quantity. No single fruit or vegetable provides all of the **nutrients** you need to be healthy. The key lies in the variety of different fruits and vegetables that you eat.

When you buy fruits and vegetables that are in season, you'll pay less for them. Local fruits and veggies have far less distance to travel and will always be fresher than those that have a long journey to your store. You won't find a local pineapple in Maine, but if you love pineapple, I think you should buy it. How do you know what's in season? Shop at local farms and farmers' markets, or ask for help. The rising and dropping prices of produce will also tell you what's coming in and going out of season.

So start by listing all of the fruits and vegetables that you like. If you give this a chance you'll find that you really do like some, especially if you use creative recipes. One patient refused to eat salads at all, until she tried adding grapes and a few pistachios to one and liked it. With that one simple recipe, she made a major change in her diet.

Buying Fresh Fruit and Cooking Veggies

Learning how to buy fresh fruit and cook fresh vegetables takes some time and practice. Sometimes it's hard to find ripe fruit in supermarkets. It can be easier in natural food stores or at farmers' markets, but not always. When you're new at this, you'll often be disappointed with what you bring home. Shopping once a week means that some of it will go bad, and it will bother you to be wasting money.

Here are some tips. Buy your bananas mostly yellow, with a little green. They'll ripen quickly and by the end of your week they'll be incredibly ripe and sweet—it doesn't matter that the peel is black if you're adding it to your cereal. Oranges and apples are usually sold already ripe, just don't buy ones that are too squishy or smell bad.

Summer fruits are the hardest to buy. A peach that looks perfect today may be a mushy mess by tomorrow. How to avoid that waste of money? Be flexible about your menu planning. If you wanted to eat your peaches tomorrow, eat them today instead. Save the plums for tomorrow. Watch these fruits closely and remember that everybody loses a little summer fruit to ripening sometimes.

Berries are delicate and don't keep well, so you should buy them when you're about to use them, especially raspberries and straw-

REAL LIFE FACT: Some Veggie Tips

Cilantro and flat parsley look similar. You have to learn to smell them to tell them apart. And if a recipe calls for fresh ginger, you have to buy a little branch of it in the veggie section, not the ground version in the spices, which is used in baking.

berries. Don't wash them until you eat them either, or they'll go soggy. Blueberries last a little longer. Whenever you buy berries, look through the package for any sign of mold. Don't buy any fruit that has the slightest sign of it. It spreads very quickly and can ruin a pineapple in an afternoon.

Melons take a little more expertise. Eventually, you will know how to smell a melon and tell if it's ready for eating. In the meantime, ask the people in the fruit section of your grocery store or the grower at your farmers' market for help. In a pinch, buy the melons already cut up. It's more expensive, but if you're hosting a morning meeting and want to be sure the fruit is ripe, it might be worth it.

Should you refrigerate fruit? I think it depends on your climate. Chefs have strong opinions on the subject, but if you live where it's hot, refrigerate. (Except for tomatoes. Leave them out because refrigeration kills the flavor and they won't mind the heat.) If you want something to ripen faster, keep it in a brown paper bag on your countertop and check it twice a day to see how it's doing.

Buying vegetables is simpler than buying fruit. Look for any signs of rotting and avoid it. If the vegetable is supposed to be crisp, like celery, buy it crisp. If a potato is mushy before you buy it, it's going to taste gross after you cook it. Unlike fruit, vegetables in the store are usually already ripe, except for avocados, which are actually a fruit. If an avocado is hard when you press it gently, it's not ripe. Don't plan a fancy dinner around avocados unless you have time for them to ripen, which can take up to a week!

Once you have your vegetables home, put them away without washing them because washing encourages mold. You can store your vegetables in the fridge (except your tomatoes, which are really a fruit).

How do you prepare veggies? Steaming is the healthiest way to cook them, but the most important thing is to use just a little bit of water with a dash of salt to bring out the flavor. (And cook them for far less time than your grandma did.) How soft or crunchy do you like your veggies to be? Think about that and then cook them that way. For green vegetables and corn, cook them gently until they are tender and turn bright green (well, except for the corn). Don't overcook! Stop cooking when they are still a little crisp. For veggies like squash and potatoes, it's the opposite. You want to cook them until they are soft and a fork goes in easily.

Now start to have some fun and get a veggie cookbook or download recipes online. If you are groaning because you don't find it fun to cook, you can make the routine of it less boring by trying new things. It really can be fun to cook. Sometimes.

Anything you can do to help you eat more vegetables is good—except deep-frying them or adding a ton of butter. Ignore people who tell you to only buy fresh and never frozen, because they clearly have more time than you do to shop and cook. And you don't have to spend half an hour trimming artichokes for a weeknight dinner. Keep it simple and do what works best for you.

Prodigious Protein

It doesn't take much protein to meet your basic daily needs—about 50 grams of protein daily, or a little less than half a cup! In the United States and other developed countries, getting the minimum daily requirement of protein is fairly easy: Cereal with milk for breakfast, a turkey sandwich for lunch, and a piece of fish for dinner add up to about 70 grams of protein. Actually, the typical adult in the United States eats from 75 to 110 grams per day.

Good protein choices include chicken, fish, and vegetarian sources like nuts and beans. Eat less red meat and choose low-fat or nonfat dairy products.

The Right Protein for You

Although you'll have no problem filling your protein requirement, you should try to get protein from heart-healthy sources that are low in saturated fat and cholesterol. It's never too early to practice heart-healthy eating habits by choosing proteins that are low in saturated fats. Beef and whole-milk dairy products contain saturated fats. Heart-healthy alternatives include fish, skinless poultry, beans, nuts, tofu, quinoa, low-fat or nonfat dairy products, and soy milk.

Beef is not forbidden, it just makes good sense to limit your intake to once per week. Choose the lean varieties and trim the fat before cooking. If I had a big problem with

REAL LIFE FACT: Protein Malnutrition

Millions of people around the world don't get enough protein. Protein malnutrition leads to the condition known as kwashiorkor. Lack of protein can cause growth failure and serious health problems.

REAL LIFE FACT: Some Problems with Protein

Too much protein, such as in a low-carb/high-protein diet, can cause some health issues. Digestion of protein releases acids that your body neutralizes with calcium, some of which may be pulled from your bones. Over many months, a high-protein diet can weaken your bones, because your bones serve as a reservoir for calcium in your body. So it's not a good idea to go overboard on protein in your diet.

those restrictions, I would limit my beef to a really fabulous once-a-month steak or burger, and I wouldn't worry about the nutritional value. I would just plain enjoy it.

That's one of the pleasures of a healthy life: you can blow it at a restaurant occasionally and not ruin your body when you do, because you've got such a good base. See? You're not on a diet, you're building a new way of life. The truth is, this is how people live and maintain a healthy weight. They eat a good everyday base so that a restaurant dessert now and then doesn't matter.

So, for everyday eating, serve chicken with the skin removed. It lowers the saturated fat content. Try to use beans in cooking. They are heart-healthy and cheap. Eat fish at least twice a week. Fish and shellfish are low in fat and cholesterol compared to beef, chicken, and dairy products. To save money, buy whatever low-mercury fish is on sale, like salmon, canned light tuna, pollock, catfish, and anchovies.

Although shellfish, like lobster, have a reputation for being high in cholesterol, that's changing. The American Heart Association now considers shrimp, with about 150 mg of cholesterol in 3½ ounces, an acceptable alternative to red meat. Even lobster, which many cholesterol-limited diets have forbidden, has only 70 to 95 mg of cholesterol per 3½ ounces. Compare that with an egg, with about 200 mg of cholesterol, or 3½ ounces of hamburger, with 100 mg. The key here, as always, is moderation. And the occasional restaurant splurge!

Protein for Vegetarians

Complete proteins contain all of the essential **amino acids**, which are the building blocks of protein needed by your body. Incomplete proteins lack one or more amino acids that your body can't make. Animal sources of protein tend to be complete, while vegetarian proteins are often incomplete and therefore need to be combined to complete the amino acid profile.

Incomplete proteins usually come from fruits, vegetables, grains, and nuts. Rice and beans, for example, are each high in the essential amino acid that the other is low in. That's very interesting, given how much of the world eats rice and beans together for many meals. Other plant proteins, such as quinoa and soybeans, are complete proteins by themselves.

To get all the amino acids needed in order to keep your body running well, you must eat a variety of protein-containing foods every day. You don't need to eat them at the same meal to complete the protein! We used to think so, but it's been disproved.

A vegetarian diet can be a very healthy diet when a variety of foods are eaten. Vegetarians and vegans need to be mindful of getting enough protein if it all comes from vegetable sources. You may need to eat more than the recommended amount of protein because you'll need extra protein in this case.

Go Nuts

Nuts are a terrific source of protein. An ounce of nuts contains about 8 grams of protein, and they are rich in healthy unsaturated fats. Studies show that people who regularly eat nuts are less likely to have heart attacks or die from heart disease than people who rarely eat them. The unsaturated fats in nuts help lower **LDL** (bad cholesterol) and raise **HDL** (good cholesterol).

Nuts are rich in arginine, an amino acid needed to make a molecule called nitric oxide, which relaxes constricted blood vessels and eases blood flow. They also contain vitamin E, folic acid, potassium, fiber, and other healthy nutrients. Walnuts, in particular, are rich in healthy omega-3 fatty acids.

You need to be a little careful with nuts, as they are also high in calories. Don't add nuts to what you're already eating, substitute nuts for other protein sources. Simply adding a serving of nuts a day will add too many calories and you'll gain weight. This increase in weight will increase your risk of heart disease and offset any health benefit you obtain from consuming them.

If you are one of the rare few who can eat a few nuts and not a whole bagful, go ahead! Otherwise, use them to supply protein.

Soy Solutions

Tofu, soybeans, edamame, soy milk, and other soy products are excellent and versatile protein choices. Soy is growing in popularity and general acceptance as our knowledge about its health benefits grows. Soy foods are good for your heart and blood vessels because they usually replace less healthful choices, like red meat, and because they deliver plenty of polyunsaturated fat, fiber, vitamins, and minerals and are low in saturated fat.

Sometimes soy products take a little getting used to. But one great thing about tofu is that it takes on the flavor of whatever you cook it with. Try marinating it in your favorite sauce and it'll taste like that sauce. Remember that most tofu cooks better if you drain it first. Put a heavy plate on top of it and let the liquid run off.

How Fat in Your Diet Affects Your Health

The fat content of your diet affects your blood cholesterol level—up or down—which in turn affects your risk of developing coronary artery disease, up or down. Cholesterol can be left on the walls of your blood vessels and lead to heart disease and circulatory problems. A high blood-cholesterol level (200 mg or more) is a well-established risk factor for heart disease.

Although cholesterol comes from your diet, it's also produced in your **liver**. This synthesis happens no matter what you eat, but it can also be influenced by the amount of saturated and trans fats in your diet. The amount your body makes is often genetically inherited, so you can't completely control your cholesterol level through your diet. But your diet can strongly affect it.

During digestion, fats are joined with other proteins for distribution to the rest of your body from your **intestines**. Fats are combined with proteins for their journey in the blood. These lipid-protein complexes, called **lipoproteins**, come in a few varieties: high-density lipoproteins (HDL) and low-density lipoproteins (LDL). High levels of HDL, which carry cholesterol to the liver, are associated with a lower risk of heart disease, while high levels of LDL are associated with a higher risk of heart disease. We think of HDL as the "good cholesterol" and LDL as the "bad cholesterol." Checking your cholesterol and lipid levels starts with checking your HDL level as well as your cholesterol level, beginning at age twenty and every five years after that. Levels of LDL and **triglycerides** may be added to the test list if your cholesterol is high or your HDL is low.

Feel like you've heard all this before? I'm stressing this message so strongly that I've included it in a few different chapters.

REAL LIFE FACT: Breast Cancer Risk and Dietary Fat

More confusion! There has been a great deal of news about the role of fat in your diet and future risk of breast cancer. Recent scientific studies suggest that rates of breast cancer are increased in women when they eat a diet high in saturated fat, but not a diet high in unsaturated fat like olive oil and canola oil. It's the *type* of fat, not the total fat content in the diet that affects breast cancer risk. However, much more research is needed to understand this connection more clearly. **(See more about this in chapter 12, Your Breasts.)**

REAL LIFE FACT: Where's the Beef?

If you're hooked on having a great steak a couple of times a week, try having it less often—and make sure it's a really great one. Beef can still be part of a heart-healthy diet if you eat it about once a week. Certain cuts of beef are lower in saturated fat than others. Leaner choices for beef include tenderloin, sirloin, flank steak, and hamburger with less than 12 percent fat. Trim all the visible fat from any beef you cook. And always remember portion size—a good rule of thumb is to have your portion size about the size of a deck of cards. Savor the taste and eat it slowly.

Not All Fat Is Bad! Here's How to Tell the Difference

There is now clear scientific evidence that it's not the total amount of fat in your diet, but the type of fat you eat, that determines your risk of heart disease and ill health. The latest data suggests that not all fats are bad and, in fact, many fats should be included in a healthy diet. These include monounsaturated and polyunsaturated fats found in such foods as nuts, avocados, fish, olives, and vegetable oils. (This is a shift from the previous popular view, in which a reduction in the total percentage of calories from fat to 30 percent was the number one nutritional priority.)

Eating unsaturated fats (both monounsaturated and polyunsaturated) has been shown to protect against the development of heart disease and is now considered part of a heart-healthy diet.

To eat healthy fats, you need to replace saturated fat—found mainly in animal products such as meat, butter, whole milk, and cream—with unsaturated fats. Safflower oil, sunflower oil , corn oil, and soybean oil are high in polyunsaturated fats. Canola oil and olive oil are good sources of monounsaturated fats.

To make the majority of fat in your diet the healthy type, you will need to make the right choices in the types of meats, dairy products, and other proteins in your diet. Choose the majority of your protein from fish, beans, skinless chicken, and tofu instead of beef, which is high in saturated fat. When choosing dairy products, choose nonfat milk and yogurt and low-fat cheeses instead of whole-milk products—the nutritional benefits from protein and calcium are the same without the saturated fat. Some people switch easily to skim milk, others need to adjust gradually. Just mix your whole milk with a little skim milk, and gradually add more skim until you've changed completely. Once you get used to skim, whole milk tastes like cream. Substitute nuts for some or all of the beef or other meat in your favorite recipes. Use beans and tofu liberally as protein sources instead of, or to partially replace, beef and pork.

It's never too early or too late in life to think about the saturated fat and cholesterol levels in your diet. **Atherosclerosis** (clogged **arteries**) starts to develop even in young people and can lead not only to heart attack but also to stroke. It therefore makes good sense to keep your diet low in saturated fat and cholesterol, and to include healthy mono- and polyunsaturated fats.

Trans Fats and Hydrogenated Fats—The Bad Guys

Trans fats and hydrogenated fats are two types of unhealthy fats found in food as a result of chemical processing. These fats have been found to promote heart disease even more than saturated fats do.

What are they? In hydrogenated fat, hydrogen has been added to the fat to make a liquid into a solid (margarine is an example). If you are interested in chemistry, this means that unsaturated bonds—the forces that hold atoms together—are changed to saturated bonds. Poof! Solid fat.

Trans fat is also a chemically processed fat; in this case, the natural position of hydrogen (called cis) is changed to an unnatural position (called trans). It's mainly used to prolong the shelf life of baked goods. Fast food is loaded with trans fats.

NOTE TO SELF

Trans fat may be the most dangerous of all fats, because there are studies showing that it lowers good cholesterol and increases bad cholesterol.

Recent evidence has shown that eating trans and hydrogenated fats is really bad for you. They have adverse effects on your cholesterol, meaning that they raise LDL (the bad

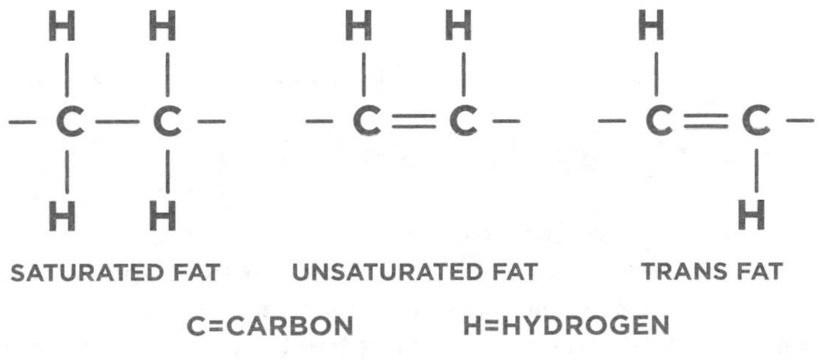

```
 H   H        H   H        H
 |   |        |   |        |
-C — C-     - C = C -    - C = C -
 |   |                         |
 H   H                         H
```

SATURATED FAT UNSATURATED FAT TRANS FAT

C=CARBON H=HYDROGEN

Fat chemistry 101: The type of fat you eat—not the total amount—is what determines your risk of heart disease and ill health. On a chemical level, saturated fats contain carbon (C) atoms filled with hydrogen (H) atoms. Trans fats are created by moving the hydrogen atoms to an unnatural position relative to the carbon atoms. Unsaturated fats are the good ones and are part of a heart-healthy diet.

REAL LIFE QUESTION: Are açai berries a weight-loss miracle?

Açai berries are a good source of antioxidants, but please don't take any supplements that promise weight loss for life. "Miracle" supplements get popular every year and then fade away. It's fine to take it if it's healthy. Otherwise, skip it. It won't work.

cholesterol), lower HDL (the good cholesterol), and increase triglycerides. This terrible trio—high LDL, low HDL, and increased triglycerides—is a bad combination for your heart.

Check the labels of any processed food you buy. That energy bar? Its chocolate may be held together by hydrogenated oil. The snack aisle at the grocery store? Ouch. As one patient says, "I know I'm in trouble when the snack bags start to talk to me. They tell me they have no trans fats, but then it turns out they still have hydrogenated oils or maybe Mother Nature's killer plan, palm and coconut oil. The only way I can avoid this mess is to walk away. I skip the snack aisle entirely. Pretty soon, the grocery stores will figure this out. They'll start putting something I need, like toilet paper, right in the middle of the snacks."

By the way, don't believe all of the Internet hype saying that palm and coconut oils are good. Many of these claims are found on websites selling these oils. While there are studies finding some benefits, the hype is way ahead of the science. Avoid them until an independent, scientific research project on humans is complete.

REAL LIFE FACT: Consumer Warning

Avoid any website that says, "You can try it for one month absolutely free"—no matter what "it" is. They will ask you for your credit card number "just to cover the shipping and handling." And at the end of one month, you will find yourself signed up for monthly delivery for the rest of your life. They will never let you cancel. One friend of mine had to change her credit card—it was the only way to stop the monthly charges.

If you do an Internet search for "açai," you'll even find one site that claims to be a scam report. The web address says that it's CNN, but it's not CNN at all—it's another scam site! Right now there are scams for açai berries and colon cleansers, but there will be new ones coming soon.

REAL LIFE QUESTION: Does a can of tuna count?

Tuna is a good thing to eat, but it doesn't count much toward your omega-3 goal. The fatty acids are reduced during the cooking process. Still, enjoy it as a healthy meal. Choose "light" tuna to reduce the amount of mercury.

Omega-3 Fatty Acids—The Good Guys, and Not Only for Your Heart!

Omega-3 fatty acids have many health benefits. There are three principal omega-3 fatty acids: alpha-linolenic acid (ALA), eicosapentaenoic acid (EPA), and docosahexaenoic acid (DHA). ALA is found in large amounts in flaxseed and flaxseed oil, and in smaller amounts in soybean and canola oils. EPA and DHA are found mainly in fatty, cold-water fish, such as salmon, tuna, swordfish, mackerel, anchovies, bluefish, and striped bass. Eating one to two servings of fatty fish a week has been shown to significantly lower LDL (bad cholesterol), raise HDL (good cholesterol), and lower levels of triglycerides. That's good fat.

The health benefits from omega-3 fatty acids can be seen for heart disease, cancer, **arthritis**, depression, and **diabetes**. Omega-3 fatty acids appear to decrease heart disease because they are natural blood thinners. They also appear to decrease **cardiac arrhythmias**. Eating omega-3 fatty acids can also help prevent the buildup of cholesterol-laden **plaques** that can clog the arteries and lead to heart attack and stroke.

The proposed theory for the protective effect in cancer prevention is that omega-3 fatty acids affect **prostaglandins** in a way that improves the immune response, blood supply, and cell membrane integrity, decreasing cancer cell growth. Keep in mind that this is a new field of study and the reasons for some of the other omega-3 health benefits are not totally clear.

Although there has been some recent concern about contaminants in fish, such as mercury and PCBs (a group of toxic industrial waste products that can contaminate fish), the overwhelming evidence suggests that the proven health benefits of fish consumption are much greater than the potential for harm. And eating fish may help prevent heart disease by replacing red meat or other less healthy sources of protein. Eat at least two servings of fish a week.

The main exception to this recommendation is for women who are or might become pregnant, nursing mothers, and young children. These groups should still include fish in their diets, but should not eat fish high in mercury (see page 351). They should instead limit seafood to two servings per week of fish that have low mercury levels yet are good sources of omega-3 fats, such as salmon, canned light tuna (light albacore tuna has more mercury than canned light tuna, according to the U.S. Food and Drug Administration), pollock, catfish, and anchovies. (I've never actually seen a child eat an anchovy, but maybe yours will.)

If you're a vegetarian and don't eat fish, you can get omega-3 fatty acids from canola oil, walnuts, and omega-3-enriched eggs. Omega-3 fatty acids are also found in flaxseed and flaxseed oil. Be aware that flaxseed has a hard outer coating, so it needs to be ground before you consume it, or it will pass through your body undigested. You can also take a DHA supplement to get that fish-specific omega-3 fatty acid (but read the sidebar on taking fish oil supplements, above, for some things to consider before you start).

NOTE TO SELF

No matter what the fad diets say, some carbs are good for you!

The Anticarb Craze

The popularity of the Atkins diet and the South Beach diet has created a lot of confusion when it comes to carbohydrates. Although it's true that refined carbohydrates such as white bread, white rice, sweets, and other highly processed foods may be a factor in weight gain and ill health, that doesn't mean all carbohydrates are bad. No matter what you read or hear about the evils of carbohydrates, they still are an important part of a healthy diet. Carbohydrates give your body fuel.

REAL LIFE QUESTION: Should I take fish oil supplements to get my omega-3s?

I don't recommend routine supplementation with fish oil. Instead, I recommend eating fish, particularly fatty fish (mackerel, trout, herring, sardines, albacore tuna, or salmon), at least twice a week.

The American Heart Association states that people who have high triglycerides (blood fats) or coronary heart disease may benefit from taking a fish oil supplement. These people should talk to their doctors about taking supplements to reduce heart disease risk. But caution is needed, because high intakes of fish oil supplements can cause serious internal bleeding problems.

If you find it difficult to eat the beneficial amount of fish, speak to your doctor about whether you should take a fish oil supplement. Pregnant women need to use caution in consuming fish, because of worries about mercury. Now some authorities are starting to recommend low doses of omega-3 supplements for pregnant women.

REAL LIFE FACT: Ingredients for a Healthy Diet

Fats: safflower, sunflower, corn, and soybean oils (polyunsaturated); canola and olive oils (monounsaturated)

Protein: fish, chicken, beans, nuts, and soy foods

Dairy: nonfat milk and yogurt and low-fat cheese

So let's look at the good carbs and the ones you should put the brakes on.

The best sources of carbohydrates are fruits, vegetables, and whole grains. I know it can be a shock to many of us that fruits are carbs, but they are. They also provide fiber and many of the essential vitamins, minerals, and nutrients your body needs for health. We'll need to go back to some basic chemistry to help you understand the different carbohydrates. The basic building block of a carbohydrate is a sugar molecule, which is a union of carbon, hydrogen, and oxygen. Carbohydrates are basically chains of sugar molecules.

Your digestive system handles all carbohydrates by breaking them down into **glucose**, which is in units small enough to be absorbed from your intestines into your **bloodstream**. Your body's cells use glucose as their preferred energy source. So what makes refined carbohydrates bad for you, when whole grains and unrefined carbs are good for you, if they all are eventually broken down into glucose?

The answer lies in the **glycemic index** of different foods. The glycemic index measures how fast your blood sugar rises and how high

C=CARBON H=HYDROGEN
O=OXYGEN

Carbohydrate chemistry 101: A carbohydrate is a compound made up of carbon (C), hydrogen (H), and oxygen (O). Carbs in the form of sugars have small and more basic chains of molecules (like glucose, the chain pictured) while grains, vegetables, legumes, and beans are made up of large and complex chains.

it goes after you eat a food that contains carbohydrates. White rice, for example, is converted very quickly into glucose in your blood stream, causing your blood sugar level to rise rapidly. So white rice is classified as having a high glycemic index. Brown rice is digested more slowly, causing a lower peak and a more gradual change in blood sugar. It has a low glycemic index. Diets filled with high-glycemic-index foods, which cause quick and pronounced increases in blood sugar levels known as spikes, have been linked to an increased risk for both diabetes and heart disease.

When it comes to digestion, slower is better. The speed of digestion is caused by the chemical nature of the carb itself and by how resistant it is to your digestive **enzymes**. A simple sugar is usually much less resistant than a starch, and so it's digested much faster. Fiber in a food slows down digestion.

Generally, the more a food is processed, the higher its glycemic index. Processing removes the fiber-rich outer bran layer from wheat, for example, and its vitamin- and mineral-rich inner germ. That leaves mostly the starchy stuff. The wheat loses its fiber power, which protects the starchy carbohydrates from the digestive enzymes. Fiber slows the release of sugar into the bloodstream. True whole-grain bread, for example, is digested slowly and gradually absorbed into your bloodstream. White bread is digested and absorbed into your bloodstream quickly. Finely ground cereals and grains are more rapidly digested, so they have a higher glycemic index than more coarsely ground cereals and grains.

Work on replacing highly processed grains, cereals, and sugars with less processed whole-grain products, brown rice, and whole wheat breads. And hold the potatoes—or at least keep them to a minimum, because they quickly break down into glucose in your body. These changes are easy for some people to make and harder for others. If it's hard for you, keep eating potatoes but buy smaller ones. Don't like brown rice? Try mixing a little brown rice into your white rice. Make these changes one day at a time, and soon you'll be following them for life.

Your Weight: The Never-Ending Battle Can Be Won

Do you know what the result is of all those fad diet plans that are clamoring for your money? Zip. A precious few people lose weight and keep it off. Most gain back the weight and then add a little more. The latest research tells us what common sense said all along: burn more calories than you consume, and you'll lose weight. The composition of your diet—the ratios of carbs to fat to protein—isn't a big player in weight loss.

What diet plan will work for you? The solution is the same whether you are obsessed with weight loss or not—whether you are a group exerciser or a loner, have been heavy your whole life or are fighting postbaby weight gain, and whether you eat to ease stress, are hooked on high-fat desserts, or consider green popsicles to be a vegetable. Why? Because most of the programs out there are extreme in some way.

Some weight-loss programs *are* better than others. If you have time to do a program like Weight Watchers and you like having group support, then give it a shot—but I want you to eat more than they recommend. It's not enough. And I want you to eat the calories it would take to sustain you at your ideal weight, and no less.

What's extreme about the weight-loss programs that deliver food? Well, that's not real life. How about the diet frozen food section at the supermarket? Most of those meals are gross. And what about insane programs like the cabbage soup or all-grapefruit diets? Again, these aren't real life solutions, they are crazy concepts, and they will give you gas. Finally, any diet with the name *Hollywood* in it has got to be crazy. Now let's get back on a positive route to a more healthy you.

How to Get in the Habit of Good Eating

It takes three weeks to establish a new habit. Let's start on day one by eating one piece of fruit in the afternoon, in that hungry time between lunch and dinner. When you have done that for a week, add another vegetable serving to your lunch or dinner. And when you get to week three, add another piece of fruit whenever you are still hungry—evening perhaps?

Try to add fruit to your diet as a side at meals or add it to other dishes, such as your cereal. Give this plan another week and you will have made wonderful new habits.

Vitamins and Nutrients Women Need: Calcium, Iron, and Folate

Eating a varied diet with lots of fruits and vegetables will almost automatically get you the vitamins and nutrients you need. Most women, however, should also pay particular attention to calcium, vitamin D, iron, and folate and may need a supplement to ensure that they get enough.

- **Calcium and vitamin D:** To keep your bones strong and to prevent bone loss, you need calcium as well as vitamin D. It's recommended that young women take 1,000 mg of calcium and 400 IU of vitamin D daily. Women who don't get enough calcium and vitamin D through foods could benefit from taking a supplement. (Mom, if you are reading this, you need more after **menopause**.) Read more about calcium and vitamin D in chapter 7, Your Bones and Joints, especially for advice on increasing your vitamin D intake above the official recommended dose.
- **Iron:** If you have heavy menstrual bleeding, you may need more iron to replace the iron lost. Iron deficiency can lead to anemia, a condition in which blood is low in **hemoglobin**, the substance that carries oxygen to tissues. The recommended daily amount of iron

for women is 18 mg. If you are anemic from iron deficiency, your doctor may recommend an iron supplement. (Still here, Mom? Talk to your doctor about stopping the iron supplements after menopause!)

- **Folate:** If you're trying to become pregnant, be certain to get enough folate. You need 400 mcg daily. Folate is needed very early in pregnancy to help protect your baby against neural tube birth defects, such as incomplete closure of the spine (spina bifida). It's a good idea to take a folic acid supplement when you are trying to conceive, because many women don't get enough folate in their diets. (Please see chapter 16, Your Fertility, for more about folate.)

Are You Getting Enough Fiber?

Dietary fiber is the indigestible portion of plant foods and an important nutrient for health. Many American women do not have enough fiber in their diet. A diet high in fiber reduces the risk of heart disease, diabetes, diverticular disease (see page 167), and constipation. Scientific studies find that a high total dietary fiber intake is linked to a lower risk of heart disease and diabetes. Fiber has long been used in the prevention of **diverticulitis**, an **inflammation** of the intestine that is one of the most common disorders of the **colon** in Western societies. A high-fiber diet reduces this risk by about 40 percent.

Fiber also makes you feel full, which can prevent overeating. Fiber has little, if any, effect on the risk of colon cancer, even though you may have heard the opposite. For many years, scientists thought that a high-fiber diet reduced the risk of colon cancer. However, recent well-designed studies have failed to show a link between fiber and reduced colon cancer risk. This new and surprising finding may be in contrast to what your doctor may have told you and what you may have read. But you need fiber for so many other reasons that you can forget about one study—and eat your fiber!

There are two forms of fiber: soluble and insoluble. Both have health benefits. Soluble fiber attracts water and turns to gel during digestion. This slows digestion and the rate of nutrient absorption from the stomach and intestine. It's found in oat bran, barley, nuts, seeds, beans, lentils, peas, and some fruits and vegetables. Insoluble fiber is not digested by the body and is found in foods such as wheat bran, all vegetables, and whole grains. It appears to speed the passage of foods through the stomach and intestines and adds bulk to the stool. This keeps your bowel movements soft and regular. To read more, see chapter 8, Your Stomach and Intestines.

Fresh fruits and vegetables are excellent sources of fiber, as are whole-grain breads, cereals, pastas, brown rice, and beans. Peeling can reduce the amount of fiber in a food, so leave the skin on fruits such as apples to increase the quantity of fiber you eat. Flaxseed provides another rich source of fiber—you can simply grind it (remember, it has to be ground or it will pass through you undigested) and sprinkle it on your yogurt or cereal for a quick fiber boost (not to mention omega-3s). The fiber content of foods is the same whether they are cooked or raw—not the vitamin content, but the fiber content.

The Science of Salt

It's a good idea to limit your intake of sodium to about 2,400 mg per day—about the amount in one teaspoon of salt. If you have high blood pressure, or **hypertension**, restricting salt may give you up to a 4-point drop in your blood pressure.

Salt may not deserve its bad reputation, however, since limiting salt has little impact on people with normal blood pressure. Salt makes a real difference to about half the people with high blood pressure, and about one in five of those with normal blood pressure. The effects of salt on blood pressure are stronger on those in middle age than in younger people. In my home, we use salt in our recipes and we're all at a healthy weight. We don't have high blood pressure, we don't eat many prepared foods, and we rarely eat fast food.

So where do we get most of our salt? Not from the saltshaker. Salt added in cooking or at the table makes up just 15 percent of the salt in the average diet. It's in processed, ready-to-eat, and restaurant foods that we get most of our salt—about 75 percent. For most people, the vast majority of salt in their diet comes from these hidden sources.

So the best way to eat less salt is to cut the amount of chips, prepared dinners, and other processed and ready-to-eat foods. You can't always go by taste in judging the salt content of an item, especially in restaurants, where food doesn't have an ingredient label.

There is a great deal of individual variation in how salt-sensitive the body is, with some people being more sensitive to salt than others. Remember, several studies show that a reduction in salt in the diet may not help everyone lower their blood pressure, because of this individual difference.

REAL LIFE FACT: Conquer Constipation

Constipation is a problem for many people who eat a typical Western diet, which is often low in fiber. Fiber in the diet is the best way to manage constipation naturally. The fiber provides bulk for stool formation and helps move wastes more quickly through your colon. Low-fiber diets have caused us to become big consumers of laxatives and stool-softening agents. Most of these pills wouldn't be needed if we added more fiber to our diets. (See chapter 8, Your Stomach and Intestines, for more.)

REAL LIFE QUESTION: Which of the following has more salt? A small order of McDonald's french fries, a McDonald's Quarter Pounder with cheese, or Campbell's chicken noodle soup.

1. McDonald's Quarter Pounder with cheese (1,250 mg)
2. Campbell's Chicken Noodle Soup (890 mg)
3. McDonald's french fries (135 mg)

So what can you do? The best approach to controlling blood pressure includes limiting salt, eating a diet rich in fruits and vegetables, keeping weight under control, and exercising regularly. Although salt is important, it's only one factor in blood pressure control and general health. A good approach to healthy salt intake is to minimize processed foods in your diet, but go ahead and use some salt in cooking to enhance the flavors of whole foods and vegetables.

Can I Have a Glass of Wine with Dinner?

A small amount of alcohol may actually be good for you. After noticing that the French have low heart disease rates despite having high-fat diets, scientists began investigating whether the red wine enjoyed with meals in France could be the reason. Research now supports the idea that, for most adults, alcohol in moderate amounts is part of a heart-healthy lifestyle. And more new research shows that the benefits from alcohol are not limited to red wine. Red and white wine, beer, and spirits all appear to cut the risk of heart attacks to a similar degree.

The problem with recommending alcohol as part of a healthy lifestyle is that the exact definition of "moderate drinking" is still not totally clear. Some people are unable to restrict their drinking to one or two drinks. Crossing the line into heavier drinking brings a host of other big problems. It's very important to realize that with alcohol, more is not better, and too much can be extremely harmful.

The problem is that moderate alcohol intake as it is defined for men—one to two drinks a day—has been shown to increase a woman's breast and colon cancer risk. And for men as well as women, alcohol can poison heart cells, **kidney** cells, and brain cells and cause liver cancer. And, of course, alcohol is an addictive substance.

If you are a woman in her reproductive years who is not using birth control, avoid alcohol. Alcohol consumed by pregnant women causes birth defects, cognitive defects in babies exposed to alcohol in the womb, and other serious pregnancy complications.

Anyone with a history of addiction or family history of alcoholism should be very wary of alcohol. And anyone who is taking any medication with which alcohol can interact, or who has any disease process in which alcohol can cause additional problems, should avoid it.

Remember, too, that alcohol contains calories, and any heart-healthy benefits will be canceled by your weight gain if you just add on calories from alcohol to your daily total without some decrease in how much you eat or some increase in extra energy burned.

But for healthy adults, one drink a day for women and one to two drinks a day for men can be part of a healthy lifestyle. Why the difference? Women need to balance the risk of breast cancer with the heart health benefits and enjoyment of alcoholic beverages. If you have a strong family history of breast cancer, you should considering drinking even less.

NOTE TO SELF

Latte alert! Moderate caffeine use is not bad for your health—but watch what you add to your coffee.

No, You Don't Have to Give Up Caffeine . . . Completely

There's a wide range of opinions about caffeine. And despite what you may have heard, caffeine is not bad for your health. Most major health organizations, including the American Medical Association and the U.S. Food and Drug Administration, have said that moderate coffee or tea drinkers are fine as long as other lifestyle habits (diet, alcohol) are okay. Moderate consumption is considered to be about 300 mg of caffeine, which is about three cups of coffee daily. If that much caffeine keeps you awake at night, you may have to cut back. A cup of coffee is considered an eight-ounce drink.

Yes, caffeine is a drug. Caffeine may increase your alertness when you are tired and enhance the performance of certain tasks. But people differ greatly in their sensitivity to caffeine. Caffeine temporarily stimulates the central nervous system and **cardiovascular system**, increasing heart rate and blood pressure, stimulating muscles, and increasing urination. Some people can drink several cups of coffee within an hour and not notice any effect, but others will feel stimulating effects after one cup. Caffeine does not build up in the bloodstream and is gone within several hours after you eat or drink it. Yet some people find they are very sensitive to caffeine and have trouble sleeping even if they have it early in the day or have chocolate for dessert.

There are side effects to getting too much caffeine. If you have more than usual, it may cause jitters, anxiety, and diarrhea. If you eat or drink caffeine regularly and suddenly stop, you may have withdrawal symptoms, including jitters and headache. And remember that caffeine has been linked to stomach trouble and increased calcium loss from your bones. This is serious. But moderate amounts of caffeine, up to 300 mg per day, don't seem to harm bone health. And you've heard the rumors, but there's no evidence that caffeine increases the risk of developing cancer or heart disease.

Should I Be Taking Vitamins?

That's one of the most common questions I'm asked. In general, it's best to get most of the nutrients you need through your diet. Vitamin supplements are relatively new, so we don't know if supplements work differently from food in your body.

However, almost 80 percent of us don't eat the recommended amounts of fruits and vegetables to get the key vitamins and minerals we need for good health. Recent evidence has shown that a lack in these vitamins and minerals can be risk factors for **chronic** diseases such as cardiovascular disease, cancer, and **osteoporosis**.

I currently recommend taking a multivitamin as insurance. Think of a multivitamin not as a substitute for eating a healthy diet, but rather as a complementary therapy. No multivitamin will make up for a poor diet. By eating a healthy diet and taking a supplement, you'll get the best of both worlds. There are some recent well-done studies that support this advice.

But remember, more is not better! It's important to avoid megadosing on vitamin supplements. In some cases, too much of a good thing can be toxic, so you should take only the recommended doses. For example, higher-than-recommended vitamin A intake during pregnancy is linked to certain birth defects. Also, one size does not fit all with supplements. To prevent the possibility of overdose, remember that your current diet already contains some vitamins and minerals. Ask your health care provider to help you choose what is best for you. Some people take a children's vitamin to get a small dose.

Multivitamins can also interact with other medications and disease conditions. The way your body uses a pill can also vary, depending on many things—your eating habits, genetic factors, your physical condition, disease states, and medications. Sometimes it's necessary to take your multivitamin at a separate time from your other medications. When taken together, they might have a negative impact or even make it hard for you to absorb the medication. For example, taking a multivitamin at the same time as **thyroid** medication can impair your body's absorption of the thyroid medication. Taking them at different times of day can often avoid this.

Sometimes, though, you actually need to raise the dosage of your thyroid medication to ensure adequate levels in your body when you are also taking a multivitamin. If you take

NOTE TO SELF

The evidence is in: The latest diet won't help you lose weight. Changing your habits gradually, controlling your portions, and exercising (even mildly!) will.

other medications, speak to your physician about this, to ensure that they don't interact with a vitamin supplement!

Always try to take your medicines and supplements with water, unless a health care provider recommends otherwise.

Now That I'm Eating Well, How Do I Drop These Pounds?

There are hundreds of plans and books about losing weight and most of them ask you to eat a restricted-calorie diet that will drive you crazy. If you absolutely, positively have to have a diet plan to follow, choose one knowing that you will probably need to add more healthy calories. The best possible way to lose weight is to learn to eat the number of calories that will maintain your goal weight. When you eat less than that, your body is going to give up on you! You won't be getting enough nutrients and your body will think you are starving.

So let's look at the big picture of successful weight management. Start with the seven habits of healthy eating. People who have achieved weight loss do these things:

1. **Eat five meals a day.** Sound funny? People who eat small meals plus two snacks seem to do a better job of not gorging themselves when they get too hungry. You're less likely to supersize it if your stomach is partially full.
2. **Exercise.** No surprise here. Set aside thirty minutes for planned exercise daily. It's hard to keep pounds off through dieting alone.
3. **Be active.** Work little bits of activity into your daily routine—five minutes here and there add up. If you work a few floors up, take the stairs every workday for a year and you'll take off three pounds a year. Park at the far end of the parking lot if it is safe to do so. (Remember to practice safety—don't go in the stairwell if the doors automatically lock, and don't cross a large empty parking lot after nightfall if there are no lights.) Take any opportunity to add a bit of activity to your day. Try the pedometer approach—clip one to your waist to measure the number of steps you take every day. It's a good way to set gradual goals for increased activity.
4. **Eat breakfast.** Breakfast eaters are consistently lower in weight.
5. **Don't give up.** Prepare for a bumpy road, but keep trying. Most dieters have tried and failed many times before they finally succeed.
6. **Weigh yourself often.** Buy a scale for your bathroom and use it regularly. Studies show that this keeps you on track with your weight. But if you live on the scale, throw yours out instead!
7. **Don't deny yourself.** Eat out, and indulge from time to time. You need to

enjoy food and the eating experience. You can learn to eat moderately one week when you know you have a lot of events to go to the following week.

Anyone who tries to deprive herself week after week and doesn't even eat her own birthday cake is headed for failure. Have you gone to a gourmet restaurant famous for its desserts and just asked for a piece of chicken breast broiled without skin? There's too much anxiety involved in this way of life, and your body won't let you do it for long. Your body can't stand anxiety or starvation, and it will make you stop. It will make you gain weight. So when in Rome, eat! When it's your birthday, have your favorite cake. Then get back to your normal healthy base. This is how people with a healthy weight eat.

One patient treats her calorie intake as a bank. For example, she and her husband really love going to the movies once a month. She loves popcorn as much as the movie. Her "diet" plan told her two things: stop going to the movies, or cut up celery and other salad vegetables into small pieces and take them to eat like popcorn.

She tried it. She lasted two months. On the third month, she'd had it. She ordered a jumbo popcorn with extra butter and free refills, a frozen candy bar, and a box of candy mints.

She learned an important lesson: life doesn't mean constant sacrifice, and neither does good health. Her evening with her husband and popcorn was precious to her. Her new plan: She eats a light breakfast and a light lunch, plus a small snack in the afternoon. See? Very small withdrawals from her bank. At the movies, she withdraws the rest of her calories for the day. She has popcorn—for dinner! If she did that every night, I'd be terrified for her health. But occasionally? It will help her to stay on a healthy path.

Healthy Eating Tools

Let's look at portion size. You may be eating a diet whose parts are all healthy, but if your portions are large and you're gaining weight, it's time to check up on how much you're eating. Anything you eat in moderate amounts is okay. But large amounts of even the healthiest foods will add too many calories to your diet.

Our portion sizes have been growing along with our waistlines. We have supersized our fries, made our muffins giant, and added 30 percent more to virtually everything you can think of. This has to stop. We need to relearn our portion sizes and keep our bodies moving.

Keep some basic portion control ideas in your mind as you make or buy your meals. Use smaller plates and cutlery. Don't invest in new stuff, just go with the salad plate and salad fork. Having small bowls in the house will help if you have foods you find hard to limit—for some people, it's ice cream—and the small bowl lets you indulge safely for your arteries.

If you are serving dinner for guests at home, you may feel these portions are too small. If these are good friends, ask them—they will probably say they would appreciate a portion-controlled dinner. If not, have extras on hand for hungry guests who may not be on your path yet.

If you use portion control, you can eat delicious foods of any kind. Without it, you'll be eating a skinless broiled chicken breast and broiled cod with lemon juice even at restaurants. Which way of life would you like better? As long as it's not too often, have a small filet mignon instead of the chicken. Share a dessert if you can—or save up for dessert by skipping the appetizer and rolls and cocktails. Is it the rolls you love? Then save up for those.

Wait, where's the portion control chart? There isn't one, but it's easy to keep the right portions in mind. Your meat should be about the size of a deck of cards and a teaspoon is about the size of your thumb. If you are overweight now, count everything that contains fat as two portions, because it probably is. Start to cut those fatty portions in half. Craving fast food? Order a kids' meal. It's bad for kids but perfect for your craving, and the portion size is right—half of a full-size meal.

If you are underweight, you'll be doubling healthy fats. If you are at your ideal weight, keep converting your food to healthy choices: olive oil instead of butter, skim milk instead of whole, less frequent beef dinners, more fruits and vegetables.

Body Mass Index: How Much Is Just Enough?

Keeping your weight in the healthy range is the most important measure of your health. Body mass index (BMI; see page 116), provides a guideline based on weight and height to determine whether your weight is appropriate for your height. (The mathematical formula is: weight [in kilograms] divided by height [in meters] squared.)

Many studies have found that keeping your BMI under 25 will decrease your risk of

REAL LIFE FACT: Dietary Inflation

It can be difficult to eat smaller portions, because we've become accustomed to seeing larger amounts of food on our plates today. For example, twenty years ago a McDonald's hamburger was just 333 calories. Today a McDonald's burger is almost twice the size, at 590 calories. And you can't just blame Ronald McDonald. At home, the average burger weighs in at eight ounces.

Bagels today are just about life preserver size. Twenty years ago a bagel was three inches in diameter and 140 calories. Today's bagel is six inches in diameter and 350 calories. You'd have to run two miles to burn those extra 210 calories, because maintaining a healthy weight is a matter of balancing the calories you take in with the calories you burn. Eating just 100 calories more per day—about two Oreos per day—adds up to ten pounds by the end of a year.

premature death, mainly from heart disease and cancer. Most experts agree that BMIs from 25 to 30 should be considered overweight, and BMIs over 30, obese. Almost one-third of Americans are now in the obese range, and obesity among children is rising at an alarming rate. You can make a huge difference in your health by controlling your weight.

Calculating BMI by itself does not diagnose your health, and it does have some limitations. For example, very muscular people may fall into the overweight category when they are actually healthy and fit. People who have lost muscle mass, such as the elderly, may be in the healthy weight category according to their BMI, when they may not be eating enough.

Let's say you were five feet four inches tall and weighed 130 pounds when you graduated from high school. At this height and weight, your BMI was in the healthy range at 22. You go off to college and gain the "freshman 15"; now you weigh 145, and you have officially joined the ranks of the overweight at a BMI of 25. You have your first child a few years later, and gain 50 pounds (more weight than you should), have a hard time losing it all, and end up one year later weighing in at 175. You have now joined the ranks of the obese. The slippery slope of weight gain can catch up with you when you don't pay close attention.

So how many calories should you eat? No simple formula is going to work for everyone. I've heard many formulas and most of them are just not enough food. For example, eating a number of calories equal to ten times the body weight you want to be is a diet and not a way of life. Twelve times your goal weight makes more sense. Try that method and adjust it if you're not getting the results you want.

There Are No Shortcuts When It Comes to Simply Healthy Eating—Just Great Benefits!

Your diet is more than a matter of taste—it can be a matter of life and death. You live in a time of an obesity epidemic. Whether you have pounds to lose or not, a healthy diet is for you. Stick with it most of the time, splurge occasionally, and your other issues start to take care of themselves.

You can still celebrate food—it's part of our culture, our religions, and our family life. Learn to cook and spend some time stocking a kitchen where you can make delicious and healthy meals. Educating yourself about a healthy diet, using portion-control eating, and staying active can be the most important factors in your long-term health and well-being. This is the simply healthy way of life. It's fun, it feels normal, it works, and it lasts.

By now we've looked at all of the major systems of your body, from your brain down to your reproductive system. But there's a lot more to learn about major issues that don't happen to fit into one neat category. That comes next.

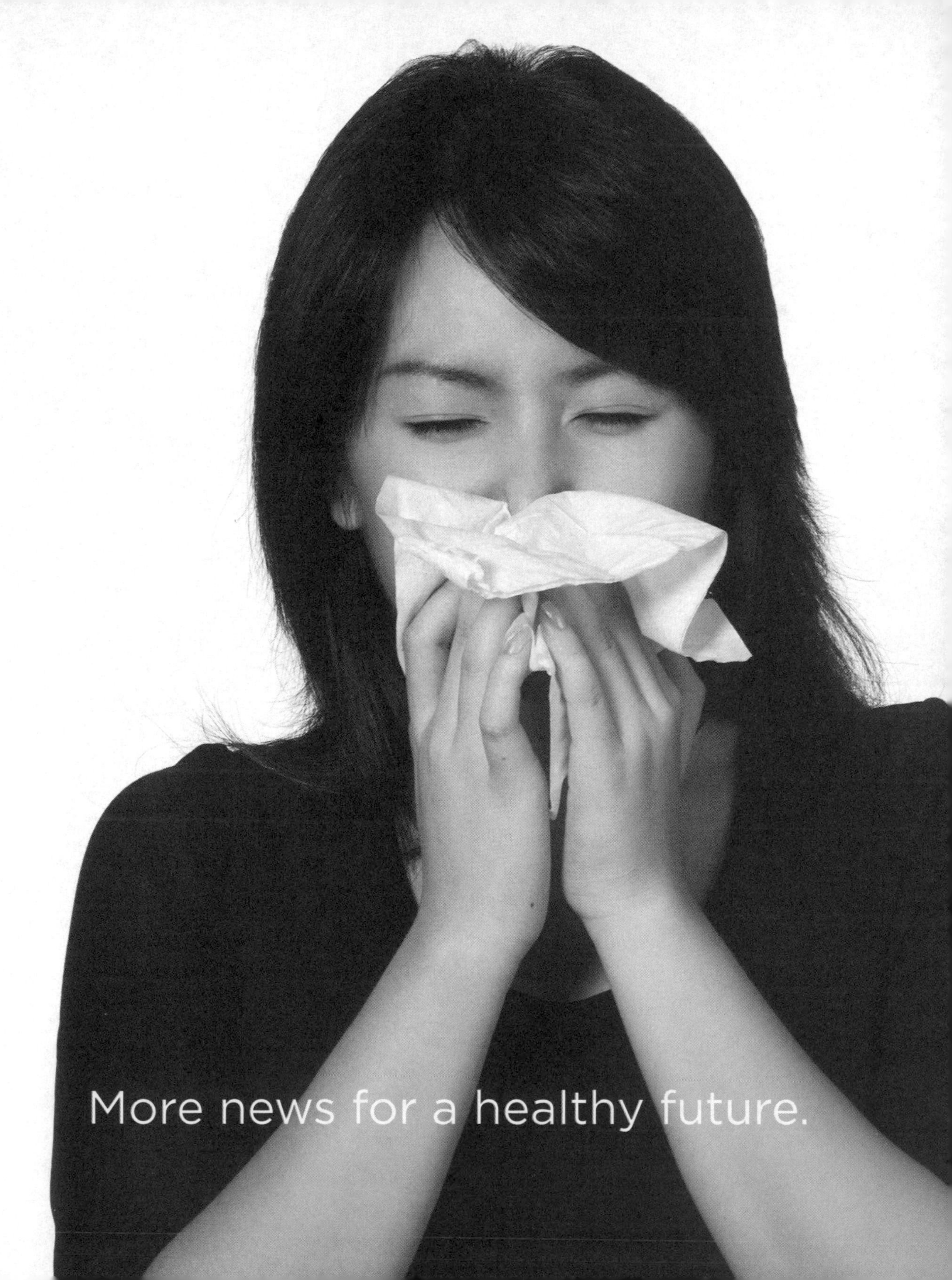
More news for a healthy future.

your body's other issues

We've finished looking at the major systems of your body that are most important for your future health. As your doctor, I care about countless other issues, and so should you. Although I can't discuss *everything* that could possibly go wrong with your body, I've covered some of the most common things here:

- Allergies
- Asthma
- Beauty treatments
- Colds and flu
- Foot trouble
- Organ donation
- Sports injuries and conditions
- Violence

Ah-choo! Allergies

Grandma was wrong. You didn't "grow out of your allergies," and you may even have a few new ones. If you occasionally sneeze when you don't feel sick, get rashes that you can't explain, and have diarrhea after eating certain foods or hives that suddenly appear on your skin, chances are you have allergies. And you have plenty of company. The Asthma and Allergy Foundation of America estimates that about fifty million people have allergies.

Here's what happens when you have an allergic reaction: Your body runs into something it doesn't like. It might not bother other people, but to you it's an allergen. The allergen activates your immune system and causes it to go on red alert. You start producing histamines, which are chemicals that give you most of your symptoms.

Although allergies can be pretty uncomfortable, the occasional reaction is something most of us can manage. But for some people, having an allergic reaction can be life threatening because it causes a very severe response called anaphylaxis. If you have severe allergic reactions, you need to see an allergist, which is a doctor who specializes in treating allergies, to manage them. Common allergens that cause severe allergies include shellfish, nuts, medications, and bee stings. To treat anaphylaxis quickly, you need a kit containing epinephrine (EpiPen is a common brand). You carry this kit with you at all times and then give yourself a shot of epinephrine in the thigh when you need it.

Most allergies—dust, pollen, mold, latex, perfume and other fragrances, and cockroach droppings—can be managed in two ways: you stay away from the allergen, or you take antihistamines or other medications as prescribed by your doctor. If you are allergic to dust, for example, you need a vacuum cleaner with a special HEPA filter to suck up the dust in your house, and mattress and pillow covers that protect you from dust mites. HEPA filters are specially designed with filter fibers that can catch small particles such as dust.

If you are allergic to tree pollen, get an air conditioner and an air purifier and keep the windows closed. You might also want to shower or rinse your hair every night so you don't get pollen in your bed. If your efforts don't make any difference, you may want to get tested for other allergies. Your doctor can do a simple skin test to figure out exactly what you are allergic to.

Your doctor may also recommend that you take medication. Sometimes it can take time to find the best medicine, because many of them make you sleepy. Some people may also choose to have regular allergy shots. But because you might have to commit to five years of shots ranging from weekly to every

REAL LIFE QUESTION: What's dander?

When you are allergic to cats or dogs, it's not normally the hair that's making you sneeze. Dander and saliva can be the culprits. Dander is flaking skin, like dandruff. It's everywhere, and not just where there are pets. Dander sticks to pet owners and travels wherever they go, often staying there. If you buy or rent a home from a pet owner, you may react to dander for several months after moving in.

> **REAL LIFE FACT: Time for an Ambulance**
>
> **Anaphylaxis means a trip to the emergency room, or for many people, a shot you give yourself. If you start getting hives that are spreading all over your body, have trouble breathing, or feel like your throat is tight or your mouth is swelling, or you even have tingling feelings, it's serious. The risk is that you'll go into anaphylactic shock, because your tissue and organs are not getting enough oxygen. Your heart starts pumping faster and faster. What to do? Call an ambulance. Don't spend any time wondering if you should. Just call.**

few weeks, most people only do this if they have allergies all year round (for example, if you marry a cat lover, but are allergic to pet dander).

Asthma

The National Heart, Lung, and Blood Institute says that **asthma** now affects twenty-two million Americans, including six million children. Boys are more likely to have asthma than girls, but women are more likely to have it than men.

The rate of asthma in African Americans is higher than for any other racial or ethnic group, and they experience more asthma-related hospitalizations and emergency room visits. There are many studies in the works to find out why that's true. One new study, for example, is searching for genetic links. Other experts are studying possible environmental links, but these tend to be focused on urban living. Urban living is bad for everybody's lungs, so I don't think a simple connection will be found. It's a complex problem and there is no magic answer. (For more statistics and information, check out the NIH website at www.nhlbi.nih.gov and www.blackhealthcare.com.)

So what is asthma? You breathe in oxygen and breathe out **carbon dioxide** through your lungs. Your airways carry the oxygen. If you have asthma, your airways don't work as well. They swell up, and if you could touch them, they'd feel sore. Once your airways are in this condition, they react much more sensitively to the world around you. Allergies, colds, infections, exercise, cold weather, pollution, smoke—all of these will make your airways swell, become narrower, and eventually trigger an asthma attack. Having an attack means you have more trouble breathing and your body doesn't get enough oxygen.

Although we don't know exactly what causes asthma, asthma and allergies are clearly linked. Many people experience asthma symptoms caused by their allergic response to pollen, dust mites, and pet dander. In people with untreated asthma, an attack can be fatal. Asthma is especially dangerous for children, who have smaller airways. Asthma keeps kids home from school more than any other **chronic** condition, and children's hospitals usually admit more kids for asthma than for any other cause.

Asthma Symptoms

When you're having an asthma attack, you might feel as if you are wheezing or struggling to breathe. Coughing is a symptom, along with a feeling of tightness in your chest. You may notice that certain things trigger your asthma, or that it seems to act up at certain times of the day. If you are having any of these symptoms, it's time to see the doctor. Your doctor will run tests to see if you have asthma and to rule out other possible causes. (Kids have more symptoms than adults. If you notice that your child is breathing faster than normal or coughs a lot, especially after being active, call the pediatrician.)

Asthma Treatment

There are both short- and long-term treatments for asthma. In short-term treatments, we try to help you when your asthma is triggered or you have a full-blown attack. The most common short-term treatment is an inhaler. Long-term treatments try to keep your airways stable over the long haul.

You know how your doctor is always on your back about taking your medication? Well, triple that for asthma. If you treat your asthma, you can live a long and healthy life. If you don't, you won't. Any day that you don't feel like taking your medicine is like subtracting a day from your life. It's not worth it. Please—have a plan and stick to it. And if you aren't sticking to it, be honest with your doctor or nurse and ask for help. You need a caregiver who will help you develop a plan that you can follow and who will share experiences about what works and what doesn't. If all you get is a "tsk," you need more help.

NOTE TO SELF

Don't treat your asthma by watching TV commercials. See your doctor to be sure that what you have is asthma and then work with him or her to create a whole plan for treatment, management, and prevention of attacks.

Finding the Causes of Your Asthma

You can help reduce the symptoms of your asthma by getting rid of triggers:

- When there's pollen outside, keep your windows closed. Change and wash your pillowcase daily during pollen season, and if you collected a lot of pollen in your hair during the day, shampoo it out at night before you go to bed.
- If you can afford air-conditioning, it will help to filter the air. You can often find free or cheap air conditioners on www.craigslist.com or www.freecycle.org. Be sure to have your unit serviced—replace

the filters and make sure it has no mold. If you spend some money at the repair shop, you could have a great machine for a bargain. If you can't afford the electric bills, keep the AC on only when and where you need it most.

- Clean the house, especially the floors, with very gentle cleaners.
- Cats and dogs are a big problem if you have allergies and asthma. There are some nonallergenic dogs, including poodles, wheaten terriers, Yorkies, bichon frises, properly bred labradoodles and goldendoodles, Malteses, Portugese water dogs, and westies. However, among cats, you've got very few choices. There are some hairless cats, and Siberians are reportedly nonallergenic even though they have a full coat. If you buy an animal, make sure you can return it if you discover that you are allergic. No matter how much you wash your cat or filter the air, you could still be sneezing and wheezing. And if you already have pets or "marry into" a pet, consider having regular allergy shots.
- To control dust mites, which are tiny critters who love mattresses and trigger allergies, you can buy special mattress pads that don't let the mites get to you.
- You already know that the worst indoor air problem is smoking. If you're not the culprit in your home, be sure everybody else knows it's a nonsmoking area, and enforce it.
- When it's cold outside, during high pollen season, or if there's a lot of pollution in your neighborhood, exercise indoors.
- If allergies keep triggering your asthma, ask your doctor to refer you to an allergist. S/he can help you to figure out what's causing your symptoms.

Beauty: What We Do in the Name of It

Women are beautiful with very little help, but that doesn't stop us from seeking a little extra edge. Some women are happy using a gentle soap and no makeup on their face and leaving their hair its natural color. Others start to pant when the new eye shadow colors come out and always have at least two treatments done during a routine visit to the hair salon.

Let's look at common beauty habits and what they mean—both positively and negatively—for your health.

The Danger of Mani-Pedis

Everyone has a nail salon horror story. Ask a podiatrist, a doctor who specializes in feet, if it's safe to have a pedi and s/he'll just conk you on the head. You should never go to those places! But . . . we do.

Here's the problem: You sit down where hundreds of women have sat before you. The person about to do your nails does not come from your germaphobic world. S/he brings out a towel for your hands. Is it clean? Maybe. Are the tools clean? Maybe. S/he cuts your cuticles, which Grandma thinks is for showgirls. What are your chances that **bacteria** from dirty tools or towels or tables are going to zip through those cuticles and give you a nice infection? Actually, pretty high. And do you really like having your feet done where hundreds of strangers feet have been done before? Ick.

But there's something satisfying about looking at your hands and feet and seeing a perfect world. Freshly done nails are the sign of a beautiful, organized woman. Getting your nails and toes done is a treat many of us love. You're going to hit that salon anyway, right? So what can you do to keep yourself safe?

Keep it clean. Bring your own tools. Or at least make sure the tools your nail tech uses come from a sterilizer and not her table. Ask her to change the towel on the counter for a new one. If you can stand it, ask her to push your cuticles back instead of cutting them. This is true: if you push your cuticles back every time you wash your hands or take a shower, you won't need to have them trimmed. And once you trim, you'll be addicted to it. You might also try putting antibiotic ointment on your cuticles when you get home for a little self-protection.

NOTE TO SELF

If you push your cuticles back every time you wash your hands or take a shower, you won't need to have them trimmed.

Eyelashes— When Is Enough, Enough?

More women are getting eyelash extensions than ever before. In this temporary procedure, an eyelash tech will extend your lashes using synthetic fibers attached to your real lashes. It's like have fake lashes put on by somebody who knows what they're doing. They last for a couple of weeks if cared for—ironically, you can't wear mascara—and they can cost up to several hundred dollars. As with all beauty procedures, your health is in the hands of the tech. Be sure that everything, especially his or her hands and tools, is freshly cleaned.

And have you heard this? People noticed that a brush-on liquid used for treatment of glaucoma increased lash growth on patients. And presto! Another new lash treatment is born. The U.S. Food and Drug Administration has approved its use as a cosmetic treatment, but I don't know if this is actually a safe, long-term option. The brand name is Latisse and you apply it yourself.

Having your eyelashes tinted is another popular beauty treatment. Vegetable dye is applied to the lashes, which dyes them to a dark color that lasts for several weeks. Most women who have their lashes dyed do it so they can skip the mascara. Lash dyeing is only done in professional salons. It has been banned in some areas due to fears of eye damage, though I have not seen a patient with that experience.

Permanent Makeup

I've seen so many disasters with permanent makeup treatments that I can't say I know what a good job looks like. This is a tattoo method to give you eyebrows, bigger lips, and even blush with permanent color. I don't like the idea of sticking needles in your face because of the risk of infection. But if you really want to do this, make sure you get references—and check them! Otherwise you may find that when you say, "Make my lips just a little bit bigger," your tech hears, "Give me those giant wax lips that you see around Halloween."

The Search for Perfect Hair

No matter what I do, I will never have three feet of swinging, shiny hair. Hair models are hair models—and they are that tiny percent of the population who have power hair. So is it safe to burn, tease, straighten, extend, curl, and everything else we do to turn our average locks into power hair? Yes—as long as you use some common sense.

If you use a straightening iron to get a sleek and smooth look, iron your hair as little and as lightly as possible if you want to keep healthy hair. If you want extensions to get that long hair look, go for high-quality extensions. Bad extensions will make you look like a man playing a woman in a comedy skit. Again, to keep hair healthy, use common sense and see a professional for weaves and extensions. These connect to your natural hair, which you want to leave undamaged.

You already know that putting chemicals in or on your body isn't a great idea, so avoid chemical straightening, coloring, bleaching, or perming. If you must, try to use healthier versions of the chemicals and use as little as possible. Insist on a well-ventilated area, which is also good for your stylist. While the amount of chemical that gets absorbed by your body is small, you may be breathing in ammonia. Ammonia is highly toxic, which you can tell by how it burns your eyes when you're near it. It will also irritate your lungs.

And every once in a while, treat yourself to a deep conditioner—one from the drugstore

REAL LIFE FACT: Foot Razoring

Many women want to have their feet razored when they have a pedicure. In razoring, the pedicurist uses a razor blade in a handle to get rid of your calluses. This technique removes more of the rough skin than scrub brushes or abrasion alone. In some places, razoring has been banned because cuts could allow bacteria to enter the skin.

REAL LIFE QUESTION: I have a dry mouth all the time. Why? And what can I do about it?

There are so many medications that cause dry mouth that you should talk with your doctor if you have this. It's important to take care of a constantly dry mouth because saliva is so beneficial to your mouth and teeth. A dry mouth breeds cavities and other problems. Until you can talk with your doctor, suck on sugarless candy or chew sugarless gum. Both help your mouth make saliva.

is fine. It doesn't make your body any healthier, but it's a nice stress buster.

Getting a Great Smile

Americans are famous around the world for our teeth. Bright white, perfect smiles. No doubt there are people who really come by those teeth naturally, but there are just as many who have cosmetic dentistry or other type of treatments done.

To keep your mouth, gums, and teeth healthy, have your teeth professionally cleaned twice a year or more often if necessary. Floss before bedtime. Use alcohol-free breath rinses and a gentle toothpaste with as few ingredients as possible. Be sure it has fluoride.

Most Americans get fluoride from the public water supply, which protects against cavities. If you don't know whether your neighborhood has water with fluoride, check with someone in the city or town water department. Fluoridated water doesn't help you or your kids if you're all drinking bottled or delivered water. So if your kids like drinks mixed with water, be sure to use water from the tap. Cook with tap water, too.

Veneers are an expensive but good-looking way to have the perfect smile. But even Hollywood has bad dentists; you can sometimes spot their work on the red carpet. (Sorry, Hillary Duff.) The teeth are now either too big for the person's mouth or too white for the person's age. So ask around and find out who does the best work.

Whitening your teeth by bleaching is increasingly popular. You can either buy the strips that you use at home or have the professional service done at the dentist's office. Both of these methods are based on peroxide-containing agents that penetrate into your teeth, which is why they take up to several weeks to work.

Bleaching appears to be safe and doesn't harm your teeth. Some people get a bit of gum irritation or tooth sensitivity from the bleach solution, especially when they first start the process. When you get this done professionally, the dentist will make a bleaching tray that is an exact mold of your teeth and gums, so it lessens the chances that the irritating bleach will get on your gums. The dentist has access to a stronger bleach solution than the over-the-counter white strips, but the dentist costs a lot more. Don't go too far and make them *too* white, or you'll look like you have false teeth, and you can't go back and make them less white. New whitening methods are being developed all the time, so ask your dentist which one is best for you.

Sweat and Body Odor

You know you're not having hot flashes! You just sweat more than everyone else at the gym—and after you leave the gym. Most excessive sweating happens under your arms, in your palms, and on the bottoms of your feet, but some people have spots of sweat or sweat all over their body. There's even a name for excessive sweating—hyperhidrosis.

If this is you, talk with your doctor because excessive sweating can have a medical cause: an overactive **thyroid** or low blood sugar. Luckily, there are many treatments available to give you relief. One quick one to try: Before you go to bed tonight, use an antiperspirant (not a plain deodorant) on the soles of your feet, your palms, and your armpits. See what happens.

What if you've tried everything—deodorants, wiping your pits during the day, folk remedies—but you still smell more than everybody else? If sweating isn't your problem, but body odor is, it's time to call your doctor. First, it's important that your doctor rule out medical causes. If you do have a medical cause, treatment will focus on the problem and the odor can resolve. If not, you'll try some lifestyle changes such as reducing stress and anxiety and thinking *dry*. Next, showering and changing your clothing often will really help. Your doctor may also prescribe prescription deodorants, which are strong and effective.

Waxing and Shaving (the Sensitive Parts)

Is it okay for you to wax or shave . . . well, anywhere? If you don't mind excruciating pain and ingrown hairs, go ahead. As a **gynecologist**, I have a unique perspective on the latest trends in waxing. These days, nearly every young woman I see has "gone Brazilian." Years ago, daring young women would have a bikini wax. This mainly meant cleaning up down there so no hair peeked out when you wore a bikini. You might also have had your eyebrows done, or had your chin, moustache, or legs waxed. A Brazilian is much more—or, really, much less—than that. It means you have hot wax smeared over the hair starting at your **anus** and working all the way up and around the **vulva**. Once the wax is removed, all of the hair is gone and you look like a little girl. That makes me a little squeamish, sociologically, but there's no question that this trend has taken off.

You've got to be really committed to go through this, bending over in many different positions so the waxer can reach all of you. The pain involved? It's horrible but it's short, and it's followed by irritation that can last a few days. I'm no longer shocked or even surprised by Brazilian waxing, now that I've seen so much of it. Only you can decide whether you'll do it—or some other version.

If you want to wax your bikini area, you can keep it conservative, go the completely naked way described above, or go the decorative way. Decorating might involve waxing the hair on the vulva into festive shapes such as hearts and stars or lightning bolts. Or you might like the basic landing strip—a narrow strip of hair that runs north to south. And, of course, the smooth skin on either side of the landing strip gives you room for glue-on gems.

The most common complications I see from waxing and shaving are infected hair follicles (folliculitis). Here's what happens: Each hair follicle has an oil **gland** at its base. When you wax or shave, sometimes dead skin, the blunt end of the hair, or both, clog the hair **follicle**. The oil gland keeps pumping, but the opening to the skin is clogged, so you get what looks like a pimple there. Sometimes these get infected and turn red and painful, and occasionally they become very large. Women with coarse, curly hair and women of color tend to get folliculitis more often than other women, probably because coarse hair clogs the follicle more easily.

Lots of women mistake these bumps for sexually transmitted infections, and they come in to see me, very worried. Look closely. If you've recently removed hair from the area of the bumps and you can see a hair follicle, it probably is not sexually transmitted. Go see your doctor if you're not sure, though.

The best treatment for folliculitis is to put a hot cloth over the area and get the hair follicle to drain on its own. Try not to scrub or squeeze (well, maybe just a gentle squeeze—see page 79 for the proper technique to pop pimples), or it will get very sore and sometimes there can be some scarring. Occasionally, these infections need to be drained by a physician, or you might even need to take **antibiotics** if they don't go away on their own. To prevent folliculitis:

- Every time you shower, gently rub the area you waxed or shaved with a natural loofah sponge to remove dead skin. This exfoliates and keeps the dead skin from clogging the hair follicles.
- If you shave, use a new razor or blade each time to minimize the bacteria on the razor.
- Consider clipping rather than shaving your pubic area if you get recurrent folliculitis.

If you do decide to wax, please follow my usual advice: ask your friends for recommendations on the best place to go, and find someone who is very experienced. When you arrive for your appointment, think clean. Insist on it. The last thing you want is a cute but infected vulva.

Colds, Flu, and More

Catching a cold is often uncomfortable and can keep you from work or leisure, but it is rarely serious and usually goes away on its own without treatment. Understanding what causes colds—and respiratory infections, which are even worse—can help you know what to do when you get one. I'll also cover how to prevent them.

NOTE TO SELF

Keep your cold or flu to yourself by sneezing into your sleeve—not your hand.

The All-Too-Common Cold

The common cold is caused by a virus, and when you have it, you might have a sore throat, nasal stuffiness, a cough, a low-grade fever, headache, and mild fatigue. A virus is a tiny organism that you catch from someone else, and the viruses that cause colds are usually highly contagious. Viruses are different from bacterial infections, and antibiotics don't work on them, no matter how much we want them to!

Viruses that cause the common cold are spread by *droplets*, which are little bits of spit that contain the virus. When someone coughs or sneezes into the air (or onto his or her hand) and you come in contact with the droplets, then the virus infects you. Usually, the viruses that cause colds can't live on objects, like doorknobs or towels, but need to be spread from human to human by close contact. So be a kind friend or family member by coughing or sneezing into your sleeve, and by using a hand sanitizer, or soap and water, any time you cough or sneeze, especially before you eat. Avoid touching your mouth and face with your hands as a general rule, to prevent spreading infection to yourself.

When you get a viral infection, your body fights it off by activating your immune sys-

REAL LIFE QUESTION: When should I see a doctor if I have a cold?

See your doctor if you have any of these symptoms:

- **A cough with colored phlegm that looks like a thick greenish gel**
- **Ear pain**
- **Difficulty breathing**
- **No improvement after ten to fourteen days**
- **Persistent fever of 102 degrees Fahrenheit or higher**
- **Severe sinus pain (pain in your face just under or over your eyes)**

tem. Many of the symptoms that make you feel awful are actually signs that your immune system is working.

Nasal Stuffiness

A stuffy nose, or nasal congestion, is caused by tissues in the inside of your nose becoming filled with blood and fluid in response to a virus. You can also get a stuffy nose from allergies or the flu. Nasal stuffiness is not dangerous, but it can be really annoying.

Nasal decongestants, which can be bought over the counter, work by decreasing the **inflammation** inside your nose. They don't make the cold go away any quicker, but they do make you feel better while your body fights the virus. Be careful of overusing nasal decongestants. Using them more than three to four days in a row can result in rebound hypercongestion, which is when your nose gets even stuffier when the medicine wears off.

NOTE TO SELF

Alcohol-based hand sanitizers allow you to keep your hands pretty free from germs, even when you aren't near soap and water. Unless your hands are clearly dirty, hand sanitizers actually do the job better than soap and water. And they are different from antibacterial soaps, which just foster the growth of antibiotic-resistant bacteria. Buy some small bottles or wipes, keep them in your bag, and use them frequently. You'll be amazed what a difference such a simple step can make in preventing colds, flus, and other infections.

Saline nasal spray is another option for relief of nasal stuffiness. The spray is simply salt water, and it can clear your nose of **mucus**. It works well for clearing pollen out of your nose if your stuffiness is due to allergy, but it may also make you feel better if you get a cold. You can buy it at the drugstore. Some people make their own by using a cup of warm boiled water mixed with a teaspoon of salt, preferably kosher salt or sea salt.

Ear Infections

An ear infection (otitis media) is an inflammation of the middle ear usually caused by the same viruses (or sometimes bacteria) that cause sore throats and colds. Although you might think only infants and young children get ear infections, they can also happen to adults.

Your ear has three main parts: outer, middle, and inner. The outer ear is the visible part of the ear and the ear canal. At the end of the ear canal is the eardrum, which separates the outer ear from the middle ear. The middle ear is an air-filled space that contains tiny bones that transmit sound from the eardrum to the inner ear. The inner ear controls hearing and balance and connects to the brain.

When you have an ear infection, it's usually in the middle ear. Outer ear infections, called "swimmer's ear," are caused by water filling the ear canal and irritating it. Swimmer's ear may be treated with antibiotics, but prevention is just as important. Using white vinegar ear drops before and after swimming can help. Add a few drops to one ear at a time, let them sit for a moment, and then tilt your head to let them drain out.

Middle ear infections often start with the symptoms of a cold, and then develop into ear pain, a feeling of blockage in the ear, and even hearing loss. If you have those symptoms, it's time to see a doctor. S/he will look into your ear with an instrument called an otoscope and can usually tell just by looking if you have an ear infection.

Sometimes the doctor will recommend waiting to see if the infection clears on its own, and sometimes s/he will prescribe antibiotics. The treatment depends on your health history and the infections that are circulating in your community at that time. Taking acetaminophen (Tylenol) will help with the ear pain. Untreated, ear infections can become serious and may cause permanent hearing loss.

Influenza (the Flu)

The seasonal flu is a viral respiratory infection that is caused by a more serious virus than the one that causes the common cold. The symptoms can include fever, cough, sore throat, stuffy nose, body aches, headache, chills, and fatigue. Some people may also have vomiting and diarrhea.

Flu season usually arrives in November and lasts until March each year. It spreads like the common cold through respiratory droplets from coughs and sneezes. Like with colds, hand hygiene can really make a big difference in decreasing the spread of influenza.

With the flu, most people are sick for five to seven days and then recover. However, some people can get very ill from the flu and even die. If you suspect you have the flu, call your doctor right away. If you are at risk, as you might be if you have asthma, your

REAL LIFE FACT: How to Avoid Airplane Ear

If you ever have to fly when you have a cold or sinus infection, you are in danger of getting what's called airplane ear. There you sit quietly, in head-splitting agony, while the other passengers read. Airplane ear happens when the pressure has built up from the change in altitude and your ears haven't popped. This can be really painful, and chances are, you're begging for that plane to land. This is certainly a miserable way to start a vacation.

There are a few ways to prevent or avoid airplane ear: take decongestants before you fly, swallow during takeoff to clear your ears, chew gum to force swallowing, never fly with an ear infection or cold, or use a filtered ear plug (called EarPlanes). These give you a gradual change in air pressure and may save you from airplane ear. Buy them *before* you go to the airport. The drugstore usually has them. The airport shops often don't. Use all of the preventive measures and you will get relief.

REAL LIFE QUESTION: What will make me feel better when I have the flu?

Take acetaminophen (Tylenol) to help lower your fever and decrease the discomforts of sore throat and body aches. To stay hydrated, drink plenty of fluids, since the high fever that can come along with the flu can dehydrate you. You will feel too tired to do much of anything except rest. Rarely, you might get sick enough to need hospitalization. But for many people, the worst is over when you finally feel well enough to get up and shower!

immune system is suppressed, or you are pregnant, there is a critical window in the first forty-eight hours when antiviral medications can shorten the duration or severity of your symptoms.

Ask your doctor if you should have a flu shot. The flu virus changes each year, and so do the recommendations for who should get a flu shot. But the strains tend to be closely related, so if you had a flu vaccine last year, you may still have partial immunity this year.

The process by which flu vaccine is made takes many months. Sometimes by the time the vaccine reaches the general public, the virus has changed (mutated), and the vaccine doesn't work as well or at all. Because the influenza virus is constantly changing, you may still catch it even if you received a vaccine. Still, most of the time the vaccine works, and it can make a big difference in the number of people who suffer through the flu.

If you have coexisting issues like asthma, a compromised immune system, pregnancy, or **diabetes**, you are most at risk from the flu. But even healthy people can get dangerously sick. Get your flu vaccine when it is recommended for you! To find out more about the flu from the Centers for Disease Control, log on to www.flu.gov.

Bronchitis

To understand bronchitis, let's start with your respiratory anatomy. The goal of breathing is to inhale oxygen and exhale the waste product carbon dioxide. When you take a breath, the air goes in your nose and mouth, down your trachea, and into the bronchi of your lungs. Then it moves into the branches of the bronchi known as bronchioles, and from there into small sacs known as alveolar sacs, where oxygen is absorbed into your body and carbon dioxide waste is picked up.

Viruses or bacteria can infect the bronchi. These infections are called bronchitis, and symptoms often include a cough that brings up mucus. Mucus is a slimy substance made by the lining of the bronchial tubes. Bronchitis also may cause wheezing, fever, and shortness of breath. Usually, the same viruses that cause colds and the flu often cause acute bronchitis. Smokers and people with asthma are more at risk for bronchitis.

Most bronchitis goes away on its own within a week. It is usually caused by a virus that's similar to the viruses that cause the common cold. The cough is typically dry.

Occasionally, however, bacteria can cause bronchitis, and often you have this bacteria on top of the viral infection. You start with a viral infection, and then while your body is busy trying to fight this, a bacterial infection sneaks in and you suddenly get worse. Often the cough worsens, and the bronchial tubes make more yellow or even green mucus. This is when you should call your doctor to see if you need antibiotics, which work against the bacteria, but not against the viruses. Sometimes the cough lasts several weeks, even after the infection is gone.

Pneumonia

Pneumonia is an infection in your lungs. Viruses, bacteria, or, more rarely, fungi or parasites can cause it. It can be mild or it can become life threatening. Pneumonia symptoms vary greatly, depending on any underlying conditions you may have and the type of organism causing the infection. Pneumonia often mimics the flu, beginning with a cough and a fever, so you may not realize you have a more serious condition. Smokers are more at risk than nonsmokers.

Symptoms of pneumonia may include fever, chills, cough, shortness of breath, and pain when you breathe. See your doctor if you have this combination of symptoms. Antibiotics can be used to treat the bacterial causes of pneumonia, but lately there are some superbugs developing that can be resistant to antibiotics. Your doctor will listen to your lungs and may want to do an **X-ray** or a test on the mucus you cough up in order to pick the best treatment. Most young and healthy people can be treated with oral antibiotics, but sometimes hospitalization is required for intravenous antibiotics and oxygen therapy.

Foot Trouble

Ever seen the feet of a woman who has worn high heels with pointy toes for a lifetime? That huge **joint** of her big toe is a bunion, by the way. And that pain in her back? You can blame it on her shoes.

But, oh yes, those sweet little strappy sandals can do wonders for your mood on a bad day . . . in moderation. If you want to avoid bunions and back pain later in life, start by having good shoe health now. Save the heels for special occasions and wear shoes with real support the rest of the time

Young people tend to think that only old ladies go to podiatrists, but *you* should go to one if you have problems with your feet. Ask your doctor for a referral.

Plantar Warts

Warts on the bottom of your feet are caused by a virus and are known as plantar warts. This kind of virus is spread from direct foot-to-foot contact, but it can also live on mats, rugs, and tiles, often in gyms and locker rooms. Usually you can get rid of the warts pretty easily by wearing an over-the-counter salicylic acid pad on the wart (per the package instructions) until the wart falls off or dissolves. This can take a long time—weeks or even months. Occasionally, plantar warts can be deep, stubborn, and painful. In this case, see a dermatologist to have them removed with a more high-tech method such as freezing or with a minor surgical procedure. Plantar warts *can* eventually go away on their own.

To help prevent plantar warts, wear flip-flops on your feet in the locker room and in public showers at the gym or in dormitories.

Ingrown Toenails

An ingrown nail happens when your nail grows into the skin a little bit. It makes it painful to walk and it can easily become infected. If your toe often feels sensitive, that's one clue that you might be prone to them.

Podiatrist Dr. Michael Haas has a few ideas about how to prevent ingrown toenails. Take a look at the top of your foot, so you can really see the shape of your nail. It is either straight or curved. All of the advice you hear about nail care tells you to cut straight across the nail. If your nails grow straight across,

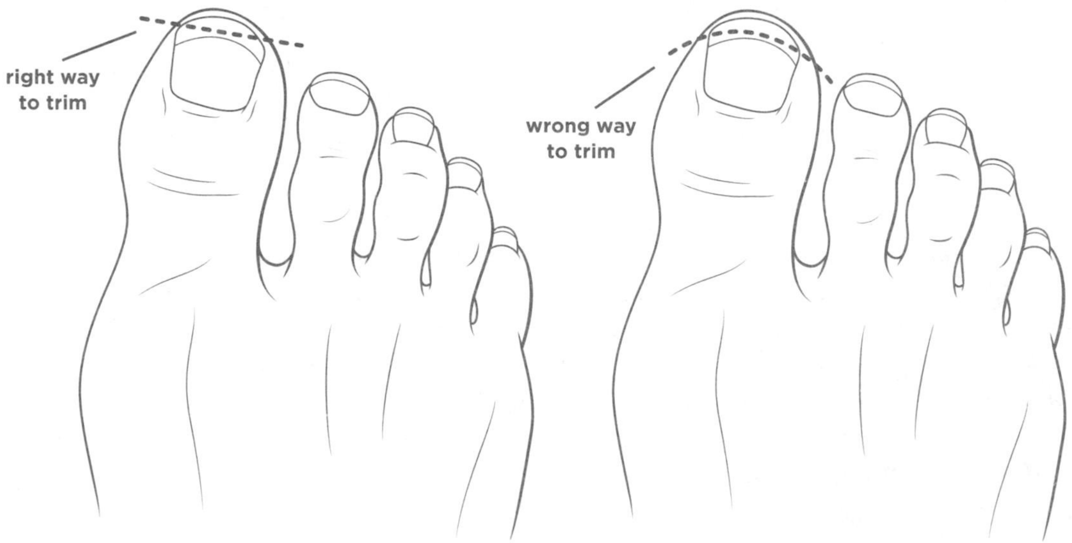

To prevent ingrown toenails, trim your nails straight across (or straight across with the corners rounded off if you have curved nails). Don't cut deeply down the side of the nail.

great. But if your nails are curved, the straight cut nail is going to keep digging straight into the toe and you will be in a lot of pain. What to do? First give it a straight cut right across the top. Then make two more cuts: one at each corner of your toenail to cut the corners off. Don't cut deeply down the side of the nail; just trim the sharp corners to round them off. Dr. Haas says if you have curved nails you want the corner to be "like a butter knife, not a steak knife."

Dry Feet

Unlike dry skin, which can be treated with moisturizers, dry feet require a lot more help. If you have painful, dry, cracked feet—but you don't have athlete's foot—try this method to get some relief.

Buy some stretchy cotton socks. Soak your feet in warm water with a mild soap or foot bath solution for about fifteen minutes. Pat them dry. If you have cracks, apply a little antibiotic ointment to them. Now apply goop. Goop is any cream that does not get absorbed easily! Products intended for diaper rash are usually good. Your favorites might include Balmex, the thickest Eucerin cream (in a jar), Vaseline, Bag Balm, or Aquaphor. Smear it on. Rub some in, and then smear again. Put your socks on and go to bed. In the morning, be careful in the shower, as your feet may be slippery. Shower as normal. You'll be amazed by the softness of your feet. You can repeat this treatment as often as you need to. Don't use a regular body lotion for this treatment if you want to see results.

You can do the same thing with your hands, using cotton-Lycra gloves. All-cotton gloves are also fine, they just have no flex, so people are more likely to be bothered by them and take them off in their sleep.

Smelly Feet

That distinctive stinky foot smell is caused by moisture and bacteria, so *think dry* again. Panty hose and synthetic materials, including what your shoes are made of, will make odor worse. Change your socks and shoes at least every day. Make sure your feet are dry after you shower, and then apply a foot powder to keep them that way.

If your problem is severe, a podiatrist can help with prescription creams and other measures. Foot odor can also be caused by hormonal changes and certain medications. So don't suffer forever. Talk with your doctor and see what can be done, and get a referral to a good podiatrist.

Organ Donation

The number of people in the United States, including kids, who need an organ transplant has grown to more than 100,000 for the first time. Most of them need a new **kidney**. **Livers** are in a distant second place, followed by the **pancreas**, heart, lungs, and **intestine**. And that's not counting all of the donations needed for major improvements in quality of life, including skin, cornea, and bone, and lifesaving bone marrow transplants.

The U.S. Department of Health and Human Services reports that seventy-seven people receive transplants every day, yet nineteen people die every day waiting for an organ.

Should I Be a Donor?

Becoming an organ donor gives you the chance to save a life. Imagine a grieving family, one of those 100,000 in the United States. Their loved one needs a kidney, but nobody in the family has the right match. If you have just been in a car accident and are dying, you might be able to help. If you haven't signed an organ donor card, guess what happens? The doctors come in and ask your sobbing parents if they will give permission to harvest your organs. If they are like most people, they will be far too upset to make a decision at a time like that—and the person who needs a kidney will probably die.

Once you've seen that happen firsthand, you sign an organ donor card right away. Here's what I don't get: why are there so many people who don't donate their organs?

I've heard some people say that their church is against it. Many people have researched that objection and found that unless you are Roma (a gypsy) or Shinto (Japanese), your church supports donation or leaves it to the individual. Jehovah's Witnesses have some restrictions, but no prohibition. Among ultraorthodox Jews, there are rabbis who are for donation and rabbis who are against it.

You have every right to be against organ donation, but if you could see the impact it has on survivors, you'd feel blessed by the opportunity. All I ask is that you don't leave the decision to your grieving family. Make it for them, by signing and carrying a card, or not, and making your wishes clear. They shouldn't have to choose for you. And whatever you do, don't let your organs go to waste because you didn't have time to sign up. Do it now.

To become an organ donor, sign up when you renew your driver's license, or download a card for your wallet at http://organdonor.gov/donor/index.htm.

Sports Injuries and Athletic Conditions

Sports injuries happen when athletes and nonathletes alike are overdoing it or aren't conditioned, hydrated, or paying attention. If you want to stay active in sports, be sure to make these good practices part of your training:

- A conditioning plan and strength training to build the muscles you need and keep them strong to be safe playing your sport
- A healthy, plentiful diet that will allow you to have enough energy and continue your period
- Enough hydration to keep you steady
- Stretching, stretching, and more stretching, before and after you play
- Having the right equipment and shoes and replacing them when they wear out
- Conditioning in the off-season

We've already covered a few of the health concerns that apply to the serious athletes among you—chiefly that **amenorrhea** (having no period) can increase your chances of a having a stress fracture (see chapter 6, Your Bones and Joints). So now let's cover a few of the other issues that athletes commonly face.

Athlete's Foot

First let's look at the most common conditions that affect those workhorses, your poor feet.

The single most common problem of any athlete—athlete's foot—is caused by a fungus. I would call it harmless except that it drives most people a little crazy with the itching and scratching. The best treatment: think *dry*. Keep your feet, your socks, and your shoes dry. Use antifungal powders and sprays. Check the label and follow the directions daily. And don't wear your athletic shoes without socks.

Don't use moisturizer on your feet for now—the cracked skin could be athlete's foot, not dryness. Wear socks made of cotton or those synthetic yarns designed to wick moisture away, and switch to a clean pair every day and for every game or practice. If the problem doesn't go away, talk with your doctor.

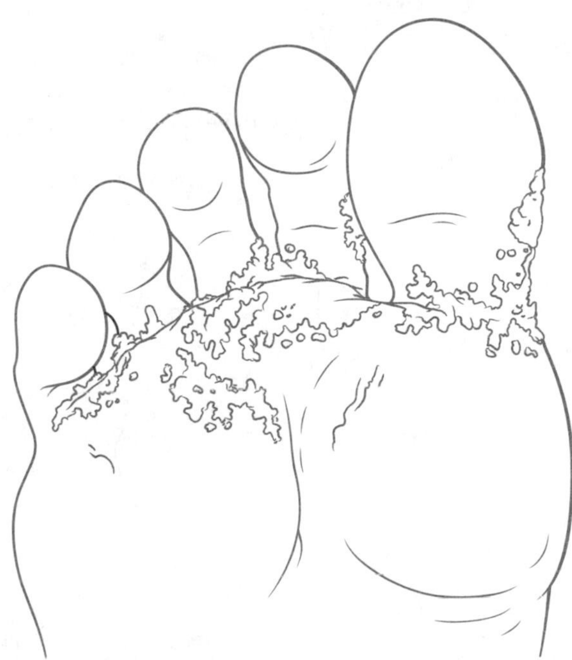

Athlete's foot is caused by a fungus. To treat it, keep your feet, socks, and shoes dry.

Plantar Fasciitis

Ouch. Plantar fasciitis hurts, especially when you first get out of bed. Usually the pain is right under the front of your heel. The plantar fascia is your arch tendon—a wide structure from the toes all the way back to the heel (see the illustration below left).

Athletes who pronate (see the illustration below right) are more likely to strain or rupture the plantar fascia. This is typically considered an overuse injury, often seen in runners or those who are on their feet a lot, especially if there is a sudden increase in your usual amount of physical activity. Because your feet handle your body weight, women who are overweight are more likely to get plantar fasciitis, though anyone can develop it if they spend enough time on their feet or if their body mechanics put them more at risk.

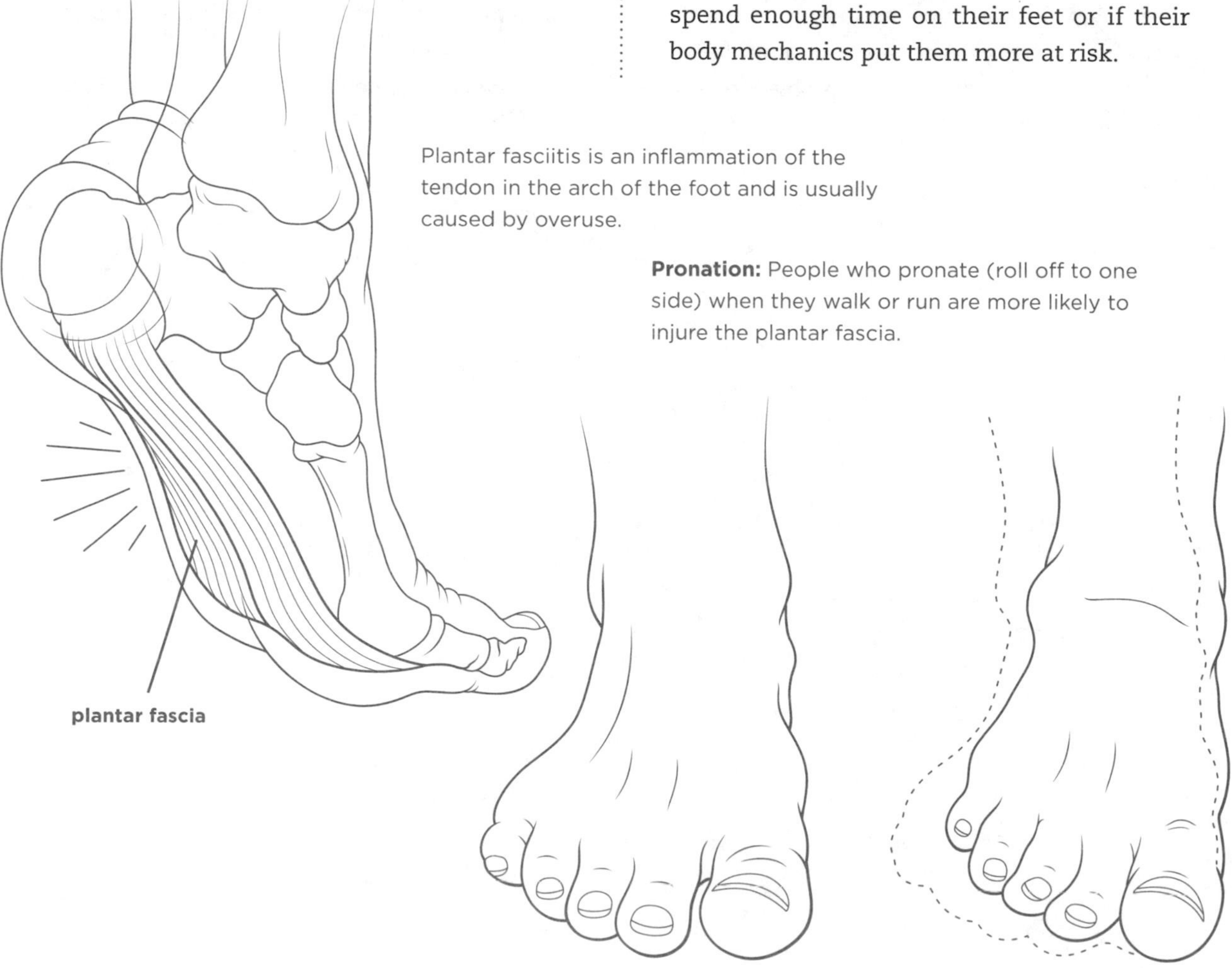

Plantar fasciitis is an inflammation of the tendon in the arch of the foot and is usually caused by overuse.

Pronation: People who pronate (roll off to one side) when they walk or run are more likely to injure the plantar fascia.

Treatment includes rest until the pain disappears, physical therapy and heel stretching exercises, ice therapy, anti-inflammatory medications (ibuprofen), and wearing night splints. Some people end up needing a steroid injection to quiet the inflammation if more conservative measures don't work. Resting alone is not going to heal your plantar fascia, and it is worth having it seen whether you are a long-term athlete or not.

Torn Ligaments in the Knee

One of the most common knee injuries is a tear of the anterior cruciate ligament (ACL). The ACL is one of four ligaments in your knee. Athletes injure the ACL more often than nonathletes, and women injure it more often than men, probably because of the way we are built and how we jump and land.

If you damage your ACL, see your doctor right away. ACL tears don't usually happen through contact. Instead, you might twist wrong as you land from a jump or your knee might simply give out on you. Your knee could feel as if it popped out of the socket. Symptoms include pain and swelling and the feeling that your knee is unstable.

Get expert help right away. I say expert help because there is a lot of debate about treating an ACL tear, especially about whether you should have surgery or not. Make sure you have a discussion about nonsurgical options if the injury is mild (wearing a brace, physical therapy) and have an MRI if the injury is thought to be severe enough for surgery.

Any of your ligaments or muscles can be injured playing sports. Seek expert help in all cases. While your coach or trainer may be very familiar with injuries, you want to be sure that the right tests are done and a doctor is consulted.

Patellofemoral Syndrome

Men's knees and women's knees are designed differently. Unfortunately, our knees don't get as much support from other bones, such as the femur, as men's do. If you have patellofemoral syndrome, it means that you have pain behind your kneecap (the patella). You will need a treatment plan that includes exercises, icing, and possibly changing to a lower-impact sport.

I can almost guarantee that you need new sneakers and possibly orthotics (custom-made shoe inserts). They appear to be such thin little things that you won't believe they can help, but you'll be amazed by the difference they can make when they are fitted properly.

Head Injuries

Concussions and head injuries are skyrocketing among female athletes. Lots of people love to try to figure out why; that the women's movement has made young women more aggressive is one popular statement that gives me hives.

The truth as I know it? When you play contact sports, you have contact. And certain contact sports require you to wear a helmet, whether you are a man or a woman. But the experts say the opposite: that putting on a helmet makes the sport more violent. That might be true. I don't know, but I do know this: Ice hockey old-timers make the same argument against helmets and face protection. They say it made the sport more violent. But take a look at the old-timers compared to the young'uns. Hmm. Today's pro hockey players look, well, normal. The old-timers? I don't know how they get out of bed. They have suffered more body injuries, facial scarring, and dental disasters than nearly anyone on earth. To me, they prove the pro-helmet argument. Put every woman in a helmet. And if she gets violent, suspend her.

Please have a head injury looked at if you have any of these symptoms: confusion, nausea, dizziness, amnesia, blurred vision, or headache. Do not try to diagnose a concussion yourself, and don't return to play until you are symptom free, no matter how much you want to.

If you are hurt while playing and you pass out, you should be taken to an emergency room for evaluation. Scans will help the doctor rule out serious problems in which you have fluid in the brain. Many sports teams take a baseline brain test before the season starts. It's not an IQ test, it just maps out what is normal for your brain while taking this test. If you have a concussion, you will have to get back to your previous score before you can play again, which can take weeks or months. Remember that concussions cause depression, and sometimes it can be quite severe. If ever you feel you've been seriously injured in your sport, trust your instincts. You either have a coach or trainer who will take care of you for the future or have one who doesn't know when to call an ambulance—or worse, one who just wants you to get back in the game. Trust yourself when you feel you should get help right away, and get the best help you can find. Be sure you are closely cared for and that you know when to call your doctor.

Violence

Rape happens when one (or more) people force someone to have sex when they've said no or have in some other way not agreed to it. This could mean forced intercourse in the vagina or forced anal or **oral sex**. Rape—including date rape—is a felony offense and can happen to both women and men.

What is date rape? It's rape. The only difference between rape and date rape is that the victim agreed to spend time with the attacker. The victim may have been on other dates with the attacker, or may have known the attacker from prior acquaintance. Either way, date rape is still rape. In fact, I think the phrase "date rape" was invented by defense attorneys to make it sound better than what it is—a felony.

Often, but not always, rape is violent. Fear alone can be used to force rape without physical violence. In some cases, rapists use drugs, including alcohol, to make you less able to fight, or even to knock you out. This is called drug facilitated sexual assault, and alcohol is the most common drug used (yes, alcohol is a drug). Another is flunitrazepam (Rohypnol), a fast-acting benzodiazepine (like a powerful tranquilizer). It works quickly, causing a loss of inhibitions, muscle relaxation, and amnesia for events that occur under the influence of the drug. Alcohol adds to its effects. Rape causes both physical and emotional harm.

NOTE TO SELF

Rape is a felony.

Why should you report a rape to the police? You already know why you should—to protect other women, to make the streets safer, and to give yourself a sense of justice—but I'm not going to lecture you about it. You do have the right *not* to report rape, but try not to make that decision while you are still in crisis. I'll ask only that you give yourself a little time to make your decision.

And while you make that decision, try to leave any evidence in place. Don't shower, douche, or soak in a tub, and don't wash your clothes. Put your clothes in a plastic bag with nothing else in it. I know that goes against every instinct you have at that moment—you want to be dunked in a giant vat of soap if it would clean you of every tiny atom of this incident. But if you can possibly wait, please do.

It's true: women often hesitate to report rape. They don't want the incident to be public, or often they are afraid to give their name and address, even to a police officer. Very often, women feel shock, fear, and anger all at once and can't make any decisions about what happened to them. If your home was robbed, you wouldn't hesitate to report it, but we all know this feels different.

Find some good friends to talk to. Choose understanding people who will listen to you, without judging your decision. You might also go to the hospital and have tests taken. The staff at the hospital can help you to avoid the

REAL LIFE FACT: If You Have Been Raped . . .

- **Don't wash, bathe, shower, or douche. This can wash away evidence.**
- **Call the police and report what happened. If you don't want to call the police, the next best choice is to call your local rape crisis center (more about this below).**
- **Go to an emergency room. The staff there is trained to care for your physical and emotional health, collect evidence, and provide you with emergency contraception and protection from sexually transmitted infections.**

REAL LIFE QUESTION: Where do I find my local rape crisis center?

Call toll-free, 1-800-656-HOPE, to reach the hotline number for the Rape, Abuse, and Incest National Network (RAINN). They can connect you with a center near you. They'll keep all of your information confidential, and you do not have to give your name or any other information. (If you are under the age of eighteen, however, and you volunteer your information, they are required by law to report the crime.)

risk of pregnancy. You don't have to give your correct name and contact information. Does this sound like bad advice from a doctor? Yes, it probably is. But I want you to have time to make the decision to report this crime without losing evidence. Just please remember the name and address you gave at the hospital. Believe me, the doctors and nurses there have seen countless Ann Jones-Smiths. The hospital can also help you to avoid the risk of pregnancy by providing emergency contraceptive pills.

You may also want to consult a therapist. Ask around for referrals, especially from a rape crisis center. You want an experienced person who will help you to put this in the rearview mirror and get on with your life, not someone who's going to explore your early childhood!

Are you to blame? No! It's impossible for rape to be your fault. It's common to wonder if you did something to cause it, or to feel embarrassed and ashamed. But no matter what, there is absolutely, positively, no way that you are to blame. It's important that you get counseling to deal with this event, as you will have many different reactions to sexual violence, and it can take a long time to work through it. If you aren't sure what happened to you, a therapist or health care provider can help you sort it out.

Do you know people who keep asking you stupid questions about the rape, such as "What were you wearing?" or "Why were you out alone at night?" No matter what happened to you, people are going to ask you dumb questions to make themselves feel better about it. They think that by asking these questions they can figure out what you did "wrong" and avoid being raped themselves. Don't waste one minute of your life on people like this. Just excuse yourself and walk away. If they persist, ask them why they want to ask these questions and tell them they're not welcome. You don't owe people a response, or anything else.

It may feel like your life will be never-ending pain. But you *will* recover from this. Life really will feel normal again, but it's going to take time. Give yourself the time you need and don't let anyone push you faster than you need to go. But make sure you are moving forward, which is the same advice I give for every difficult and painful medical problem. Take the time you need to restore your body and spirit, so you can make the choice to press on.

Conclusion

Throughout this book, I've given you lots of gradual ways to lead a healthy and active life. In the appendix, I'll cover a few more practical matters, like how to know when to call the doctor at 2 a.m., how to keep track of your PMS symptoms or your digestion problems, how to tell if someone you love is having a heart attack or **stroke**, and what to do if you can't afford all the health care I've advised you to get.

To get more information about the topics in this book, or to contact us, check out our website at www.thereallifebodybook.com. Take care and be well!

REAL LIFE FACT: Protect Yourself from Rape

Rape can't always be prevented. But there are a few things you can do to decrease your chances of ending up in a risky situation. They may seem like common sense, but let's review them:

- **Go to parties with friends you know, and be sure someone is the designated driver. Don't get left behind.**
- **Don't go home with someone you don't know.**
- **Stay in control by not drinking or doing drugs, or only drinking moderately.**
- **Don't accept a drink from someone you don't know. Order your own drink and keep your eye on it. Don't leave a drink at your table to go to the bathroom or to dance and then come back and drink it.**
- **Don't walk alone at night.**
- **Say no if you mean no. Be clear in your communication.**
- **Trust your instincts. If someone makes you uncomfortable, walk away.**
- **Always have enough money to get yourself home or to use a pay phone to call for a ride if you need to.**
- **Violence comes in many forms. If your partner is abusive, please see chapter 3, Stress and Your Body, for information.**

appendix: tools to use

Everything else you need to be healthy for life.

When you're sick, I don't want you to spend a lot of time diagnosing yourself before calling the doctor. But I know that sometimes you'll hesitate. When I ask patients why they didn't call me when the problem started last night, they often say that they were afraid of bothering me.

So here's a list that tells you when it's time to call 911, when to call your doctor right away, when you can wait until morning, and when you can wait for an appointment.

When to Call 911

First, check to make sure that 911 is your town's emergency number—check that right now. Seriously—stop reading and find out the number, because 911 does not work everywhere. Call 411 and ask.

Next, prepare an emergency list that you keep in your wallet or purse. It should include:

- Your name, address, and telephone number
- A reliable family member's contact information
- Your health insurance numbers (your member number plus the customer service telephone number)
- Any allergies you have to medications or other things
- All medications you take, including over-the-counter drugs and vitamin supplements, with the dosage
- Any medical conditions you have
- Your doctor's name, address, and telephone number
- The address and telephone number of your pharmacy

NOTE TO SELF

Make a promise to yourself to write your emergency list out tonight. Pick one day each year (at least) when you will update it, such as your birthday or when you turn your clocks back. That can also be the day you schedule your physical.

Call 911, right now, without discussing it to death—*just call*—if you have any of these symptoms.

Heart Attack Symptoms

- Chest pain
- New, unexplained pain in the back, stomach, arms, neck, or jaw
- Shortness of breath
- Nausea, dizziness, or cold sweats

For women, the stomach pain, back pain, jaw pain, nausea, dizziness, and cold sweats are particular heart attack symptoms. Remember: Heart attacks don't always look like they do on TV. They can come on slowly.

Stroke Symptoms

Learn the following symptoms of stroke and you could save your own or someone else's life someday. The American Stroke Association and the National Stroke Association have both created campaigns to help people remember the signs of stroke. Call 911 if you or someone else is experiencing one or more of these symptoms.

GIVE ME 5	
W—Walk	Are you off balance?
T—Talk	Is your speech slurred or is your face droopy?
R—Reach	Is one side of you weak or numb?
S—See	Is your vision completely or partly gone?
F—Feel	Do you have a severe headache?

Source: American Stroke Association, www.strokeassociation.org

ACT F.A.S.T.	
Face	Ask the person to smile. Does one side of the face droop?
Arms	Ask the person to raise both arms. Does one arm drift downward?
Speech	Ask the person to repeat a simple sentence. Are the words slurred? Can s/he repeat the sentence correctly?
Time	If the person shows any of these symptoms, time is important. Call 911 or get to the hospital fast. Brain cells are dying.

Source: National Stroke Association, www.stroke.org

Other Times to Call 911

- You have an asthma attack, and despite the usual treatment, you can't catch your breath.
- You have chest pain.
- You are physically or sexually assaulted.
- You have shortness of breath without

- You have shortness of breath without exertion.
- You have an accident and seem to be injured.
- You have a combination of vomiting, headache, lethargy or confusion, neck stiffness, rash, and fever.
- A friend has taken an overdose of drugs or alcohol or is unconscious and you can't figure out why.
- You have taken an overdose and you're still able to call or have someone else call.

When to Call Your Doctor

We've all done it. You felt a little burning while peeing on Saturday but didn't want to bother the doctor, so you waited until Monday morning to call. It took an hour to get through because everybody else did the same thing. The doctor prescribed **antibiotics** for your urinary tract infection and told you that if you had called over the weekend, you'd feel a lot better by now!

So how do you know when to call the doctor? Here's a guide to use when it's 2 a.m. on the weekend and you're not sure if what you have is serious enough to call. Before you do call the doctor, make sure you know where there is a twenty-four-hour pharmacy in your area, and what the phone number is.

Call in the middle of the night or on the weekend if:

- You have had a positive pregnancy test and you have vaginal bleeding.
- You think you may have a urinary tract infection and are in severe pain, are going frequently, or have a fever.
- You have an asthma attack that is not resolving completely with your usual treatment.

REAL LIFE QUESTION: What is the best way to get to the emergency room?

If you are having any of the symptoms described here, call 911 and wait for the ambulance. The emergency medical technicians (EMTs) know what to do if you are having a heart attack, a stroke, or other life-threatening event. They can start treating you wherever you are or in the ambulance on the way to the hospital—remember, seconds count!

If you are single or your partner is often away, be sure to have an emergency friend. Promise to give each other a ride to the emergency room whenever it is needed. You'll be surprised by the peace of mind this gives you. However, don't wait for a friend when you really need an ambulance!

- You are feeling short of breath, even when at rest, especially if you've had a cough, or if you have pain when you take a deep breath or are coughing up blood.
- You have heavy vaginal bleeding that leaves you light-headed and dizzy and unable to walk securely.
- You have heavy vaginal bleeding that soaks two pads or tampons an hour for more than two hours consecutively.
- You are feeling suicidal.

When you call a doctor in the middle of the night, your call will be answered by an answering service. These are not doctors or nurses, so you should only give them a short description of your situation: "I'm a patient of Dr. Paratestes. I have severe urinary burning and would like a call back." You'll give your name and number. If you don't hear back in half an hour, call again.

Wait and call the doctor first thing in the morning, when the office opens, to make a same-day urgent appointment, if:

- You have irritating, itchy, or smelly vaginal discharge.
- You have mild pain with urination or are going urgently or frequently. Remember that strong pain with urination means you call the doctor quickly. Technically, it is unlikely to be an emergency, but if you've had a UTI before, you know you want those antibiotics right now!
- You think you've been exposed to a sexually transmitted infection.
- You have swelling in your leg, especially if it is only on one side and is uncomfortable.
- You have a cold with a stuffy nose that after about a week gets worse; you have greenish yellow discharge from your nose and a headache or your face hurts; or you have a persistent cough and you are bringing up yellow greenish globs of phlegm.
- You have had unprotected sex and want a prescription for Plan B emergency contraception called in. (You should still be seen to be sure you don't have a sexually transmitted infection, but Plan B is best started right away.) It's sold over the counter, but your insurance only covers it by prescription. *Note*: You have a limited time for Plan B to work. So if it's Friday night, don't wait until Monday morning. Call first thing Saturday morning, ask the doctor to write the prescription immediately, pick it up right away, and take it.

Wait to call the doctor for a nonurgent, scheduled appointment within a few days to a few weeks if:

- You have a breast lump, discharge, or pain that does not resolve with your period.
- You have frequent headaches.
- You have period problems—painful, heavy, irregular (more often than every three weeks, less often than every five weeks, or missing more than two

REAL LIFE QUESTION: Why isn't my breast lump an emergency?

First, because there are many types of noncancerous lumps. Second, because even a cancerous lump grows very slowly. To you, though, that lump is one big emergency. Find a way to get it off your mind while you wait a few weeks for your appointment—remember, stress is not your friend. But don't wait longer than a few weeks. Ask to be put on the cancellation list for a chance to get an earlier appointment.

in a row without the possibility of pregnancy).

- You have a skin rash.
- You need a vaccination (like the HPV vaccine).
- You have pain with sex.
- You are worried about your alcohol or drug use.
- You have a mole that is bothering you or changing.
- You have mild abdominal or pelvic pain.
- You have a new lump or bump in your labial area or vulva.
- You are feeling depressed or having mood swings or anxiety.
- You need help quitting smoking.

Call to ask a question over the phone, during business hours, if:

- You don't know how to take a medication that was prescribed.
- You don't know if it's okay to take an over-the-counter medication with your prescription medication.
- You have a cold—stuffy nose, cough, sore throat, aches—and you are not sure if you need to be seen or just let it run its course. Has it been too many days and maybe you need to come in?
- You need a refill on a prescription, and it's not on file for a refill at your pharmacy.
- You have not heard back on results from a blood test or imaging or other evaluation, or you don't understand the letter you received reporting the results.
- You don't know whether you are due for a physical or **Pap test**.

Your Preventive Care Appointment

It's a good idea to be seen once a year for a checkup. This may be the time for your Pap test, testing for sexually transmitted infections when appropriate, birth control prescription or options discussion, and a general once-over to be sure you are healthy. Schedule this well in advance, as often there can be a wait for "routine" health care, which is actually the most important kind of preventive maintenance. For more information about your preventive care appointment, see chapter 1, Meet Your Body and Your Doctor.

Emergency Phone Numbers You Should Know

The best way to make sure that an emergency has a happy ending is to be prepared in advance, when you're not stressed. Look up these numbers and keep them in your purse or wallet along with your medical information, so you always know where they are when time is important.

- Emergency number for my area (Be sure you have checked to see what number is used in your area!)
- Emergency number to call from a cell phone (In some areas, this is a different number.)
- Family member(s) to contact in case of emergency
- Fire department
- Local 24-hour pharmacy
- Poison control center
- Police department
- Primary care doctor
- Gynecologist
- Other health care specialists
- Your emergency friend's name and telephone number

How to Get Health Care When You Have Little or No Insurance

Almost 18 percent of the U.S. population under age sixty-five lives without health insurance. That's about forty-six million people, according to the U.S. Census. Advocacy groups have come up with even higher numbers.

Are you uninsured? Many younger women are. Even if offered health insurance, some women have none because they think that being young means they don't have to go to the doctor. Others don't want to spend the money. But many cannot afford it or are unemployed and have no access. If that's you, read on.

While it's true that you are less likely to fall sick than your eighty-five-year-old grandma, you are not immortal. What happens if you are hurt in a car crash?

Lucky for you, public hospitals in the United States cannot send you away from the emergency room (ER) just because you can't pay. Being treated for a car crash in the ER makes perfect sense—it's by far the best place to go. But what about your daily and long-term health care needs?

Many poor families try to get their health care from emergency departments at local hospitals. They will visit the ER for strep throat, flu, or bronchitis. Of course, the cost to the hospital is enormous when people do that. Instead of getting a quick check of a sore throat by a general practitioner, they use the resources of an expensive medical service they can't pay back. And because they don't have a life-threatening illness, they wait hours while the car crash victims—or other emergencies—are taken care of.

I mention that to encourage you to seek better health care—preventive care that will keep you healthy. There is nothing in an emergency room that will give you preventive health care. Save the ER option for accidents and emergencies, and find other options for your year-round care. Here are some ideas:

- **Hill-Burton clinics:** There are health care facilities in your community staffed by doctors who are required to give you health care regardless of your ability to pay. They are designated as Hill-Burton facilities. To find the nearest location to you, call the Hill-Burton hotline at (800) 638-0742, or (800) 492-0359 in Maryland. *Note*: There are no Hill-Burton facilities in Indiana, Nebraska, Nevada, Rhode Island, Utah, or Wyoming.
- **Federally assisted health clinics:** These clinics receive funds from the U.S. Department of Health and Human Services. They exist in every state and many, many counties. You pay what you can afford, based on your income. These clinics provide healthy checkups, sick visits, full pregnancy care, birth control, screening and treatment of sexually transmitted infections, mental health care, dental care, and prescription drugs, as well as substance abuse care. To locate a center, start online at http://findahealthcenter.hrsa.gov/. If you don't have online access at home, head for the public library. If you don't know how to go online, ask the librarian for help.
- **Hospital resources:** Your local public hospital has a financial office or a social worker who can help you find out all of the latest information on programs that are available to help you receive health care when you can't afford it.
- **Free or reduced-cost mammograms and Pap tests:** The National Breast and Cervical Cancer Early Detection Program (NBCCEDP) provides reduced-cost mammograms and Pap smears in your state. To find them online, go to www.cdc.gov/cancer/NBCCEDP/. Or call the Centers for Disease Control at (800) 232-4636 and tell them you would like to have the telephone number for the NBCCEDP's mammograms and Pap smear program in your state. You may have to be on hold for a while, so it's a good thing it's a free call.
- **Medications:** The Patient Assist Program Center (www.rxassist.org) offers information on reduced-cost and free medications. Costs are charged based on your income and ability to pay. The website offers information on many different medications. You can also ask your local pharmacist to recommend patient assistance programs in your area.

Forms to Chart Your Health

It's easy for me to ask you to chart your symptoms, but it's much more helpful if I give you some good forms and charts to help you keep track. Use the following forms to trace your family health history and record symptoms of digestion or PMS. I hope you'll use these charts every day so you can make good decisions with your doctor for your care. Make as many copies of the forms and charts as you need!

Family Health History

When you go to the doctor for your annual physical, you will be asked to fill in some forms about your family health history. Ask family members in advance if they have a history of any of the conditions listed.

Use the forms on pages 426–27 to write down who had what and at what age they had it. Your doctor's form will include some or all of these conditions, so this will help you be prepared for your appointment.

Digestion Journal

Use the Digestion Journal on page 428 for tracking your diet and any symptoms or side effects you experience after eating certain foods. Keeping a digestion journal is helpful if you are trying to figure out if you are lactose intolerant or why you keep having constipation, diarrhea, nausea, or stomach pain.

PMS Symptom Diary

Use the PMS Symptom Diary on page 429 to keep track of the symptoms you experience before, during, and after your period. It will help your doctor to know how to diagnose or treat your problem. If you want to keep track of more than one cycle, make copies of the blank form before you start filling it out.

To fill in the chart, start at Day 1 on the first day of your period and use one row for each day for an entire cycle (until the first day of your next period). Fill in the severity of your symptoms, from 1 to 3, for each symptom you experience. If you get to the end of the chart and you haven't gotten your period again, just add on days until your next period starts.

FAMILY HEALTH HISTORY			
Condition	**You**	**Family Member (Relationship to You)**	**Age When It Started**
Alcohol or drug use			
Allergies			
Alzheimer's			
Aneurysm			
Arthritis			
Asthma			
Birth defects			
Blood clots			
Cancer			
Breast			
Colon			
Endometrial			
Lung			
Ovarian			
Prostate			
Other			
Colon polyps			
Depression			
Diabetes: adult or type 2			
Diabetes: juvenile or type 1			
Epilepsy or seizures			
Eye problems			
Hearing loss			
Heart disease			
High blood pressure (hypertension)			
High cholesterol			
Infertility			
Kidney disease			
Mental illness			
Mental retardation			
Miscarriages			

FAMILY HEALTH HISTORY			
Condition	You	Family Member (Relationship to You)	Age When it Started
Obesity			
Osteoporosis			
Sleep disorders			
Stroke			
Thyroid problems			
Ulcer			
Vision loss			

Major Surgeries	What	When

Medications	Trade and Generic Names	Purpose	Dosage and Number of Times/Day	Special Instructions

DIGESTION JOURNAL				
Time	Food or Drink	Amount	Symptoms	Time Symptom Began

PMS SYMPTOM DIARY									
Symptom Rating: 1 = none 2 = mild 3 = severe									
	Bloating	Breast Tender-ness	Fatigue	Food Cravings	Anxiety	Depression	Irritability	Moodiness	Other
Day 1									
Day 2									
Day 3									
Day 4									
Day 5									
Day 6									
Day 7									
Day 8									
Day 9									
Day 10									
Day 11									
Day 12									
Day 13									
Day 14									
Day 15									
Day 16									
Day 17									
Day 18									
Day 19									
Day 20									
Day 21									
Day 22									
Day 23									
Day 24									
Day 25									
Day 26									
Day 27									
Day 28									

glossary

acid reflux
What it's called when acids in your stomach back up into your esophagus.

adrenal glands
Hormone-producing organs located just above the kidneys.

AIDS (acquired immunodeficiency syndrome)
An immune system disease that makes people vulnerable to infections and other diseases. It's passed on through bodily fluids (such as during sex) and through blood (such as through transfusions or by sharing hypodermic needles).

amenorrhea
What it's called when you stop having periods. It can be caused by stress, undereating, heavy-duty exercising, being pregnant, or being overweight.

amino acids
The building blocks of protein. Amino acids are probably the oldest nutrients on earth and are found in ancient fossils and even meteorites. They are essential to your health. The good news: You'll get enough by eating a healthy diet.

amniocentesis
A test done by an obstetrician where s/he takes a sample of the fluid that surrounds a baby in the uterus to determine the overall health of the growing baby. It looks for major birth defects, which are caused by chromosomal abnormalities, when a possible problem is noted on genetic testing, or in older moms, in families with a history of birth defects, or after an abnormal ultrasound.

androgens
The generic name for male sex hormones.

androstenedione
A type of male hormone (androgen) that is converted to testosterone. It has a synthetic form, which Mark McGwire said he was taking when he hit all those home runs.

anorexia nervosa
An eating disorder in which you have a terrible and irrational fear of being fat. You'll need help to deal with it.

antibiotics
A class of drugs that attack bacteria.

antibody
A protein made by the body and sent by the blood or the lymphatic system to attack foreign invaders, such as viruses, bacteria, parasites, or an organ transplant.

antigens
These molecules are the body's alarm system and tell the body to make antibodies to attack germs.

anus
The opening in your bottom where poop (or feces) comes out.

aorta
It's the big trunk of all of your arteries that carry blood away from the heart and to your limbs and organs. It starts in the left side of your heart.

arteries
Blood vessels that take blood away from the heart to the rest of the body.

arthritis
A usually painful condition caused by your joints being inflamed.

asthma
A breathing disorder that's triggered by allergies, cold, and exercise. It often comes with coughing and a tight feeling in your chest.

atherosclerosis
When the heart's arteries narrow because the walls are clogged, usually with cholesterol.

atria
The collection chambers of the heart. Your blood waits in the atria and is pumped out of the heart by the ventricles.

aura
A visual symptom of a migraine headache that looks like an arc or a circle of unpleasant light.

autoimmune disorder
What it's called when your body acts as if it is allergic to itself and starts making antibodies to attack healthy parts. Lupus, Addison's disease, rheumatoid arthritis, and multiple sclerosis are autoimmune diseases.

bacteria
A one-cell organism that can live freely and harmlessly in the body or in soil, water, and the environment and can also cause disease in animals, plants, and humans.

barium enema
A medical test in which your doctor puts a barium solution into your rectum and colon and then takes an X-ray to help diagnose lower intestinal problems.

benign
In medicine, this word means that something is not cancerous.

bile
A digestive fluid made in the liver.

biopsy
The process of removing a small amount of tissue from the body to diagnose diseases, especially cancers.

bladder
The sac where your body stores urine from the kidneys before you pee it out.

bloodstream
What we call your blood as it flows out of the heart, through the arteries, and back to the heart through the veins.

bowels
Your intestines, especially your large intestine (colon).

Brazilian
A type of bikini wax in which all of the hair around the genitals is removed.

bulimia nervosa
An eating disorder in which a fear of becoming fat leads someone to binge on food and then purge through self-induced vomiting, excess use of laxatives, or obsessive exercising.

cancer
What it's called when cells in a certain part (or parts) of your body or in your bloodstream multiply out of control.

capillaries
Tiny vessels (thinner than a fingernail) that carry blood to your tissues. You have zillions of them, and they are located between your arteries and your veins.

carbohydrates
One of the basic food types, in the form of sugars and starches.

carbon dioxide
An odorless, colorless gas produced from oxygen when we breathe. We breathe in oxygen and breathe out harmless carbon dioxide—not to be confused with the deadly gas called carbon monoxide. This is a good place to remind you to install carbon monoxide detectors (similar to your smoke detectors) in your home and check them annually.

carcinogen
Anything that causes cancer.

cardiac arrhythmias
What it's called when you have an irregular heartbeat.

cardiovascular system
The name for your whole circulatory system, including your heart and the blood that carries oxygen, gases, nutrients, and everything else around your body.

catheter
A tube that's inserted in the body, usually referring to a tube that drains urine when you can't pee by yourself, such as after surgery.

cervix
The little opening between a woman's vagina and uterus.

chlamydia
A sexually transmitted infection that's caused by bacteria and often shows no symptoms.

cholesterol
A fatty substance that is important to your cell structure but can also clog your arteries.

chronic
A problem that doesn't go away, sometimes even with treatment, and so must be managed for life with treatment or medication.

circulatory system
The name for your cardiovascular system plus your lymphatic system.

clitoris
A highly sensitive female organ located in front of the urethral opening that causes arousal and orgasm.

cognitive behavioral therapy (CBT)
A method of therapy that focuses on understanding and changing thoughts and behavior.

colon
Another name for your large intestine.

colonoscopy
A medical test in which a small tool with a tiny camera called a colonoscope is used to view the inner walls of the colon and bowels for polyps, adenomas, or other abnormalities, as well as diagnosing other bowel disorders such as Crohn's disease.

condom
You know what it is. The important thing to remember is to pack your own!

constipated
What it's called when you have difficult and/or infrequent bowel movements. It can be very uncomfortable.

corpus luteum
A temporary structure left behind in the ovary after you ovulate. It helps to maintain pregnancy by producing progesterone.

cortisol
A stress hormone. It pushes your blood pressure and blood sugar up, and lowers your immunity.

C-reactive protein
A protein found in the blood that signals inflammation.

Crohn's disease
An inflammatory, autoimmune disease that attacks the digestive system.

cystitis
A bladder infection.

cystoscopy
A test that allows your doctor to explore your bladder.

dehydroepiandrosterone (DHEA)
A steroid hormone that is formed naturally in your adrenal glands (in both men and women). It's an androgen (male hormone). Sometimes DHEA is used by athletes in supplement form for enhanced performance, but there's not enough data to support that.

dental dam
A sheet of plastic that is used to prevent the spread of sexually transmitted infections during oral sex.

diabetes
A condition that takes two forms. In type 1 diabetes, the pancreas is not making enough insulin, so there are high blood sugar levels. People need to take insulin in shot form to treat this. In type 2 diabetes, the body is resistant to the effects of insulin, resulting in high blood sugar levels. This may be treated with diet, oral medications to lower sugar levels, or insulin.

dialectical behavioral therapy
A type of therapy similar to cognitive behavioral therapy (CBT) that stresses mindful awareness of the world around us, the events that happen, and our feelings and responses.

diaphragm
A barrier method of contraception consisting of a rubbery cup, fitted by a health care provider, that is coated with spermicide and placed into the vagina near the cervix to prevent sperm from reaching the uterus.

diverticulitis
The diverticula become infected. Think intestinal pain and fever. An urgent problem—call your doctor now!

diverticulosis
Little pockets called diverticula form in the wall of the colon, usually as a result of the standard American diet of red meat and low fiber, which stresses the constipated bowels, causing these little outpouchings. You don't notice them much until you get diverticulitis.

DNA microarray
A new technology that allows scientists to look at a wide range of genes all at the same time, instead of one by one.

dopamine
An active neurotransmitter in the brain that is linked with many conditions, from Parkinson's disease to drug addiction. It also acts as a hormone and is involved in lactation (breast milk production).

duodenum
The first section of the small intestine where a lot of the chemical digestion and absorption of nutrients takes place.

dyspareunia
Painful sex, even when you use a lubricant. (See your doctor.)

dysthymia
A mood disorder that gives you long-term, low-grade depression.

E. coli
Bacteria found in fecal matter that can make you sick if you eat food that has been contaminated. This might be animal poop found in the field where the food was grown, human poop found in the same field, or poop from workers in the grocery store or restaurant who prepared the food without first washing their hands. Not all *E. coli* will make people sick, but some of it causes food poisoning.

ectopic pregnancy
A dangerous pregnancy that forms in the fallopian tube. Its main symptoms are pain and bleeding, and it is considered a medical emergency that requires immediate attention—even at 2 a.m. You are likely to be headed for some surgery to remove the pregnancy, which is a life-threatening problem for the mother.

electrolytes
Substances like sodium, potassium, chloride, and bicarbonate that regulate our metabolic processes and need to be balanced in the bloodstream. When your electrolytes are off balance (usually from not drinking enough water), you may feel dizzy, light-headed, confused, and irritable. For a quick treatment, have a sports drink (which often contains electrolytes) and eat a banana. If you don't feel better, call your doctor to see if you need to go in for extra hydration.

embryo
What we call the developing zygote after it implants itself in the wall of the uterus. At the end of eight weeks doctors will call it the fetus.

endometriosis
A condition in which cells of the uterine lining—the endometrium—grow in the pelvis outside of the uterus. These cells are still controlled by the hormones controlling the endometrium. The main symptom of endometriosis is pain, especially with intercourse, the menstrual cycle, and bowel and bladder functions. For some women, endometriosis can result in an infertility problem.

endometrium
The lining of your uterus, which sloughs off and comes out during your period and then rebuilds itself.

endorphins
Peptides in the brain that cause that wonderful feeling you get at a certain point during exercise, excitement, and even orgasm.

endoscopy
A medical test in which your doctor looks inside your body through a natural opening such as your mouth or rectum using an endoscope, a long, flexible tube with a light and camera at the end. Sometimes the procedure is diagnostic, and other times it can be used to remove polyps, as in a colonoscopy.

enzyme
Complex proteins that facilitate chemical reactions.

esophagus
The muscular tube that carries food from the back of your throat to your stomach using peristalsis, or waves of motion, to move food along. It is why, theoretically, you could eat upside down, but please don't try.

estrogen
The main female hormone.

fallopian tubes
The tubes that connect your ovaries to your uterus. Your eggs travel through them.

follicle
This has two meanings, depending on the part of the body you're talking about. On the skin, it refers to a small dip where your hair grows. In your ovaries, it's a group of cells that house one egg.

foreplay
The sexy, romantic, and playful ways that a couple interacts before sex to increase arousal.

free radicals
Atoms or molecules that have a single electron instead of a pair; they have been linked to aging and cell damage.

gallbladder
The organ that sits near the liver and concentrates your bile. If you develop large gallstones (small stones usually don't have symptoms), the gallbladder may or may not need to be removed.

gastroenterologist
A doctor who specializes in the digestive system, also called a GI doctor.

gastrointestinal
A word used to describe conditions or symptoms that involve your stomach or intestines.

gastroparesis
A condition in which your stomach loses the ability to empty itself completely. Symptoms include nausea, vomiting, bloating, blood sugar levels that bounce all over the place, and losing your appetite. It can be treated with medicine and changes to your diet.

gland
An organ that produces hormones, saliva, breast milk, and other substances that the body needs, and then excretes the substances either within or outside of the body. Think sweat.

glucose
A simple sugar. Glucose is found in the blood. When you have a diabetes test, the doctor is measuring the concentration of glucose, also called blood sugar.

gluten
A protein found in grains such as wheat, barley, and rye. People with celiac disease are allergic to gluten and usually must follow a lifelong gluten-free diet.

glycemic index
A measurement that describes how slowly or quickly foods release glucose in the bloodstream. Foods made from refined carbohydrates, such as candy bars and white bread, have a high glycemic index. Fruits and vegetables have a low glycemic index, except for especially sugary or starchy foods such as watermelon and potatoes.

gonorrhea
A sexually transmitted infection that often shows no symptoms.

G-spot
A sexually charged area rumored to be located at the front of the vagina. Is it real? I don't believe that we have such a thing, but have fun with your partner trying to find it!

gynecologist / "gyn"
A doctor who specializes in female reproductive and breast health.

HDL (high-density lipoprotein)
The "good" cholesterol fat that reduces your risk of developing heart disease.

heartburn
What we call it when stomach acid comes up the esophagus and burns your throat.

heart disease
Any heart problem that damages the heart or the blood vessels that feed the heart or causes heart attack or heart failure.

hematocrit
A test that measures the percent volume of red blood cells in your blood.

hemochromatosis
A condition in which the body hangs on to too much iron. It tends to run in families and can be diagnosed through blood testing. If caught early, it can be treated. With delayed diagnosis it can become very serious. The symptoms include generally not feeling well, stomach pain, fatigue, skin darkening, losing weight, and losing hair.

hemoglobin
The part of your red blood cells that carries oxygen through your circulatory system.

hemoglobin electrophoresis
A blood test that looks for problems with your hemoglobin.

hemorrhoids
The swelling and inflammation of veins in your rectum and anus, usually caused by eating a low-fiber diet, though also common in pregnancy and after childbirth. Some hemorrhoids can't be felt, but others can be extremely painful lumps. One sure symptom of hemorrhoids is seeing bright red blood on the toilet paper when you wipe yourself. If they don't go away on their own, talk to your doctor.

herpes
A disease that is transmitted through human-to-human contact that can appear as cold sores on your lips (simplex 1) or as sexually transmitted lesions in the genital area (simplex 2). Teenagers love to mix the two up.

HIPAA
The Healthcare Insurance Portability and Accountability Act (HIPAA) is the law passed in the United States in 1996 that protects your medical privacy.

HIV (human immunodeficiency virus)
The virus that causes AIDS.

human papillomavirus (HPV)
A sexually transmitted virus that can cause cancer of the cervix (the narrow passageway between your vagina and uterus).

hymen
A fold of mucous membrane that partly covers the entry to your vagina. People used to think that a woman must have an intact hymen to be a virgin, but now we know that there are many ways that your hymen can tear. (If yours is intact, your first sexual experience may be painful, but it won't continue after the first time.)

hyper- and hypoactive sexual desire disorders
The media calls a person with hyperactive disorder a sex addict. A person who is not interested in sex for the short or long term is said to have hypoactive sexual desire disorder. If you identify with either group, please see your doctor. These are real conditions.

hyperinsulinemia
What we call it when you have too much insulin in your blood, especially in type 2 diabetics.

hypertension
Another word to describe high blood pressure.

hyponatremia
When the salt concentration in your blood is too low and your body holds too much liquid relative to salt. This problem can happen to athletes and others who drink too much water. This is a serious condition that must be managed by your doctor.

hysterectomy
A surgery in which the uterus is removed.

inflammation
The body's response to infection. When you see a red area around a wound, that's inflammation.

inner labia
(see *labia*)

insulin
A hormone that helps your liver, fat cells, and muscle cells store glucose and use it as an energy source. If your insulin is out of control, you have diabetes. (Favorite trivia question: Where are the Isles of Langerhans? Answer: In the pancreas! They are clusters of cells that produce insulin.)

insulin resistance
A condition in which the normal amounts of insulin made in your body are not enough to maintain a healthy balance, a problem in type 2 diabetes.

intestines
The general name for your small intestine and large intestine (colon).

joint
The junction where bones meet, such as at the arm and shoulder, that generally enables movement.

Kegel exercises
A type of squeezing exercise that strengthens the pelvic floor, the vagina, and the urethra.

kidneys
The organs (you have two) that filter your blood and send salts, waste, water, and toxins to the bladder through the ureters. They are located on either side of your body on the back side of your abdomen, and are each about the size of a fist.

labia
The inner lips (also called labia minora) and the outer

lips (also called labia majora) that form the border of the vulva.

lactobacillus
The active ingredient in some yogurt. The hype about the benefits of this natural bacteria has not been proven, but yogurt is good for you anyway.

large intestine
Another name for your colon, the part of your digestive system where the body draws water from what you have eaten and forms poop.

LDL (low-density lipoprotein)
The "bad" cholesterol fat that increases your risk of developing heart disease.

liver
The critical, filtering organ that makes bile, helps to digest food, and is a part of many complex processes in your body. The liver is the filter for many of the unhealthy things we do to our bodies, such as drinking alcohol and abusing drugs.

lower gastrointestinal series
A series of medical tests, such as a barium enema, that looks at your lower digestive system.

lymphatic system
One part, along with the cardiovascular system, of your body's circulatory system. It consists of many small channels that carry lymphatic fluid through the body to help fight germs. It can also carry cancer cells.

lymph node
You have many of them; they carry lymph, a clear fluid that helps to remove bacteria and wastes from your tissues, around your body. Lymph is also believed to carry cancer cells.

malignant
A word that means something in your body contains cancerous cells.

menopause
The period during middle age when a woman's cycle of ovulation and menstruation gradually ceases. Many women have few symptoms during this hormonal transition. Others are plagued with hot flashes, vaginal dryness, and mood swings.

metabolic rate
The number of calories you burn per hour for every square meter of your body's surface.

micturition reflex
The reflex that makes you relax your urethral sphincter when your bladder is full to allow you to empty your bladder.

migraine
A particular type of severe and often chronic headache that requires attention from your doctor.

mitral valve
The valve in your heart that controls blood flow between the left atrium and the left ventricle.

mucous membrane
The lining of the parts of your body that are exposed to the outside world and that produce mucus, including your nose, mouth, and vagina.

mucus
A slippery coating secreted by mucous membranes.

musculoskeletal
The parts of your body that work together to make you move, including your muscles, tendons, ligaments, bones, and joints.

neurotransmitter
Chemical substances that help the brain communicate by transmitting nerve impulses across synapses. Neurotransmitters include dopamine, norepinephrine, and serotonin.

neutrophils
The common white blood cells that form the body's front line in fighting infection by racing to the scene where germs are, eating the threatening foreign germs, and immediately dying.

nitrosamines
Chemical compounds used to cure and preserve some foods, most commonly bacon. Some nitrosamines are thought to be carcinogenic (cancer causing) in animals and possibly in humans. The U.S. government has restricted the level of nitrites (which convert to nitrosamines through high-temperature cooking such as frying) in foods to keep risks at a minimum while maximizing food safety.

norepinephrine
A hormone and neurotransmitter that kicks off your flight-or-fight response.

nutrients
Substances obtained from food that we need to be healthy.

obstetrician
A doctor who specializes in fertility, pregnancy, and childbirth.

obstetrician-gynecologist (ob-gyn)
A doctor who specializes in female reproductive health, as well as fertility, pregnancy, and childbirth.

oral sex
Using your mouth on your partner's genitals to cause arousal or orgasm.

orgasmic disorder
The inability to have an orgasm, among women or men. (Women are often uncomfortable talking about this, but your doctor can help.)

orthotics
Inserts that you slip inside of your shoes to relieve pain by changing your balance and gait. They can be custom made (go this route if your insurance covers it) or bought over the counter, and can make a big difference in your life if you have pain with walking.

osteoblast
A cell that makes bone.

osteoclast
A cell that eats bone.

osteoporosis
A condition in which you begin to lose your normal bone density and strength and your bones become more fragile.

outer labia
(see *labia*)

ovary
The organs where women's eggs are developed and released. We have two of them.

ovulation
The part of your monthly cycle when you release an egg from your ovary, which happens about once a month. You are at your most fertile during this time.

oxygenated
A word used to describe something that has been supplied with oxygen.

pancreas
The organ behind your stomach that produces insulin and digestive enzymes.

panic attacks
Episodes marked by an overwhelming feeling of anxiety and fear. (See your doctor if you have a chronic problem with recurrent attacks.)

Pap test or Pap smear
The process of examining cells from the cervix to look for changes that signal early signs of pre-cancer.

Parkinson's disease
A complicated and serious brain disorder that gets worse over time. Symptoms include tremors and difficulty walking.

pelvis
The girdle of bones connecting your upper body to your legs. Your pelvis contains your intestines, your internal sex organs, and your bladder.

peristalsis
The involuntary, wavelike muscular movements that move food through the esophagus, stomach, and intestines.

plaque
A substance that forms on a body part or surface. Plaque accumulated on the teeth will form tartar and create tooth decay and gum disease. On your arteries, plaque increases your risk of heart attack.

plasma
The yellowish liquid part of your blood that carries the blood cells.

platelets
Small bodies that help your blood to clot when, for example, your skin is cut.

PMS (premenstrual syndrome)
A set of symptoms shared by many women in the days leading up to their period, including bloating, headache, fatigue, acne, insomnia, anxiety, cramps, mood swings or breast swelling and tenderness. (Nobody gets all of these symptoms. If your PMS is too much to handle, see your doctor for help.)

polyps
Benign growths.

postpartum depression

A hormone-driven depression that many women experience after childbirth, made worse by sleep deprivation and the complete upheaval a new baby causes. (It has nothing to do with how much you love your baby or your partner. Please tell your obstetrician if you think you have postpartum depression.)

premenstrual dysphoric disorder (PMDD)

A very severe form of PMS that deserves your doctor's attention.

progesterone

A major female hormone that prepares your body for pregnancy, helps maintain a pregnancy, and also controls your monthly cycle.

progestin

A synthetic ingredient that mimics natural progesterone; used in birth control pills and hormone therapy.

prolactin

A hormone produced by the pituitary gland that gets your breast milk started up and maintains it after childbirth.

prostaglandins

Hormonelike substances found in many cells in our bodies. We don't know everything about them, but we know they are involved in calcium movement, making us more sensitive to pain, bowel contractions, uterine contractions, stomach acid production, and many other physical functions.

protein

An essential building block of a healthy body, found in meat, fish, poultry, tofu and other soybean products, eggs, dairy products, nuts, beans, and grains.

psychopharmacologist/psychopharm

Someone who specializes in prescribing and managing medicines for mental health and mood disorders.

rectum

The tail end (the last six to eight inches) of your large intestine, where your poop waits until you go to the bathroom.

red blood cells

The majority of your blood cells; their specific job is to carry oxygen.

remodeling

This can refer to a surgical procedure, such as reconstructive surgery, or it can mean the body's natural process of making bones.

resorption

What we call it when your body takes calcium from your bones, resulting in bone loss.

restless legs syndrome

An aching, fidgety feeling in your legs (and sometimes the arms) that usually happens when you're trying to fall asleep. (There are tests to determine whether you have it and treatments that you can try, so be sure to tell your doctor if you have this.)

reticulocyte

An immature red blood cell.

saliva glands

The glands around your mouth and throat that make your spit.

saturated fat

Fat from animals, dairy, and coconut or palm oils that tends to increase cholesterol levels and heart disease risk.

scintillating scotoma

A kind of aura associated with the beginning of a migraine.

selective serotonin reuptake inhibitors (SSRIs)

A common form of antidepressant medication.

sensory adaptation

A way to describe the body's method of getting used to things, such as when your eyes adapt to the dark or your nose adapts to a bad smell.

serotonin

A neurotransmitter in the brain that scientists believe is involved in the causes of depression.

sex hormone-binding globulin (SHBG)

A protein produced by the liver that binds the sex hormones estrogen and testosterone, making them inactive. Once these hormones are bound to this protein, they are not active in the body.

sexual arousal disorder

I hesitate to name these disorders, because I wonder if it's fair. What if it's a woman's choice to be sexually inactive? If that's you, this won't need exploring, just like the other so-called disorders we've talked about. This one means a condition in which the body does not respond to arousal with the usual signs, such as tightening of the nipples and lubrication of the vagina.

sexual pain disorder
(See *vaginismus*)

sleep apnea
A sleep disorder caused by abnormal pauses in breathing as you sleep. (Your partner may notice that you have periods of silence followed by loud snoring.) Untreated, apnea can cause other serious problems, including heart conditions.

small intestine
The long, narrow part of the intestine where nutrients are absorbed.

speculum
A hinged tool shaped like a duck's bill used to hold the vagina open while cells are taken for a Pap test.

sphincter
A round muscle that opens and shuts parts of the body, such as the anus, the urethra, and the esophagus.

spironolactone
A diuretic and antiandrogen medicine, used to treat heart failure, high blood pressure, and both hair loss and excessive hair growth.

STI/STD
A sexually transmitted infection or disease.

stomach acid
The solution in your stomach that breaks down food. It also causes heartburn.

stones
Crystal-like balls of calcium or salt that may build up in your body, especially in the gallbladder, kidneys, or bladder. (Contact your doctor if you suspect that you have stones.)

stroke
Disruption of the blood supply to the brain because a vessel is blocked or ruptured. A mild stroke may barely be noticed, while a severe stroke can be fatal. Learn the warning signs for strokes on page 419 so that someday you may save someone's life. Early treatment makes a huge difference.

testosterone
The primary male hormone, found in both men and women.

thalassemia
A genetic blood disorder in which the body cannot produce enough red blood cells and hemoglobin, resulting in anemia. There are treatments available, but if you have this problem, it will be very important to work at having good health.

thyroid
A hormone-producing gland located in the neck.

trachea
The tube that connects your nose and mouth to your lungs, also called the windpipe.

trans fat
One of the "bad" fats that increases heart disease risk. It is used by manufacturers to make liquid fats solid and stable so food products don't melt or go bad in the store.

trapezius
The group of muscles that run across the back of your shoulders.

triglycerides
The most common type of fat found in your body. Having a high number of blood triglycerides may be part of a series of health problems called metabolic syndrome, which increases your chances of having heart disease, stroke, and diabetes.

triptans
A medicine that is commonly used as a treatment for migraine headaches.

tubal ligation
The process of surgically cutting or sealing the fallopian tubes so eggs can't travel to the uterus. It is a permanent form of sterilization for women. See also "vasectomy."

ulcer
A deterioration of the mucous membrane in the stomach, lower esophagus, or the beginning of the small intestine.

ureters
The tubes that carry urine from the kidneys to the bladder.

urethra
The opening in your body that carries pee from the bladder to the toilet.

urinalysis
A medical test in which we look at your urine for signs of health problems.

urinary tract infection (UTI)
Urinary tract infections can be very painful. If it hurts to pee, call your doctor. This needs to be treated. The faster you call, the faster that pain is going to go away.

uterus
The womb, the muscular and hollow organ where a fertilized egg is implanted and grows into an embryo and then a fetus.

vagina
The birth canal, which connects the uterus to the outside world. During sex, semen is ejaculated into the vagina and then travels through the cervix into the uterus to fertilize an egg.

vaginismus
A treatable condition characterized by vaginal tightness that causes pain and burning during sex and can even make sex impossible.

vas deferens
The tube in men that connects the testes and the urethra and carries semen.

vasectomy
The process of sealing the vas deferns (the tube that carries sperm). It is a permanent form of sterilization for men. See also "tubal ligation."

veins
The vast network of vessels that return blood to the heart from the rest of your body. They may look blue under your skin.

ventricles
The pumping chambers of the heart. Your blood waits in the atrium and is pumped out of the heart by the ventricles.

vertigo
A feeling of dizziness or loss of balance. (Having vertigo can signal other problems, so always check in with your doctor if you have this.)

villi
Tiny, fingerlike projections in the small intestine that help the body to absorb nutrients.

vulva
A woman's genital area, including the vaginal opening, the clitoris, the labia, and the urethral opening.

white blood cells
The infection-fighting cells in your blood.

X-ray
The process of taking a picture of your bones and other inner parts of your body using electromagnetic radiation.

yeast infection
An itchy vaginal infection with a discharge caused by an imbalance of *Candida albicans*, a normal yeast that lives in the body all the time.

bibliography

CHAPTER 1: MEET YOUR BODY AND YOUR DOCTOR

American Heart Association. Risk Factors and Coronary Heart Disease. www.americanheart.org.

Barton MB, Harris R, Fletcher SW. 1999. Does this patient have breast cancer? The screening clinical examination: should it be done? How? *Journal of the American Medical Association* 282:1270–80.

Centers for Disease Control and Prevention, National Center for Health Statistics. 2006. Deaths and Mortality. www.cdc.gov/nchs/fastats/deaths.htm

Centers for Disease Control and Prevention. Sexually transmitted diseases treatment guidelines. 2002. *Morbidity and Mortality Weekly Report* 51 (No. RR-6):1–80.

Laumann EO, Paik A, Rosen RC. 1999. Sexual dysfunction in the United States: prevalence and predictors. *Journal of the American Medical Association* 281:537–44.

Miller AB, To T, Baines CJ, et al. 2000. Canadian National Breast Screening Study-2: 13-year results of a randomized trial in women aged 50–59 years. *Journal of the National Cancer Institute* 92:1490–99.

Thomas DB, Gao DL, Ray RM, et al. 2002. Randomized trial of breast self-examination in Shanghai: final results. *Journal of the National Cancer Institute* 94:1445–57.

Weinstock SH, Berman S, Cates, W Jr. 2004. Sexually transmitted diseases among American youth: incidence and prevalence estimates, 2000. *Perspectives on Sexual and Reproductive Health* #36:6–10.

CHAPTER 2: YOUR HEAD

Aetna Intelihealth. Migraine. www.intelihealth.com/IH/ihtIH/WSIHW000/9339/10344.html.

American Psychiatric Association. 2000. *Diagnostic and Statistical Manual of Mental Disorders,* fourth edition. Washington, DC: American Psychiatric Association. Eating Disorders.

American Psychiatric Association. 2000. *Diagnostic and Statistical Manual of Mental Disorders,* fourth edition. Washington, DC: American Psychiatric Association. Premenstrual Syndrome.

Bertone-Johnson ER, Hankinson SE, Bendich A, et al. 2005. Calcium and vitamin D intake and risk of incident premenstrual syndrome. *Archives of Internal Medicine* 165:1246–52.

Blehar MC, Oren DA. 1997. Gender differences in depression. *Medscape Women's Health* 2:3.

Claman F, Miller T. 2006. Premenstrual syndrome and premenstrual dysphoric disorder in adolescence. *Journal of Pediatric Health Care* 20:329–33.

Culpepper L. 2002. Generalized anxiety disorder in primary care: emerging issues in management and treatment. *Journal of Clinical Psychiatry* 63:35–42.

Cyranowski JM, Frank E, Young E, et al. 2000. Adolescent onset of the gender difference in lifetime rates of major depression. *Archives of General Psychiatry* 57:21–27.

Dictionary.com. 2008. Migraine. http://dictionary.reference.com/browse/migraine.

Edwards VJ, Holden GW, Felitti VJ, et al. 2003. Relationship between multiple forms of childhood maltreatment and adult mental health in community respondents: results from the adverse childhood experiences study. *American Journal of Psychiatry* 160:1453–60.

Fava M, Alpert J, Nierenberg AA, et al. 2005. A doubleblind randomized trial of St John's wort, fluoxetine, and placebo in major depressive disorder. *Journal of Clinical Psychopharmacology* 25:441–47.

Feuerstein M, Shaw WS. 2002. Measurement properties of the calendar of premenstrual experience in patients with premenstrual syndrome. *Journal of Reproductive Medicine* 47:279–89.

Ford O, Lethaby A, Mol B, et al. 2006. Progesterone for premenstrual syndrome. *Cochrane Database of Systematic Reviews* CD003415.

Fosberg S, Lock J. 2006. The relationship between perfectionism, eating disorders and athletes: a review. *Minerva Pediatrica* 58:525–36.

Freeman EW. 2002. Evaluation of a unique oral contraceptive (Yasmin) in the management of premenstrual dysphoric disorder. *European Journal of Contraception and Reproductive Health Care* 3:27–34.

Jones R, Britten N, Culpepper L, et al. 2003. *Oxford Textbook of Primary Care*. Oxford, UK: Oxford University Press. Chapter 9: Depression, 952–54.

Jones R, Britten N, Culpepper L, et al. 2003. *Oxford Textbook of Primary Care*. Oxford, UK: Oxford University Press. Section 9.10: Psychological treatments for mental health problems, 983–88.

Kennedy SH, Eisfeld BS, Dickens SE. 2000. Antidepressant-induced sexual dysfunction during treatment with moclobemide, paroxetine, sertraline, and venlafaxine. *Journal of Clinical Psychiatry* 276:276–81.

Kornstein SG. 1997. Gender differences in depression: implications for treatment. *Journal of Clinical Psychiatry* 58(supplement 15):12–18.

Kroll R, Rapkin AJ. 2006. Treatment of premenstrual disorders. *Journal of Reproductive Medicine* 51:359–70.

Lanteri-Minet M, Valade D, Geraud G, et al. 2005. Migraine and probable migraine: results of FRAMG 3, a French nationwide survey carried out according to the 2004 HIS classification. *Headache* 25:1146–58.

Laurn L, Nordheim LW, Ekeland E, et al. 2006. Exercise in prevention and treatment of anxiety and depression among children and young people. *Cochrane Database of Systematic Reviews* 3:CD004691.

Lewisohn PM, Hyman H, Roberts RE, et al. 1993. Adolescent psychopathology: prevalence and incidence of depression and other *DSM-III-R* disorders in high school students. *Journal of Abnormal Psychology* 102:133–44.

Loj J, Solomon GD. 2006. Migraine prophylaxis: who, why, and how. *Cleveland Clinic Journal of Medicine* 73:793–4, 797, 800–801.

Mayo Clinic. 2004. Women and depression: understanding the gender gap. www.mayoclinic.com/health/depression/MH00035.

McGrath E, Keita GP, Stickland BR, et al. 1990. Women and Depression: Risk Factors and Treatment Issues. www.apa.org/ppo/issues/pwomenanddepress.html.

Mortola JF, Girton L, Beck L, et al. 1990. Diagnosis of premenstrual syndrome by a simple, prospective, and reliable instrument: the calendar of premenstrual experiences. *Obstetrics and Gynecology* 76:302–07.

National Institute of Mental Health. 2000. *Depression: What Every Woman Should Know*. Bethesda, MD: National Institutes of Health, US Department of Health and Human Services. NIH Publication No. 00-3679.

National Institute of Mental Health. 2009. Depression. www.nimh.nih.gov/health/publications/depression/what-are-the-different-forms-of-depression.shtml.

National Mental Health Information Center. Eating Disorders. http://mentalhealth.samhsa.gov/publications/allpubs/ken98-0047/default.asp.

National Stroke Association. www.stroke.org.

Parry BL, Sorenson DL, Meliska CJ, et al. 2003. Hormonal basis of mood and postpartum disorders. *Current Women's Health Reports* 3:230–35.

Pearlstein T. 2002. Selective serotonin reuptake inhibitors for premenstrual dysphoric disorder: the emerging gold standard? *Drugs* 62:1869–85.

Pearson NJ, Johnson LL, Nahin RL. 2006. Insomnia, trouble sleeping, and complementary and alternative medicine: analysis of the 2002 National Health Interview Survey data. *Archives of Internal Medicine* 166:1775–82.

Perkins SJ, Murphy R, Schmidt U, et al. 2006. Self-help and guided self-help for eating disorders. *Cochrane Database Systematic Reviews* CD004191.

Roland, LP. 2005. *Merritt's Neurology*. Philadelphia: Lippincott Williams & Wilkins. Chapter 159: Mood Disorders, 1125–32.

Ruhrmann S, Kasper S, Hawellek B, et al. 1998. Effects of fluoxetine versus bright light in the treatment of seasonal affective disorder. *Psychological Medicine* 28:923–33.

Taylor MJ, Freemantle N, Geddes JR, et al. 2006. Early onset of selective serotonin reuptake inhibitor antidepressant action: systematic review and meta-analysis. *Archives of General Psychiatry* 63:1217–23.

Trivedi MH, Greer TL, Grannemann BD, et al. 2006. Exercise as an augmentation strategy for treatment of major depression. *Journal of Psychiatric Practice* 12:205–13.

U.S. Food and Drug Administration. Center for Drug Evaluation. www.fda.gov.

Weiss EL, Longhurst JG, Mazure CM, et al. 1999. Childhood sexual abuse as a risk factor for depression in women: psychosocial and neurobiological correlates. *American Journal of Psychiatry* 156:816–28.

Wyatt K, Dimmock P, Jones P, et al. 2001. Efficacy of progesterone and progestogens in management of premenstrual syndrome. *British Medical Journal* 323:776–80.

CHAPTER 3: STRESS AND YOUR BODY

Domar AD, Dreher H. 2007. *Self-Nurture: Learning to Care for Yourself as Effectively as You Care for Everyone Else*. New York: Penguin Group.

Domar AD, Kelly AL. 2008. *Be Happy Without Being Perfect: How to Break Free from the Perfection Deception*. New York: Random House.

CHAPTER 4: YOUR SKIN

Abdulla FR, Feldman SR, Willifor PJ. 2005. Tanning and skin cancer. *Pediatric Dermatology* 22:501–12.

Acne.org. 2009. What is acne? www.acne.org/whatisacne.html.

Bolognia JL. 2006. Too many moles. *Archives of Dermatology* 142:479–83.

Burrall B. 2006. The relationship of diet and acne. *Dermatology Online Journal* 12:25.

Draelos ZD. 2002. Self-tanning lotions: are they a healthy way to achieve a tan? *American Journal of Clinical Dermatology* 3:317–18.

Environmental Protection Agency. 2006. Sunscreen: The Burning Facts. Publication No. 430-F-06-013.

Freedberg IM, Eisen AZ, Wolff K, et al. 2003. *Fitzpatrick's Dermatology in General Medicine*. New York: McGraw-Hill. Chapter 6: Structure and Development of Skin, 59–86.

Freedberg IM, Eisen AZ, Wolff K, et al. 2003. *Fitzpatrick's Dermatology in General Medicine*. New York: McGraw-Hill. Chapter 73: Diseases of the Sebaceous Glands, 672–87.

Freedberg IM, Eisen AZ, Wolff K, et al. 2003. *Fitzpatrick's Dermatology in General Medicine*. New York: McGraw-Hill. Chapter 251: Other Topical Medications, 2363–68.

Gallagher RP, Spinelli JJ, Lee TK. 2005. Tanning beds, sunlamps, and risk of cutaneous malignant melanoma. *Cancer Epidemiology Biomarkers and Prevention* 14:562–66.

Huber J, Walch K. 2006. Treating acne with oral contraceptives: use of lower doses. *Contraception* 73:23–29.

Johnson MA, Kimlin MG. 2006. Vitamin D, aging, and the 2005 Dietary Guidelines for Americans. *Nutrition Reviews* 64:410–21.

Petitjean A, Mac-Mary S, Sainthillier JM, et al. 2006. Effects of cigarette smoking on the skin of women. *Journal of Dermatological Science* 42:259–61.

Rao S, Malik MA, Wilder LJ, et al. 2006. Clinical inquiries: what is the best treatment for mild to moderate acne? *Journal of Family Practice* 55:994–96.

Sharpe G. 2006. Skin cancer: prevalence, prevention and treatment. *Clinical Medicine* 6:333–34.

Yin L, Morita A, Tsuji T. 2001. Skin aging induced by ultraviolet exposure and tobacco smoking: evidence from epidemiological and molecular studies. *Photodermatology, Photoimmunology and Photomedicine* 17:178–83.

CHAPTER 5: YOUR HEART

American Heart Association. 2004. Physical Activity. www.americanheart.org/presenter.jhtml?identifier=4563.

American Heart Association. 2006. Alcohol, Wine, and Cardiovascular Disease. www.americanheart.org/presenter.jhtml?identifier=4422.

American Heart Association. 2006. Diet and Lifestyle Recommendations Revision 2006. *Circulation* 114:82–96.

American Heart Association. 2006. Homocysteine, Folic Acid, and Cardiovascular Disease. www.americanheart.org/presenter.jhtml?identifier=4677.

American Heart Association. 2007. Inflammation, Heart Disease and Stroke: The Role of C-Reactive Protein. www.americanheart.org/presenter.jhtml?identifier=4648.

American Heart Association. 2008. Healthy Levels of Cholesterol. www.americanheart.org/presenter.jhtml?identifier=3045974.

American Heart Association. Smoking Is a Woman's Single Biggest Risk Factor for Heart Attack. www.americanheart.org/presenter.jhtml?identifier=2779.

American Heart Association. Women and Cardiovascular Disease Statistics. www.americanheart.org/downloadable/heart/1168614043234WOMEN07.pdf.

American Lung Association. 2009. Women and Tobacco Use. www.lungusa.org/stop-smoking/about-smoking/facts-figures/women-and-tobacco-use.html.

Ayanian JZ, Cleary PD. 1999. Perceived risks of heart disease and cancer among cigarette smokers. *Journal of the American Medical Association* 281:1019–21.

Centers for Disease Control and Prevention. 1999. Cigarette smoking among adults: United States. *Morbidity and Mortality Weekly Report* 48:993–96.

Centers for Disease Control and Prevention. 2004. Cigarette use among high school students: United States, 1991–2003. *Morbidity and Mortality Weekly Report* 53:499–502.

Centers for Disease Control and Prevention. 2005. Trends in leisure-time physical inactivity by age, sex, and race/ethnicity: United States, 1994–2004. *Morbidity and Mortality Weekly Report* 54:991–94.

Centers for Disease Control and Prevention. 2009. Smoking and Tobacco Use: Quit Tips. www.cdc.gov/tobacco/quit_smoking/how_to_quit/quit_tips.htm.

Department of Health and Human Services, National Institutes of Health. 2000. Table for Calculated Body Mass Index Values for Selected Heights and Weights. www.nhlbisupport.com/bmi.

Glaser R, Herrmann HC, Murphy SA, et al. 2002. Benefit of an early invasive management strategy in women with acute coronary syndromes. *Journal of the American Medical Association* 288:3124–29.

Hayes SN. 2006. Preventing cardiovascular disease in women. *American Family Physician* 74:1331–40.

Hyland A, Li Q, Bauer JE. 2004. Predictors of cessation in a cohort of current and former smokers followed over 15 years. *Nicotine and Tobacco Research* 3:363–69.

Li TY, Rana JS, Manson JE, et al. 2006. Obesity as compared with physical activity in predicting risk of coronary heart disease in women. *Circulation* 113:499–506.

Lichtenstein AH, Ausman LM, Jalbert SM, et al. 1999. Effects of different forms of dietary hydrogenated fats on serum lipoprotein cholesterol levels. *New England Journal of Medicine* 24:1933–40.

Maynard C, Every NR, Martin JS, et al. 1997. Association of gender and survival in patients with acute myocardial infarction. *Archives of Internal Medicine* 157:1379–84.

Medline Plus. Heart Disease and Women. www.nlm.nih.gov/medlineplus/ency/article/007188.htm.

Miller ER III, Erlinger TP, Appel LJ. 2006. The effects of macronutrients on blood pressure and lipids: an overview of the DASH and Omni Heart Trials. *Current Atherosclerosis Reports* 8:460–65.

Miller M, Byington R, Hunninghake D, et al. 2000. Sex bias and underutilization of lipid-lowering therapy in patients with coronary artery disease at academic medical centers in the United States and Canada: Prospective randomized evaluation of the vascular effects of Norvasc trial (PREVENT) investigators. *Archives of Internal Medicine* 160:343–47.

Mitka M. 2005. Obesity's role in heart disease requires apples and pears comparison. *Journal of the American Medical Association* 294:3071–72.

Mosca L, Manson JE, Sutherland DE, et al. 1997. Cardiovascular disease in women: a statement for healthcare professionals from the American Heart Association. *Circulation* 96:2468–82.

Panagiotakos DB, Rallidis LS, Pitsavos C. 2006. Cigarette smoking and myocardial infarction in young men and women: a case-control study. *International Journal of Cardiology* #16:371–75.

Pearson TA, Blair SN, Daniels SR, et al. 2002. AHA Guidelines for Primary Prevention of Cardiovascular Disease and Stroke: 2002 Update. *Circulation* 106:388–91.

Rexrode KM, Carey VJ, Hennekens CH, et al. 1998. Abdominal adiposity and coronary heart disease in women. *Journal of the American Medical Association* 280:1843–48.

Schulman KA, Berlin JA, Harless W, et al. 1999. The effect of race and sex on physicians' recommendations for cardiac catheterization. *New England Journal of Medicine* 340:618–26.

Sclavo M. 2001. Cardiovascular risk factors and prevention in women: similarities and differences. *Italian Heart Journal* 2:125–41.

Stampfer MJ, Hu FB, Manson JE, et al. 2000. Primary prevention of coronary heart disease in women through diet and lifestyle. *New England Journal of Medicine* 343:16–22.

U.S. National Institutes of Health. National Cancer Institute. Low-Tar Cigarettes: Evidence Doesn't Indicate Benefit to Public Health. www.cancer.gov/newscenter/lowtar.

Vivekananthan DP, Penn MS, Sapp SK, et al. 2004. Use of antioxidant vitamins for the prevention of cardiovascular disease: a meta-analysis of randomized trials. *Lancet* 21:662.

Von Eyben FE, Bech J, Madsen JK, et al. 1996. High prevalence of smoking in young patients with acute myocardial infarction. *Journal of the Royal Society of Health* 116:153–56.

Willett WC. 2006. Trans fatty acids and cardiovascular disease: epidemiological data. *Atherosclerosis* 7:5–8.

Willett WC, Green A, Stampfer MJ, et al. 1987. Relative and absolute risks of coronary heart disease among women who smoke cigarettes. *New England Journal of Medicine* 317:1303–09.

Willett WC, Manson JE, Stampfer MJ, et al.1995. Weight, weight change, and coronary heart disease in women: risk within the "normal" weight range. *Journal of the American Medical Association* 273:461–65.

CHAPTER 6: YOUR BLOOD

Centers for Disease Control and Prevention. 1998. Recommendations to prevent and control iron deficiency in the United States. *Morbidity and Mortality Weekly Report* 47:1–29.

Kasper DL, Braunwald E, Fauci AS, et al. 2005. *Harrison's Internal Medicine*. New York: McGraw-Hill Companies. Chapter 90: Iron Deficiency and Other Hypoproliferative Anemias.

Kasper DL, Braunwald E, Fauci AS, et al. 2005. *Harrison's Internal Medicine*. New York: McGraw-Hill Companies. Chapter 99: Transfusion Biology and Therapy—Blood Group Antigens and Antibodies.

Red Gold: The Epic Story of Blood (story of librarian Percy Oliver). 2002. PBS series.

U.S. Food and Drug Administration. 1996. Fact Sheet: Folic Acid Fortification. *FDA Consumer*, July.

CHAPTER 7: YOUR BONES AND JOINTS

Barzel US, Massey LK. 1998. Excess dietary protein can adversely affect bone. *Journal of Nutrition* 128:2529.

Borer KT. 2005. Physical activity in the prevention and amelioration of osteoporosis in women: interaction of mechanical, hormonal and dietary factors. *Sports Medicine* 35:779–830.

Cromer BA, Scholes D, Berenson A, et al. 2006. Depot medroxyprogesterone acetate and bone mineral density in adolescents—the black box warning: a position paper for the Society for Adolescent Medicine. *Journal of Adolescent Health* 39:296–301.

Gordon CM, Nelson LM. 2003. Amenorrhea and bone health in adolescents and young women. *Current Opinions in Obstetrics and Gynecology* 15:377–84.

Heller HJ, Stewart A, Haynes S, et al. 1999. Pharmacokinetics of calcium absorption from two commercial calcium supplements. *Journal of Clinical Pharmacology* 39:1151–54.

Hellman DB, Stone JH. 2006. *Current Medical Diagnosis and Treatment, forty-fifth edition*. New York: Lange Medi cal Books/McGraw-Hill Publishing Division. Chapter 20: Arthritis and Musculoskeletal Disorders.

Hooper MM. 2006. Tending to the musculoskeletal problems of obesity. *Cleveland Clinic Journal of Medicine* 73:839–45.

Isenberg DA, Maddison PJ, Woo P. 2004. *Oxford Textbook of Rheumatology*. Oxford, UK: Oxford University Press. Section 3: Bone in Health, 335–44.

Jackson KA, Saaiana DA. 2001. Lactose maldigestion, calcium intake and osteoporosis in African-, Asian-, and Hispanic-Americans. *Journal of the American College of Nutrition* 20:198S–207S.

Junnila JL, Cartwright VW. 2006. Chronic musculoskeletal pain in children: part II. Rheumatic causes. *American Family Physician* 15:293–300.

Lahita RG. 1998. Collagen disease: the enemy within. *International Journal of Fertility and Women's Medicine* 43:229–34.

Marshall TA, Eichenberger Gilmore JM, Broffitt B, et al. 2005. Diet quality in young children is influenced by beverage consumption. *Journal of the American College of Nutrition* 24:65–75.

Massey LK, Wise KJ. 1989. The effect of dietary caffeine on urinary excretion of calcium, magnesium, sodium and potassium in healthy young females. *Nutrition Research* 4:43–50.

National Fibromyalgia Research Association. ACR Fibromyalgia Diagnostic Criteria. www.nfra.net/Diagnost.htm.

National Institutes of Health. Dietary Supplement Fact Sheet: Vitamin D. Office of Dietary Supplements. http://dietary-supplements.info.nih.gov/factsheets/vitamind.asp.

Rickenlund A, Carlstrom K, Ekblom B, et al. 2004. Effects of oral contraceptives on body composition and physical performance in female athletes. *Journal of Clinical Endocrinology and Metabolism* 89:4364–70.

Sabatier JP, Guaydier-Souquieres G, Benmalek A, et al. 1999. Evolution of lumbar bone mineral content during adolescence and adulthood: a longitudinal study in 395 healthy females 10–24 years of age and 206 premenopausal women. *Osteoporosis International* 9:476–82.

Sutton AJ, Muir KR, Mockett S, et al. 2001. A case-control study to investigate the relation between low and moderate levels of physical activity and osteoarthritis of the knee using data collected as part of the Allied Dunbar National Fitness Survey. *Annals of the Rheumatic Diseases* 60:756–64.

U.S. Department of Agriculture, Agricultural Research Service. 2004. USDA Food and Nutrient Database for Dietary Studies, version 1.0. www.barc.usda.gov/bhnrc/foodsurvey/home.htm.

U.S. Department of Agriculture. 2009. National Nutrient Database for Standard References, Release 17. Calcium Content of Selected Foods per Common Measure, Sorted Alphabetically. www.nal.usda.gov/fnic/foodcomp/Data/SR17/wtrank/sr17a301.pdf.

Yates AA, Schlicker SA, Suitor CW, et al. 2003. Dietary Reference Intakes. The new basis for recommendations for calcium and related nutrients, B vitamins, and choline. *Journal of the American Dietetic Association* 98:699–706.

CHAPTER 8: YOUR STOMACH AND INTESTINES

FamilyDoctor.org. Inflammatory Bowel Disease. http://familydoctor.org/online/famdocen/home/common/digestive/disorders/252.html.

MayoClinic.com. Colon Cancer. www.mayoclinic.com/health/colon-cancer/DS00035.

MayoClinic.com. Irritable Bowel Syndrome. www.mayoclinic.com/health/irritable-bowel-syndrome/DS00106.

MayoClinic.com. Lactose Intolerance. www.mayoclinic.com/health/lactose-intolerance/DS00530.

National Heartburn Alliance. Heartburn Overview. www.heartburnalliance.org/heartburn_overview.php.

Walker R, Buckley M. 2006. *Probiotic Microbes: The Scientific Basis.* A report from the American Academy of Microbiology. http://academy.asm.org/images/stories/documents/probioticmicrobesfull.pdf.

CHAPTER 9: YOUR NECK AND SPINE

Ankrum DR. 1996. Viewing distance at computer workstations. *Workplace Ergonomics*, September, 10–13.

Becker KL. 2001. *Principles and Practice of Endocrinology and Metabolism*, 3rd edition. Philadelphia: Lippincott Williams & Wilkins. Chapter 30: Thyroid Hormone Regulation, 319–20.

Eriksson L, Kullgren A. 2006. Influence of seat geometry and seating posture on NIC (max) long-term AIS 1 neck injury predictability. *Traffic Injury Prevention* 7:61–69.

Farmer CM, Wells JK, Lund AK. 2003. Effects of head restraint and seat redesign on neck injury risk in rear-end crashes. *Traffic Injury Prevention* 4:83–90.

Hormone Foundation. 2006. Thyroid Disorders Overview. www.hormone.org/public/thyroid/overview.cfm.

Seghers J, Jochem A, Spaepen A. 2003. Posture, muscle activity and muscle fatigue in prolonged VDT work at different screen height settings. *Ergonomics* 46:714–30.

Triano, J. Office Chair: How to Reduce Back Pain? www.spine-health.com/wellness/Ergonomics/office-chair-how-reduce-back-pain.

Womenshealth.gov. Graves' Disease. www.womenshealth.gov/faq/graves-disease.cfm.

CHAPTER 10: YOUR WATERWORKS

Almond CSD, Shin AY, Fortescue EB, et al. 2005. Hyponatremia among runners in the Boston Marathon. *New England Journal of Medicine* 352:1550–56.

Digital Urology Journal. Urinary Incontinence in Women. www.duj.com/UrinaryIncontinence.html.

International Functional Electrical Stimulation Society. 2002. Incontinence: Electrical Stimulation for Management of Bladder and Bowel Incontinence. www.ifess.org/Services/Consumer_Ed/Incontinence.htm.

Jepson RG, Craig JC. 2008. Cranberries for preventing urinary tract infections. Cochrane Database of Systematic Reviews. Issue 1. Art. No.:CD001321.

Lynch DM. 2004. Cranberry for prevention of urinary tract infections. *American Family Physician* 70:2175–77.

National Kidney and Urologic Diseases Information Clearinghouse. Interstitial Cystitis/Painful Bladder Syndrome.

http://kidney.niddk.nih.gov/kudiseases/pubs/interstitial cystitis.

National Kidney and Urologic Diseases Information Clearinghouse. Urinary Incontinence in Women. http://kidney.niddk.nih.gov/kudiseases/pubs/uiwomen.

OptumHealth. 2008. How to Do Kegel Exercises. www.myoptumhealth.org/portal/Information/item/How+to+do+Kegel+Exercises?archiveChannel=Home%2FArticle&Clicked=true.

Perry S, Shaw C, Assassa P, et al. 2000. An epidemiological study to establish the prevalence of urinary symptoms and felt need in the community: the Leicestershire MRC Incontinence Study. Leicestershire MRC Incontinence Study Team. *Journal of Public Health Medicine* 22:427–34.

Santillo VM, Lowe FC. 2007. Cranberry juice for the prevention and treatment of urinary tract infections. *Drugs Today* 43:47–54.

CHAPTER 11: YOUR BEST SEX

American Psychiatric Association. 2000. *Diagnostic and Statistical Manual of Mental Disorders*, fourth edition. Washington, DC: American Psychiatric Association. Sexual and Gender Identity Disorders.

Davis SR, Davison SL, Donath S. 2005. Circulating androgen levels and self-reported sexual function in women. *Journal of the American Medical Association* 294:91–96.

Durex Global Sex Surveys. 2005. www.durex network.org/en-GB/research/faceofglobalsex/Pages/Home.aspx.

Frank, JE, Mistretta P, Will J. 2008. Diagnosis and treatment of female sexual dysfunction. *American Family Physician* 77:635–42.

Hines TM. 2001. The G-spot: a modern gynecologic myth. *American Journal of Obstetrics and Gynecology* 285:359–62.

Kingsberg S, Shifren J, Wekselman K, et al. 2007. Evaluation of the clinical relevance of benefits associated with transdermal testosterone treatment in postmenopausal women with hypoactive sexual desire disorder. *Journal of Sexual Medicine* 4:1001–1008.

Masters WH, Johnson VE. 1965, 1966. *Human Sexual Response*. Boston, MA, and Churchill, London: Little, Brown & Company.

Zolbrod A, Dockett L. 2002. *Sex Talk: Uncensored Exercises for Exploring What Really Turns You On*. Oakland, CA: New Harbinger Publications.

CHAPTER 12: YOUR BREASTS

Adebamowo CA, Hu FB, Che E, et al. 2005. Dietary patterns and the risk of breast cancer. *Annals of Epidemiology* 15:789–95.

Armstrong ML, Caliendo C, Roberts AE. 2006. Pregnancy, lactation and nipple piercings. *Association of Women's Health, Obstetric, and Neonatal Nurses Lifelines* 10:212–17.

Baer JH, Colditz GA, Rosner B, et al. 2005. Body fatness during childhood and adolescence and incidence of breast cancer in premenopausal women: a prospective cohort study. *Breast Cancer Research* 7:83.

Balluz L, Ahlumwalia IB, Murphy W, et al. 2004. Surveillance for certain health behaviors among selected local areas: United States, behavior risk factor surveillance system, 2002. *Morbidity and Mortality Weekly Review* 53(SS05):1–100.

Boetes C, Veltman J. 2005. Screening women at increased risk with MRI. *Cancer Imaging* 5:S10–15.

Collaborative Group on Hormonal Factors in Breast Cancer. 2004. Breast cancer and abortion: collaborative reanalysis of data from 53 epidemiological studies, including 83,000 women with breast cancer from 16 countries. *Lancet* 363:1001–16.

Gotzche PC, Nielsen M. 2006. Screening for breast cancer with mammography. *Cochrane Database of Systematic Reviews* CD001877.

Harris JR. 2009. *Breast Diseases*, fourth edition. Philadelphia: Lippincott Williams & Wilkins. Chapter 7: Management of breast pain, 52–57.

Holmes MD, Willett WC. 2004. Does diet affect breast cancer risk? *Breast Cancer Research* 6:170–78.

Hughes LE, Mensel RE, Webster DJT. 1999. *Benign Disorders of the Breast: Concepts and Clinical Management*, second edition. Philadelphia: WB Saunders. Chapter 7: Fibroadenoma and related tumors, 73–94.

Hunt N. 1996. Lactation after augmentation mammoplasty. *Obstetrics and Gynecology* 87:30–34.

Key TJ, Allen NE, Spencer EA, et al. 2003. Nutrition and breast cancer. *Breast* 12:412–16.

Ma H, Bernstein L, Pike MC, et al. 2006. Reproductive factors and breast cancer risk according to joint estrogen and progesterone receptor status: a meta-analysis of epidemiological studies. *Breast Cancer Research* 8:43.

Magnusson CM, Roddam AW, Pike MC, et al. 2005. Body fatness and physical activity at young ages and the risk of breast cancer in premenopausal women. *British Journal of Cancer* 93:817–24.

Marchbanks PA, McDonald JA, Wilson HG, et al. 2002. Oral contraceptives and the risk of breast cancer. *New England Journal of Medicine* 346:2025–32.

Mirick DK, Davis S, Thomas DB. 2002. Antiperspirant use and the risk of breast cancer. *Journal of the National Cancer Institute* 94:1578–80.

Morris PJ, Wood WC. 2000. *Oxford Textbook of Surgery*, second edition. Oxford, UK: Oxford University Press. Chapter 21: The Breast, 1169–72.

Morris PJ, Wood WC. 2000. *Oxford Textbook of Surgery*, second edition. Oxford, UK: Oxford University Press. Chapter 50: Principles and Practice of Plastic Surgery—Breast Surgery, 3544–47.

Pisano ED, Gatsonis C, Hendrisk E, et al. 2005. Diagnostic performance of digital versus film mammography for breast-cancer screening. *New England Journal of Medicine* 353:1773–83.

Reichman ME, Judd JT, Longcope C, et al. 1993. Effects of alcohol consumption on plasma and urinary hormone concentrations in premenopausal women. *Journal of the National Cancer Institute* 85:722–27.

Rosolowich V, Saettler E, Szuck B, et al. 2006. Mastalgia. *Journal of Obstetrics and Gynaecology Canada* 28:49–57.

Sakorafas GH. 2001. Nipple discharge: current diagnostic and therapeutic approaches. *Cancer Treatment Reviews* 27:275–82.

Souto GC, Giugliani ERJ, Giugliani C, et al. 2003. The impact of breast reduction surgery on breastfeeding performance. *Journal of Human Lactation* 19:43–49.

Thomas DB, Gao DL, Ray RM, et al. 2002. Randomized trial of breast self-examination in Shanghai: final results. *Journal of the National Cancer Institute* 94:1445–57.

Thorensen M, Wesche J. 1988. Doppler measurements of changes in human mammary and uterine blood flow during pregnancy and lactation. *Acta Obstetricia et Gynecologica Scandinavica* 67:741–45.

Trock BJ, Hilakivi-Clarke L, Clarke R. 2006. Meta-analysis of soy intake and breast cancer risk. *Journal of the National Cancer Institute* 98:459–71.

U.S. Department of Agriculture (USDA). 2005. *Dietary Guidelines for Americans*. Chapter 9: Alcoholic Beverages. www.health.gov/dietaryguidelines/dga2005/document/html/chapter9.htm.

U.S. Food and Drug Administration. 2006. News release: FDA Approves Silicone Gel-Filled Breast Implants After In-Depth Evaluation. www.fda.gov/NewsEvents/Newsroom/PressAnnouncements/2006/ucm108790.

Vargas HI, Vargas MP, Gonzalez KD, et al. 2004. Outcomes of sonography-based management of breast cysts. *American Journal of Surgery* 188:443–47.

Verlinden I, Gungor N, Wouters K, et al. 2005. Parity-induced changes in global gene expression in the human mammary gland. *European Journal of Cancer Prevention* 14:129–37.

Weiss NS. 2003. Breast cancer mortality in relation to clinical breast examination and breast self-examination. *The Breast Journal Supplement* 2:S86–89.

Yankaskas BC. 2005–2006. Epidemiology of breast cancer in young women. *Breast Disease* 23:3–8.

CHAPTER 13: YOUR VAGINA AND CERVIX

ACOG Committe on Practice Bulletins. 2009. *American College of Obstetricians and Gynecologists Practice Bulletin: Clinical Management Guidelines for Obstetrician-Gynecologists*. Number 109, December. Cervical cytology screening. *Obstetrics and Gynecology*. 114:1409–20.

Advisory Committee for HIV and STD Prevention. 1998. HIV prevention through early detection and treatment of other sexually transmitted diseases: United States. *Morbidity and Mortality Weekly Report* 47:1–24.

Ault KA. 2006. Epidemiology and natural history of human papillomavirus infections in the female genital tract. *Infectious Disease in Obstetrics and Gynecology* 14:40470.

Beutner KR, Reitano MV, Richwald GA, et al. 1998. External genital warts: report of the American Medical Association Consensus Conference. AMA Expert Panel of External Genital Warts. *Clinical Infectious Disease* 27:796–806.

Bosch FX, Manos MM, Munoz N, et al. 1995. Prevalence of human papillomavirus in cervical cancer: a worldwide perspective. International Biological Study on Cervical Cancer (IBSCC) Study Group. *Journal of the National Cancer Institute* 87:796–802.

Centers for Disease Control and Prevention. 1985. Chlamydia trachomatis infections: policy guidelines for prevention and control. *Morbidity and Mortality Weekly Report* 34:53S-74S.

Centers for Disease Control and Prevention. 1993. Recommendations for the prevention and management of *Chlamydia trachomatis* infections. *Morbidity and Mortality Weekly Report* 42:1–39.

Centers for Disease Control and Prevention. 2002. HIV and AIDS cases reported through December 2001. *HIV/AIDS Surveillance Report* 13:1–44.

Fleming DT, McQuillan GM, Johnson RE, et al. 1997. Herpes simplex virus type 2 in the United States 1976–1994. *New England Journal of Medicine* 337:1105–11.

Hatcher RA, Trussel J, Stewart F, et al. 1998. *Contraceptive Technology*, seventeenth revised edition. New York: Ardent Media.

Kuehn BM. 2006. CDC panel backs routine HPV vaccination. *Journal of the American Medical Association* 296:640–41.

Peyton CL, Schiffman M, Lorincz AT, et al. 1998. Comparison of PCR- and hybrid capture-based human papillomavirus detection systems using multiple cervical specimen collection strategies. *Journal of Clinical Microbiology* 36:3248–54.

Qualters JR, Lee NC, Smith RA, et al. 1992. Breast and cervical cancer surveillance, United States, 1973–1987. CDC surveillance summaries. *Morbidity and Mortality Weekly Report* 41:1–15.

Ries LAG, Kosary CL, Hankey BE, et al. 1999. *SEER Cancer Statistics Review, 1973–1996*. Bethesda, MD: US Department of Health and Human Services, National Institutes of Health, National Cancer Institute.

Solomon D, Davey D, Kurman R, et al. 2002. The 2001 Bethesda System: terminology for reporting results of cervical cytology. *Journal of the American Medical Association* 287:2114–19.

U.S. Food and Drug Administration. 2009. Gardasil. www.fda.gov/BiologicsBloodVaccines/ApprovedProducts/UCM094042.

Winer RL, Hughes JP, Feng Q, et al. 2006. Condom use and the risk of genital human papillomavirus infection in young women. *New England Journal of Medicine* 354:2645–54.

World Health Organization. 2002. WHO/CONRAD technical consultation on nonoxynol-9, World Health Organization, Geneva, 9–10 October 2001: summary report. *Reproductive Health Matters* 10:175–81.

World Health Organization. 2003. State of the art new vaccines: research and development. Initiative for Vaccine Research. www.who.int/vaccine_research/documents/en/stateofart_excler.pdf.

CHAPTER 14: YOUR OVARIES

Collaborative Group on Epidemiological Studies of Ovarian Cancer. 2008. Ovarian cancer and oral contraceptives: collaborative reanalysis of data from 45 epidemiological studies including 23,257 women with ovarian cancer and 87,303 controls. *Lancet* 371:303–14.

Medline Plus. Ca-125. www.nlm.nih.gov/medlineplus/ency/article/007217.htm.

National Cancer Institute. 2009. Ovarian Cancer Screening (PDQ). www.cancer.gov/cancertopics/pdq/screening/ovarian/patient.

National Institutes of Health. 2005. Questions and Answers: OvaCheck and NCI/FDA Ovarian Cancer Clinical Trials Using Proteomics Technology. home.ccr.cancer.gov/ncifdaproteomics/pdf/OvaCheckQandA.pdf.

Petricoin E, Ardekani EA, Hitt BE, et al. 2002. Use of proteomic patterns in serum to identify ovarian cancer. *Lancet* 359:572–77.

Womenshealth.gov. Infertility: Frequently Asked Questions. www.womenshealth.gov/faq/infertility.cfm.

Womenshealth.gov. Ovarian Cysts: Frequently Asked Questions. www.womenshealth.gov/faq/ovarian-cysts.cfm.

CHAPTER 15: YOUR REPRODUCTIVE SYSTEM

Centers for Disease Control and Prevention. 2009. Male latex condoms and sexually transmitted diseases. Condoms and STDs: Fact sheet for public health personnel. www.cdc.gov/condomeffectiveness/latex.htm.

Collier A. 2007. *The Humble Little Condom: A History*. Amherst, NY: Prometheus Books.

El-Refaey H, Rajasekar D, Abdalla M, et al. 1995. Induction of abortion with mifepristone (RU 486) and oral or vaginal misoprostol. *New England Journal of Medicine* 332:983–87.

Fu H, Darroch KE, Haas T, et al. 1999. Contraceptive failure rates: new estimates from the 1995 National Survey of Family Growth. *Alan Guttmacher Institute, Family Planning Perspectives* 31:56–63.

Guttmacher Institute. 2006. Facts on Induced Abortion in the States. www.guttmacher.org/pubs/fb_induced_abortion.html.

Kulier R, Gülmezoglu AM, Hofmeyr GJ, et al. 2004. Medical methods for first trimester abortion. *Cochrane Database of Systematic Reviews* 1:CD002855.

Kulier R, Helmerhorst, O'Brien P, et al. 2006. Copper containing, framed intra-uterine devices for contraception. *Cochrane Database of Systematic Reviews* CD005347.

Marchbanks PA, McDonald JA, Wilson HG, et al. 2002. Oral contraceptive and the risk of breast cancer. *New England Journal of Medicine* 346:2025–32.

National Abortion Federation. 2001. Early Options: A Provider's Guide to Medical Abortion. www.early optionpill .org.

Nelson AL. 2000. The intrauterine contraceptive device. *Obstetrics and Gynecology Clinics of North America* 27:723–40.

Planned Parenthood. Birth Control. www.plannedparenthood.org/birth-control-pregnancy/birth-control-4211.htm.

Speroff L, Darney P. 1996. *Contraception in the USA: A Clinical Guide for Contraception*, second edition. Baltimore: Lippincott Williams & Wilkins. Chapter 7: Intrauterine Contraception, 221–58.

UNDP/UNFPA/WHO/World Bank Special Programme of Research, Development and Research Training in Human Reproduction. 1997. Long-term reversible contraception: twelve years of experience with the TCu380A and TCu220C. *Contraception* 56:341–52.

World Health Organization. 1998. Randomized controlled trial of levonorgestrel versus the Yuzpe regimen of combined oral contraceptives for emergency contraception. *Lancet* 352:428–33.

CHAPTER 16: YOUR FERTILITY

Greenberg JA, Bell SJ, Van Ausda W. 2008. Omega-3 fatty acid supplementation during pregnancy. *Reviews in Obstetrics and Gynecology* 1:162–69.

Leung AM, Pearce EN, Braverman LE. 2009. Iodine content of prenatal multivitamins in the United States. *New England Journal of Medicine* 360:939–40.

U.S. Food and Drug Administration. 2004. What You Need to Know About Mercury in Fish and Shellfish. www.fda .gov/Food/FoodSafety/Product-SpecificInformation/ Seafood/FoodbornePathogensContaminants/ Methylmercury/ucm115662.htm.

CHAPTER 17: YOUR DIET

Kris-Etherton PM, Harris WS, Appel LJ, et al. 2002. Fish Consumption, Fish Oil, Omega-3 Fatty Acids, and Cardiovascular Disease. *Circulation* 106:2747–57.

Michels KB, Mohllajee A, Roset-Bahmanyar E, et al. 2007. Diet and breast cancer. *Cancer* 109:2712–49.

Svetkey LP, Sacks FM, Obarzanek E, et al. 1999. The DASH Diet, Sodium Intake, and Blood Pressure Trial (DASH-sodium): rationale and design. DASH-Sodium Collaborative Research Group. *Journal of the American Dietetic Association* 99:S96–104.

CHAPTER 18: YOUR BODY'S OTHER ISSUES

Armstrong ML, DeBoer S, Cetta F. 2008. Infective endocarditis after body art: a review of the literature and concerns. *Journal of Adolescent Health* 43:217–25.

Armstrong ML, Roberts AE, Koch JR, et al. 2008. Motivation for contemporary tattoo removal: a shift in identity. *Archives of Dermatology* 144:879–84.

Kuperman-Beade M, Levine VJ, Ashinoff R, et al. 2001. Laser removal of tattoos. *American Journal of Clinical Dermatology* 2:21–5.

Melzer DI. 2005. Complications of body piercing. *American Family Physician* 72:2035–36.

index

A

B